Teen Health Series

Alcohol Information For Teens, Third Edition

Alcohol Information For Teens, Third Edition

Health Tips About Alcohol Use, Abuse, And Dependence

Including Facts About Alcohol's Effects On Mental And Physical Health, The Consequences Of Underage Drinking, And Understanding Alcoholic Family Members

Edited by Karen Bellenir

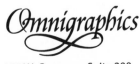

Omnigraphics

155 W. Congress, Suite 200
Detroit, MI 48226

Bibliographic Note

Because this page cannot legibly accommodate all the copyright notices, the Bibliographic Note portion of the Preface constitutes an extension of the copyright notice.

Edited by Karen Bellenir

Teen Health Series

Karen Bellenir, *Managing Editor*
David A. Cooke, M.D., *Medical Consultant*
Elizabeth Collins, *Research and Permissions Coordinator*
EdIndex, *Services for Publishers, Indexers*

* * *

Omnigraphics, Inc.
Matthew P. Barbour, *Senior Vice President*
Kevin M. Hayes, *Operations Manager*

* * *

Peter E. Ruffner, *Publisher*
Copyright © 2013 Omnigraphics, Inc.
ISBN 978-0-7808-1313-7
E-ISBN 978-0-7808-1314-4

Library of Congress Cataloging-in-Publication Data

Alcohol information for teens : health tips about alcohol use, abuse, and dependence including facts about alcohol's effects on mental and physical health, the consequences of underage drinking, and understanding alcoholic family members. -- Third edition / edited by Karen Bellenir.
   pages cm. -- (Teen health series)
 Summary: "Provides basic consumer health information for teens about the physical and mental health effects of alcohol use, with facts about alcohol abuse and underage drinking, treatment and recovery, and coping with alcoholism in the family. Includes index and resource information"-- Provided by publisher.
 Includes bibliographical references and index.
 ISBN 978-0-7808-1313-7 (hardcover : alk. paper) -- ISBN 978-0-7808-1314-4 (eISBN) 1. Alcohol--Physiological effect. 2. Alcoholism--Prevention. 3. Youth--Alcohol use. I. Bellenir, Karen editor.
 QP801.A3A4275 2013
 613.81--dc23
                                                                                          2013000216

Table of Contents

Preface

Part Three: Alcohol's Physical Effects

Part Four: Mental Health And Behavioral Risks Associated With Alcohol

Part Five: Alcoholism Treatment And Recovery

Part Six: Alcoholism In The Family

Part Seven: If You Need More Information

Preface

About This Book

Alcoholic beverages have been used around the world and throughout thousands of years of recorded history. Alcohol has been used as a medicine, in religious ceremonies, for celebrations, and to increase conviviality in social gatherings. Despite its widespread acceptance, however, negative effects associated with its misuse have also accompanied it through the ages.

Today, various forms of alcoholic beverages are known by many names, such as malts, spirits, or liquor and a host of slang terms, including booze, hooch, and sauce. Alcoholic beverages come in different forms, such as beers, wines, and mixed drinks, and servings can contain vastly different amounts of pure alcohol. But all these beverages share a common concern: Teens should not drink them.

In the United States it is illegal in all 50 states for anyone under the age of 21 to consume alcoholic beverages. But perhaps even more important than legal concerns are the potential health-related outcomes. Alcohol consumption can have negative effects on the still-maturing teen brain, and research has shown that the earlier teens begin drinking the more they risk developing alcohol dependency and other adverse conditions.

Alcohol Information For Teens, Third Edition provides updated information about the use and misuse of alcohol. It describes ways alcohol can affect mental and physical health. It discusses the special vulnerabilities of the teen brain and the changes in brain functioning that lead to dependency. A section on treatment and recovery discusses achieving and maintaining sobriety, and a section on alcohol abuse in the family addresses the special concerns of teens who live with an alcoholic relative. The book concludes with resource directories for finding help or more information about alcohol and substance abuse.

How To Use This Book

This book is divided into parts and chapters. Parts focus on broad areas of interest; chapters are devoted to single topics within a part.

Part One: About Alcohol And Alcohol Abuse explains the ways in which people use alcohol, and it addresses practices associated with alcohol misuse and the development of dependency. It identifies adult drinking patterns that have not been linked to adverse consequences, and it provides details about other patterns—such as binge drinking, underage drinking, and heavy drinking—that can seriously impact health.

Part Two: Underage Drinking offers an in-depth discussion about the various reasons teenage drinking is a significant problem. One special concern relates to brain development. Researchers now realize that the human brain continues maturing through the adolescent years and that alcohol consumption during this critical time can lead to life-long changes in how the brain functions. Other difficulties linked to underage drinking include hazards associated with typical teen drinking patterns, the relationship between teen alcohol consumption and injury, and behavioral risks associated with sexual activity, academic performance, driving, and suicide.

Part Three: Alcohol's Physical Effects explains what happens inside the body and the brain when alcohol is consumed. It describes the factors that contribute to blood alcohol concentration (BAC) and how increasing BAC plays a role in hampering physical and mental functioning. Some of the most common circumstances in which alcohol can damage other organs or contribute to cancer development are also described. The part concludes with information about the devastating ways alcohol can affect fetal development.

Part Four: Mental Health And Behavioral Risks Associated With Alcohol discusses the correlation between teen drinking and depression, bipolar disorder, schizophrenia, anxiety disorders, and other mental health concerns. It describes the process by which addiction develops and discusses how alcohol use can contribute to risky or violent behaviors.

Part Five: Alcoholism Treatment And Recovery offers facts for teens who already drink and want to quit and for teens who want to understand the challenges faced by others who are struggling to achieve and maintain sobriety.

Part Six: Alcoholism In The Family addresses teens who live in an uncertain or inconsistent home environment because they have a parent, grandparent, sibling, or other close relative or caregiver with an alcohol abuse disorder. It explains some of the challenges often experienced in relationship patterns and answers questions about the role of family history in the development of alcohol addiction. It also offers tips for discussing alcohol-related concerns in a positive way.

Part Seven: If You Need More Information provides directories of resources for additional help about alcohol and other substance abuse concerns.

Bibliographic Note

This volume contains documents and excerpts from publications issued by the following government agencies: Administration for Children and Families; Centers for Disease Control and Prevention; Federal Trade Commission; National Cancer Institute; National Institute of Arthritis and Musculoskeletal and Skin Diseases; National Institute of Diabetes and Digestive and Kidney Diseases; National Institute of Mental Health; National Institute on Aging; National Institute on Alcohol Abuse and Alcoholism; National Institute on Drug Abuse; National Institutes of Health; Office of Adolescent Health; Office on Women's Health; Substance Abuse and Mental Health Services Administration; U.S. Department of Agriculture; U.S. Department of Education; U.S. Department of Health and Human Services; U.S. Department of Veterans Affairs; U.S. Food and Drug Administration; and U.S. Office of Personnel Management. In addition, this volume contains copyrighted articles written by the following individuals: David Cooke, Lisa Esposito, Zachary Klimecki, and Laurie Lewis. Full citation information is provided on the first page of each chapter. The photograph on the front cover is © Peter Dazeley/Getty Images.

Acknowledgements

In addition to the people and organizations listed above, special thanks are due to Liz Collins, research and permissions coordinator; Lisa Bakewell, verification assistant; and WhimsyInk, prepress services provider.

About The *Teen Health Series*

At the request of librarians serving today's young adults, the *Teen Health Series* was developed as a specially focused set of volumes within Omnigraphics' *Health Reference Series*. Each volume deals comprehensively with a topic selected according to the needs and interests of people in middle school and high school.

Teens seeking preventive guidance, information about disease warning signs, medical statistics, and risk factors for health problems will find answers to their questions in the *Teen Health Series*. The *Series*, however, is not intended to serve as a tool for diagnosing illness, in prescribing treatments, or as a substitute for the physician/patient relationship. All people concerned about medical symptoms or the possibility of disease are encouraged to seek professional care from an appropriate health care provider.

If there is a topic you would like to see addressed in a future volume of the *Teen Health Series*, please write to:

Editor
Teen Health Series
Omnigraphics, Inc.
155 W. Congress, Suite 200
Detroit, MI 48226

A Note About Spelling And Style

Teen Health Series editors use *Stedman's Medical Dictionary* as an authority for questions related to the spelling of medical terms and the *Chicago Manual of Style* for questions related to grammatical structures, punctuation, and other editorial concerns. Consistent adherence is not always possible, however, because the individual volumes within the *Series* include many documents from a wide variety of different producers and copyright holders, and the editor's primary goal is to present material from each source as accurately as is possible following the terms specified by each document's producer. This sometimes means that information in different chapters or sections may follow other guidelines and alternate spelling authorities. For example, occasionally a copyright holder may require that eponymous terms be shown in possessive forms (Crohn's disease *vs.* Crohn disease) or that British spelling norms be retained (leukaemia *vs.* leukemia).

Locating Information Within The *Teen Health Series*

The *Teen Health Series* contains a wealth of information about a wide variety of medical topics. As the *Series* continues to grow in size and scope, locating the precise information needed by a specific student may become more challenging. To address this concern, information about books within the *Teen Health Series* is included in *A Contents Guide to the Health Reference Series*. The *Contents Guide* presents an extensive list of more than 16,000 diseases, treatments, and other topics of general interest compiled from the Tables of Contents and major index headings from the books of the *Teen Health Series* and *Health Reference Series*. To access *A Contents Guide to the Health Reference Series*, visit www.healthreferenceseries.com.

Our Advisory Board

We would like to thank the following advisory board members for providing guidance to the development of this *Series*:

Dr. Lynda Baker, Associate Professor of Library and Information Science, Wayne State University, Detroit, MI

Nancy Bulgarelli, William Beaumont Hospital Library, Royal Oak, MI

Karen Imarisio, Bloomfield Township Public Library, Bloomfield Township, MI

Karen Morgan, Mardigian Library, University of Michigan-Dearborn, Dearborn, MI

Rosemary Orlando, St. Clair Shores Public Library, St. Clair Shores, MI

Medical Consultant

Medical consultation services are provided to the *Teen Health Series* editors by David A. Cooke, MD, FACP. Dr. Cooke is a graduate of Brandeis University, and he received his M.D. degree from the University of Michigan. He completed residency training at the University of Wisconsin Hospital and Clinics. He is board-certified in internal medicine. Dr. Cooke currently works as part of the University of Michigan Health System and practices in Ann Arbor, MI. In his free time, he enjoys writing, science fiction, and spending time with his family.

Part One
About Alcohol And Alcohol Abuse

Chapter 1

Straight Talk About Alcohol

Booze. Sauce. Brewskis. Hard stuff. Juice. Call it what you want, but alcohol in any form—from beer to a fruity drink—can hit you really hard. Sure, alcohol may make you feel good for a little while. But it can cause so many problems. In fact, teens who drink are more likely to become victims of a crime, including a sexual attack. They are more likely to be in a drinking-related car crash. And they are more likely to have problems with alcohol later in life. Not to mention that drinking can make you act goofy, throw up, or pass out. It also can make you gain weight, become addicted, have problems in school, and otherwise mess up your life.

Be Smart About Alcohol

You may have heard that drinking alcohol at a party helps you to loosen up, talk to people, and make new friends. But the truth is that lots of teenagers know that alcohol—even a little—can make you have less control over what happens to you and your body. You can end up in uncomfortable or even dangerous situations. The safest choice is not to use alcohol at all. And remember other ways to stay safe around alcohol:

- If you're at a party with alcohol, drink something else instead, like soda or water.

- Never put your cup down and go back to finish it. Someone can spike (put alcohol in) your drink or even put a drug in it!

- Always take extra money and your cell phone anywhere that people you're with may wind up drinking. Never get into a car with someone who has been drinking. Call a taxi or ask your parents to pick you up.

About This Chapter: Text in this chapter is excerpted from "Straight Talk about Alcohol," Office on Women's Health, U.S. Department of Health and Human Services, May 18, 2010.

Alcohol Is A Drug

Alcohol can cause short-term and long-term damage to your body. This is how alcohol affects your body:

Brain: Drinking alcohol leads to a loss of coordination, poor judgment, slowed reflexes, distorted vision, loss of memory, and even blackouts.

Heart: Drinking alcohol could cause your blood pressure to rise, increase your heart rate, cause your heart to beat abnormally, and can increase the size of your heart.

Stomach: You're putting empty calories into your body, which could cause weight gain. If you drink too much, you may vomit because alcohol is toxic. Drinking alcohol can also cause stomach ulcers and cancer.

Liver: Drinking alcohol could cause diseases such as cirrhosis (pronounced sir-o-sis). It can also cause hepatitis (inflamed liver) or even liver cancer. Liver disease can weaken the liver's ability to clot and keep our blood free from poisons and bacteria.

Reproductive System: Heavy drinking can cause painful periods, heavy flow, discomfort before your period (PMS), and irregular periods (not getting your period when you're supposed to). Drinking also raises the risk of getting sexually assaulted and having unsafe sex.

The Consequences Of Underage Drinking

- A person who begins drinking as a young teen is four times more likely to develop alcohol dependence than someone who waits until adulthood to use alcohol.

- During adolescence significant changes occur in the body, including the formation of new networks in the brain. Alcohol use during this time may affect brain development.

- Motor vehicle crashes are the leading cause of death among youth ages 15 to 20, and the rate of fatal crashes among alcohol-involved drivers between 16 and 20 years old is more than twice the rate for alcohol-involved drivers 21 and older. Alcohol use also is linked with youthful deaths by drowning, suicide, and homicide.

- Alcohol use is associated with many adolescent risk behaviors, including other drug use and delinquency, weapon carrying and fighting, and perpetrating or being the victim of date rape.

Source: Excerpted from an undated fact sheet, "The Facts about Youth and Alcohol," National Institute on Alcohol Abuse and Alcoholism (www.niaaa.nih.gov), 2010.

Alcohol Can Affect Girls And Boys Differently

How fast alcohol affects you is influenced by many things, including your weight, how much you've eaten, and how fast you drink. Changes in hormones that happen throughout the month also affect how much alcohol stays in a girl's blood. And females' bodies process alcohol differently from males' bodies, so alcohol usually hits girls and women faster.

Remember, alcohol may be affecting you even if you aren't slurring words or stumbling around. And once you're drunk, the only thing that will sober you up is time. Coffee, cold showers, exercise, or other "cures" will not speed up how fast your body gets rid of the alcohol.

A 12-ounce can of beer, a 5-ounce glass of wine, and a 1.5-ounce shot of hard liquor all have the same amount of alcohol and the same effect on you. Mixed drinks can have even more alcohol. And don't be fooled by a drink's taste. A sweet or fruity drink can have just as much alcohol as a bitter one. Also, larger serving sizes are common and count as more than one drink.

"Impaired" Versus "Intoxicated"

Impairment is when the amount of alcohol you have had affects your judgment, coordination, and reaction time. It can start with your first drink. A person may not look or feel impaired even though she or he is. And because it takes time for alcohol to leave the stomach and enter the bloodstream, a person may become even more impaired following their last drink.

Intoxication is a term that is often used when discussing laws around drinking, including rules for driving and how you can act in public. These laws usually are set by your state. You may be found to be intoxicated based on your behavior or on your blood alcohol content (BAC). BAC is found through a blood, urine, or breath test and is measured in the number of grams of alcohol in 100 millimeters of blood. Different states may have different definitions and different consequences for being "impaired" or "intoxicated."

But legal definitions aside, it's important to remember that your mind and body can work less well—can be impaired—starting with your first drink. And don't forget that if you're under 21 and you drive with any alcohol in your body, you can get in serious trouble.

Binge Drinking

Binge drinking means having a lot of alcohol on one occasion, like at a party. For males, having five or more drinks in a row, and for females, having four or more drinks in a row is considered binge drinking.

Too much alcohol can cause serious physical problems, like throwing up, difficulty breathing, sleepiness, unconsciousness, and coma or even death. It also can cause you to make bad decisions that could lead to being the victim of sexual assault, being in a car accident, getting a sexually transmitted infection (STI), or getting pregnant.

And over time, if you drink too much you could develop painful or irregular periods or damage to the brain, liver, kidneys, and other parts of your body. You could also have problems with schoolwork and relationships

Legal Matters

Learn some key points to stay out of trouble:

- It's not legal to drink before you're 21. You may think this isn't fair, but the bottom line is that if you drink, you break the law.

Underage Drinking

You probably see and hear a lot about alcohol—from TV, movies, music, and your friends. But what are the real facts about underage alcohol use?

Myth: Alcohol isn't as harmful as other drugs.

FACT: Alcohol increases your risk for many deadly diseases, such as cancer. Drinking too much alcohol too quickly can lead to alcohol poisoning, which can kill you.

Myth: Drinking is a good way to loosen up at parties.

FACT: Drinking is a dumb way to loosen up. It can make you act silly, say things you shouldn't say, and do things you wouldn't normally do (like get into fights).

Myth: Drinking alcohol will make me cool.

FACT: There's nothing cool about stumbling around, passing out, or puking on yourself. Drinking alcohol also can cause bad breath and weight gain.

Myth: All of the other kids drink alcohol. I need to drink to fit in.

FACT: If you really want to fit in, stay sober. Most young people don't drink alcohol. Research shows that more than 70 percent of youth age 12 to 20 haven't had a drink in the past month.

- If you get caught drinking and you're under 21, the consequences could include getting arrested and being required to enter an alcohol treatment program. Each state has its own laws. In Pennsylvania, for example, your first underage drinking offense could mean a $300 fine, losing your license for 90 days, or going to jail.

- You can get into even more trouble if you're caught drinking and driving.

- If you're at a party with alcohol and you're not 21—even if you're not drinking—you could get arrested.

- Using a fake ID to buy alcohol can get you in serious trouble. Each state sets its own rules, but you could wind up in jail or paying big fines. You also could have a conviction on your permanent record, which can hurt your chances when you look for a job or apply to college.

Myth: I can sober up quickly by taking a cold shower or drinking coffee.

FACT: On average, it takes two to three hours for a single drink to leave the body. Nothing can speed up the process, not even drinking coffee, taking a cold shower, or "walking it off."

Myth: Adults drink, so kids should be able to drink too.

FACT: A young person's brain and body are still growing. Drinking alcohol can cause learning problems or lead to adult alcoholism. People who begin drinking by age 15 are five times more likely to abuse or become dependent on alcohol than those who begin drinking after age 20.

Myth: Beer and wine are safer than liquor.

FACT: Alcohol is alcohol. It can cause you problems no matter how you consume it. One 12-ounce bottle of beer or a 5-ounce glass of wine (about a half cup) has as much alcohol as a 1.5-ounce shot of liquor. Alcopops—sweet drinks laced with malt liquor—often contain more alcohol than beer!

Myth: I can drink alcohol and not have any problems.

FACT: If you're under 21, drinking alcohol is a big problem: It's illegal. If caught, you may have to pay a fine, perform community service, or take alcohol awareness classes. Kids who drink also are more likely to get poor grades in school and are at higher risk for being a crime victim.

Source: "Real Facts About Underage Drinking," Substance Abuse and Mental Health Services Administration (www.samhsa.gov), 2011.

Parental Drinking

Because their bodies are mature, adults process alcohol differently and it affects them differently than it does teens. Teens are still growing in many ways, so even a small amount of alcohol can affect their physical and mental development. Besides, your parents are allowed by law to drink. When they drink, they should be doing it responsibly and in reasonable amounts—which means they never drive after drinking, and they have one to two drinks a day or less. So it's okay if your parents have a glass of wine at dinner or a beer during the football game. But if they misuse alcohol for any period of time, they will also cause serious damage to their health.

Signs You're Hooked On Alcohol

If you're under 21, you're not supposed to be drinking at all. But if you are drinking, it's important to know whether you're developing a serious problem. If you can relate to any of the items listed below, think about how alcohol is affecting your life and talk to an adult you trust for help.

- Alcohol has become more important than family activities and relationships or friendships.
- Your schoolwork is suffering.
- You use alcohol to escape from feeling unhappy.

Alcohol Use Is Widespread Among Today's Teenagers

- Nearly 70% of 8th graders perceive alcoholic beverages as "fairly easy" or "very easy" to get.
- By the time they complete high school nearly 80% of teenagers have consumed alcohol, 30% report having been drunk in the past month, and 29% report having five or more drinks in a row in the past two weeks.

Alcohol Use Increases Substantially From Middle To High School

- Approximately 20% of 8th graders report having recently (within the past 30 days) consumed alcohol compared to 35% of 10th graders and almost 50% of 12th graders.
- A little over 20% of 8th graders report having been drunk at least once in their life compared to almost 45% of 10th graders and 60% of 12th graders.

Source: Excerpted from, "The Facts about Youth and Alcohol," National Institute on Alcohol Abuse and Alcoholism (www.niaaa.nih.gov), 2010.

- You drink when you're mad at your parents, family, or friends.

- You can't control your drinking once you start. Even if you decide you'll only have one or two drinks, you end up having a lot.

- You need to drink more alcohol than before to get the same effect.

- You have blackouts or events you don't fully remember after drinking.

If you're using alcohol, www.girlshealth.gov can help you quit.

Chapter 2

Questions And Answers About Alcohol

What is alcohol?

Ethyl alcohol, or ethanol, is an intoxicating ingredient found in beer, wine, and liquor. Alcohol is produced by the fermentation of yeast, sugars, and starches.

How does alcohol affect a person?

Alcohol affects every organ in the body. It is a central nervous system depressant that is rapidly absorbed from the stomach and small intestine into the bloodstream. Alcohol is metabolized in the liver by enzymes; however, the liver can only metabolize a small amount of alcohol at a time, leaving the excess alcohol to circulate throughout the body. The intensity of the effect of alcohol on the body is directly related to the amount consumed.

Why do some people react differently to alcohol than others?

Individual reactions to alcohol vary and are influenced by many factors, such as age, gender, race or ethnicity, physical condition (weight, fitness level, etc), amount of food consumed before drinking, and how quickly the alcohol was consumed. Other factors include the use of drugs or prescription medicines and a family history of alcohol problems.

What is a standard drink in the United States?

A standard drink is equal to 14.0 grams (0.6 ounces) of pure alcohol. Generally, this amount of pure alcohol is found 12 ounces of beer, 8 ounces of malt liquor, 5 ounces of wine, or 1.5 ounces (or a "shot") of 80-proof distilled spirits or liquor (for example, gin, rum, vodka, or whiskey).

About This Chapter: From "Frequently Asked Questions," Centers for Disease Control and Prevention (www.cdc.gov), October 15, 2012.

Is beer or wine safer to drink than liquor?

No. One 12-ounce beer has about the same amount of alcohol as one 5-ounce glass of wine, or 1.5-ounce shot of liquor. It is the amount of alcohol consumed that affects a person most, not the type of alcoholic drink.

What are caffeinated alcoholic beverages?

Caffeinated alcoholic beverages (CABs) are premixed beverages that combine alcohol, caffeine, and other stimulants. They may be malt-based or distilled spirits–based and usually have higher alcohol content than beer (for example, 5%–12% on average for CABs compared to 4%–5% for beer). The caffeine content in these beverages is usually not reported.

What does moderate drinking mean?

According to the *Dietary Guidelines for Americans*, moderate alcohol consumption is defined as having up to one drink per day for adult women and up to two drinks per day for adult men. This definition is referring to the amount consumed on any single day and is not intended as an average over several days. The *Dietary Guidelines* also state that it is not recommended that anyone begin drinking or drink more frequently on the basis of potential health benefits because moderate alcohol intake also is associated with increased risk of breast cancer, violence, drowning, and injuries from falls and motor vehicle crashes.

Is it safe to drink alcohol and drive?

No. Alcohol use slows reaction time and impairs judgment and coordination, which are all skills needed to drive a car safely. The more alcohol consumed, the greater the impairment.

Alcohol And It's Effects

Ethyl alcohol, or ethanol, is an intoxicating ingredient found in beer, wine, and liquor. Alcohol is produced by the fermentation of yeast, sugars, and starches. It is a central nervous system depressant that is rapidly absorbed from the stomach and small intestine into the bloodstream.

Alcohol affects every organ in the drinker's body and can damage a developing fetus. Intoxication can impair brain function and motor skills; heavy use can increase risk of certain cancers, stroke, and liver disease. Alcoholism or alcohol dependence is a diagnosable disease characterized by a strong craving for alcohol, and/or continued use despite harm or personal injury. Alcohol abuse, which can lead to alcoholism, is a pattern of drinking that results in harm to one's health, interpersonal relationships, or ability to work.

Source: Excerpted from an undated document titled "Alcohol," National Institute on Drug Abuse (www.nida.nih.gov), accessed October 27, 2012.

What does it mean to be above the legal limit for drinking?

The legal limit for drinking is the alcohol level above which an individual is subject to legal penalties (for example, arrest or loss of a driver's license). Legal limits are measured using either a blood alcohol test or a breathalyzer. They are typically defined by state law, and may vary based on individual characteristics, such as age and occupation.

All states in the United States have adopted 0.08% (80 mg/dL) as the legal limit for operating a motor vehicle for drivers aged 21 years or older. However, drivers younger than 21 are not allowed to operate a motor vehicle with any level of alcohol in their system.

It is important to realize that legal limits do not define a level below which it is safe to operate a vehicle or engage in some other activity. Impairment due to alcohol use begins to occur at levels well below the legal limit.

How do I know if it's okay to drink?

According to the *Dietary Guidelines for Americans*, people who should not drink alcoholic beverages at all include the following:

- Children and adolescents
- Individuals of any age who cannot limit their drinking to low level
- Women who may become pregnant or who are pregnant
- Individuals who plan to drive, operate machinery, or take part in other activities that require attention, skill, or coordination
- Individuals taking prescription or over-the-counter medications that can interact with alcohol
- Individuals with certain medical conditions
- Persons recovering from alcoholism

What is meant by heavy drinking?

For adult men, heavy drinking is typically defined as consuming an average of more than two drinks per day. For adult women, heavy drinking is typically defined as consuming an average of more than one drink per day. And, if you're under 21, you're not supposed to drink at all.

What is binge drinking?

According to the National Institute on Alcohol Abuse and Alcoholism binge drinking is defined as a pattern of alcohol consumption that brings the blood alcohol concentration

(BAC) level to 0.08% or more. This pattern of drinking usually corresponds to five or more drinks on a single occasion for men or four or more drinks on a single occasion for women, generally within about two hours.

What is the difference between alcoholism and alcohol abuse?

Alcohol abuse is a pattern of drinking that results in harm to one's health, interpersonal relationships, or ability to work. The following items describe what alcohol abuse might look like:

- Failure to fulfill major responsibilities at work, school, or home.

- Drinking in dangerous situations, such as drinking while driving or operating machinery.

- Legal problems related to alcohol, such as being arrested for drinking while driving or for physically hurting someone while drunk.

- Continued drinking despite ongoing relationship problems that are caused or worsened by drinking.

Long-term alcohol abuse can turn into alcohol dependence. Dependency on alcohol, also known as alcohol addiction and alcoholism, is a chronic disease. The signs and symptoms of alcohol dependence include a strong craving for alcohol and continued use despite repeated physical, psychological, or interpersonal problems. Another sign is the inability to limit drinking.

What does it mean to get drunk?

"Getting drunk" or intoxicated is the result of consuming excessive amounts of alcohol. Binge drinking typically results in acute intoxication. Alcohol intoxication can be harmful for a variety of reasons:

- Impaired brain function resulting in poor judgment, reduced reaction time, loss of balance and motor skills, or slurred speech.

- Dilation of blood vessels causing a feeling of warmth but resulting in rapid loss of body heat.

- Increased risk of certain cancers, stroke, and liver diseases (for example, cirrhosis), particularly when excessive amounts of alcohol are consumed over extended periods of time.

- Damage to a developing fetus if consumed by pregnant women.

- Increased risk of motor-vehicle traffic crashes, violence, and other injuries.

- Coma and death can occur if alcohol is consumed rapidly and in large amounts.

How do I know if I have a drinking problem?

Drinking is a problem if it causes trouble in your relationships, in school, in social activities, or in how you think and feel. If you are concerned that either you or someone in your family might have a drinking problem, consult your personal health care provider.

What can I do if I or someone I know has a drinking problem?

Consult your personal health care provider if you feel you or someone you know has a drinking problem. Other resources include the National Drug and Alcohol Treatment Referral Routing Service available at 800-662-HELP. This service can provide you with information about treatment programs in your local community and allow you to speak with someone about alcohol problems.

What health problems are associated with excessive alcohol use?

Excessive drinking both in the form of heavy drinking or binge drinking, is associated with numerous health problems:

- Chronic diseases such as liver cirrhosis (damage to liver cells); pancreatitis (inflammation of the pancreas); various cancers, including liver, mouth, throat, larynx (the voice box), and esophagus; high blood pressure; and psychological disorders

- Unintentional injuries, such as motor-vehicle traffic crashes, falls, drowning, burns and firearm injuries

- Violence, such as child maltreatment, homicide, and suicide

- Harm to a developing fetus if a woman drinks while pregnant, such as fetal alcohol spectrum disorders

- Sudden infant death syndrome (SIDS)

- Alcohol abuse or dependence

I'm still young. Is drinking bad for my health, too?

Studies have shown that alcohol use by youth and young adults increases the risk of both fatal and nonfatal injuries. Research has also shown that youth who use alcohol before age 15 are five times more likely to become alcohol dependent than adults who begin drinking at age 21. Other consequences of youth alcohol use include increased risky sexual behaviors, poor school performance, and increased risk of suicide and homicide.

Is it okay for women to drink when pregnant?

No. There is no safe level of alcohol use during pregnancy. Women who are pregnant or plan on becoming pregnant should refrain from drinking alcohol. Several conditions, including fetal alcohol spectrum disorders have been linked to alcohol use during pregnancy. Women of child bearing age should also avoid binge drinking to reduce the risk of unintended pregnancy and potential exposure of a developing fetus to alcohol.

Chapter 3

Can Some People Consume Alcohol Safely?

Overview Of Alcohol Consumption

People drink to socialize, celebrate, and relax. Alcohol often has a strong effect on people—and throughout history, we've struggled to understand and manage alcohol's power. Why does alcohol cause us to act and feel differently? How much is too much? Why do some people become addicted while others do not? Here's what researchers currently know:

Alcohol's effects vary from person to person, depending on a variety of factors, including how much they drink, how often they drink, their age and health status, and their family history. While drinking alcohol is itself not necessarily a problem—drinking too much can cause a range of consequences, and increase your risk for a variety of problems.

There are consequences associated with drinking too much. Alcohol enters your bloodstream as soon as you take your first sip. Alcohol's immediate effects can appear within about 10 minutes. As you drink, you increase your blood alcohol concentration (BAC) level, which is the amount of alcohol present in your bloodstream. The higher your BAC, the more impaired you become by alcohol's effects. These effects can include reduced inhibitions, slurred speech, motor impairment, confusion, memory problems, concentration problems, coma, breathing problems, and death. Other risks of drinking can include car crashes and other accidents, risky behavior, violent behavior, and suicide and homicide.

About This Chapter: This chapter begins text from "Overview of Alcohol Consumption," National Institute on Alcohol Abuse and Alcoholism (www.niaaa.nih.gov), 2010. "Adult Alcohol Consumption," is excerpted from "Chapter 3: Foods and Food Components to Reduce," U.S. Department of Agriculture and U.S. Department of Health and Human Services. *Dietary Guidelines for Americans, 2010. 7th Edition*, Washington, DC: U.S. Government Printing Office, December 2010. This chapter also includes "What Is a Standard Drink?" a fact sheet produced by the National Institute on Alcohol Abuse and Alcoholism, 2010; and "What Is Low Risk Drinking?" excerpted from "Rethinking Drinking," NIAAA, April 2010.

People who drink too much over a long period of time may experience alcohol's longer-term effects, which can include alcohol dependence, health problems, and increased risk for certain cancers.

Adult Alcohol Consumption

In the United States, approximately 50 percent of adults are current regular drinkers and 14 percent are current infrequent drinkers.

The consumption of alcohol by adults can have beneficial or harmful effects, depending on the amount consumed, age, and other characteristics of the person consuming the alcohol. Alcohol consumption may have beneficial effects when consumed in moderation. Strong evidence from observational studies has shown that moderate alcohol consumption is associated with a lower risk of cardiovascular disease. Moderate alcohol consumption also is associated with a total reduced risk of death among middle-aged and older adults and may help to keep the brain functions of thinking and understanding (cognitive functions) intact with age. However, it is not recommended that anyone begin drinking or drink more frequently on the basis of potential health benefits because moderate alcohol intake also is associated with increased risk of breast cancer, violence, drowning, and injuries from falls and motor vehicle crashes.

Excessive (that is heavy, high-risk, or binge) drinking has no benefits, and the hazards of heavy alcohol intake are well known. Excessive drinking increases the risk of cirrhosis of the liver, hypertension, stroke, type 2 diabetes, cancer of the upper gastrointestinal tract and colon, injury, and violence. Excessive drinking over time is associated with increased body weight and can impair short- and long-term cognitive function. For the growing percentage of the population with elevated blood pressure, reducing alcohol intake can effectively lower blood pressure, although this is most effective when paired with changes in diet and physical activity patterns.

Excessive alcohol consumption is responsible for an average of 79,000 deaths in the United States each year. More than half of these deaths are due to binge drinking. Binge drinking also is associated with a wide range of other health and social problems, including sexually transmitted diseases, unintended pregnancy, and violent crime.

There are many circumstances in which people should not drink alcohol:

- Individuals who cannot restrict their drinking to moderate levels.

- Anyone younger than the legal drinking age. Besides being illegal, alcohol consumption increases the risk of drowning, car accidents, and traumatic injury, which are common causes of death in children and adolescents.

- Women who are pregnant or who may be pregnant. Drinking during pregnancy, especially in the first few months of pregnancy, may result in negative behavioral or neurological consequences in the offspring. No safe level of alcohol consumption during pregnancy has been established.

- Individuals taking prescription or over-the-counter medications that can interact with alcohol.

- Individuals with certain specific medical conditions (for example, liver disease, hypertriglyceridemia, pancreatitis).

- Individuals who plan to drive, operate machinery, or take part in other activities that require attention, skill, or coordination or in situations where impaired judgment could cause injury or death (for example, swimming).

What Is A Standard Drink?

Many people are surprised to learn what counts as a drink. The amount of liquid in a glass, can, or bottle does not necessarily match up to how much alcohol is actually in the drink. Different types of beer, wine, or malt liquor can have very different amounts of alcohol content. For example, many light beers have almost as much alcohol as regular beer—about 85% as much. Here's another way to put it:

- Regular beer: 5% alcohol content

- Some light beers: 4.2% alcohol content

Key Definitions For Alcohol Consumption

What is moderate alcohol consumption?

Moderate alcohol consumption is defined as up to one drink per day for women and up to two drinks per day for men.

What is heavy or high-risk drinking?

Heavy or high-risk drinking is the consumption of more than three drinks on any day or more than seven per week for women and more than four drinks on any day or more than 14 per week for men.

What is binge drinking?

Binge drinking is the consumption within two hours of four or more drinks for women and five or more drinks for men.

Source: U.S. Department of Agriculture and U.S. Department of Health and Human Services. Dietary Guidelines for Americans, 2010. 7th Edition, Washington, DC: U.S. Government Printing Office, December 2010.

That's why it's important to know how much alcohol a drink contains. In the United States, one "standard" drink contains roughly 14 grams of pure alcohol. Even though they come in different sizes, the drinks listed below are each examples of one standard drink:

- 12 ounces of regular beer, which is usually about 5% alcohol

- 8 to 9 ounces of malt liquor, which is about 7% alcohol

- 5 ounces of wine, which is typically about 12% alcohol

- 1.5 ounces of distilled spirits, which is about 40% alcohol

Although the "standard" drink amounts are helpful for following health guidelines, they may not reflect customary serving sizes. For example, a single mixed drink made with hard liquor can contain one to three or more standard drinks, depending on the type of spirits and the recipe.

What Is "Low-Risk" Drinking?

A major nationwide survey of 43,000 U.S. adults by the National Institutes of Health shows that only about two in 100 people who drink within both the "single-day" and weekly limits shown in Figure 3.1 have alcoholism or alcohol abuse.

"Low risk" is not "no risk." Even within these limits, drinkers can have problems if they drink too quickly, have health problems, or are older (both men and women over 65 are generally advised to have no more than three drinks on any day and seven per week). Based on their health and how alcohol affects them, some people may need to drink less or not at all.

Low-risk drinking limits		Adult Men	Adult Women
	On any single DAY	No more than **4** ▮▮▮▮ drinks on any **day**	No more than **3** ▮▮▮ drinks on any **day**
		** AND **	** AND **
	Per WEEK	No more than **14** ▮▮▮▮▮▮▮ ▮▮▮▮▮▮▮ drinks per **week**	No more than **7** ▮▮▮▮▮▮▮ drinks per **week**
To stay low risk, keep within BOTH the single-day AND weekly limits.			

Figure 3.1. Low-risk drinking habits apply to adults only. Anyone younger than the legal drinking age (21) should not drink alcohol. Drinking alcohol is inherently more risky in young people, and according to the Centers for Disease Control and Prevention people who begin drinking by age 15 are five times more likely to abuse or become dependent on alcohol than those who begin drinking after age 20.

Chapter 4

Problems With Caffeinated Alcoholic Beverages

Caffeinated Alcoholic Beverages

Caffeinated alcoholic beverages (CABs) are premixed beverages that combine alcohol, caffeine, and other stimulants. They may be malt- or distilled spirits–based and usually have higher alcohol content than beer (that is, 5%–12% alcohol content on average for CABs and 4%–5% alcohol content for beer). The caffeine content in these beverages is usually not reported.

CABs have experienced rapid growth in popularity since being introduced into the marketplace. For example, two leading brands of CABs together experienced a 67-fold increase in sales, from 337,500 gallons in 2002 (the first year of significant CAB production) to 22,905,000 gallons in 2008.

Currently, more than 25 brands of CABs are sold in a variety of U.S. retail alcohol outlets, including many convenience stores.

CABs are heavily marketed in youth-friendly media (for example, on websites with downloadable images) and with youth-oriented graphics and messaging (for example, connected with extreme sports or other risk-taking behaviors).

Dangers Of Mixing Alcohol And Energy Drinks

Energy drinks are beverages that typically contain caffeine, other plant-based stimulants, simple sugars, and other additives. They are very popular among youth and are regularly consumed by 31% of 12- to 17-year-olds and 34% of 18- to 24-year-olds.

About This Chapter: Text in this chapter is excerpted from "Caffeinated Alcoholic Beverages," Centers for Disease Control and Prevention (www.cdc.gov), July 20, 2010.

When alcoholic beverages are mixed with energy drinks, a popular practice among youth, the caffeine in these drinks can mask the depressant effects of alcohol. At the same time, caffeine has no effect on the metabolism of alcohol by the liver and thus does not reduce breath alcohol concentrations or reduce the risk of alcohol-attributable harms.

Drinkers who consume alcohol mixed with energy drinks are three times more likely to binge drink (based on breath alcohol levels) than drinkers who do not report mixing alcohol with energy drinks.

Drinkers who consume alcohol with energy drinks are about twice as likely as drinkers who do not report mixing alcohol with energy drinks to report being taken advantage of sexually, to report taking advantage of someone else sexually, and to report riding with a driver who was under the influence of alcohol.

A Troubling Mix

Caffeinated alcoholic beverages, or CABs, are alcoholic beverages that contain caffeine as an additive and are packaged in combined form. Alcoholic beverages to which caffeine has been added as a separate ingredient have raised health concerns at the Food and Drug Administration (FDA) as well as in other federal, state, and local agencies.

According to data and expert opinion, caffeine can mask sensory cues that people may rely on to determine how intoxicated they are. This means that individuals drinking these beverages may consume more alcohol—and become more intoxicated—than they realize. At the same time, caffeine does not change blood alcohol content levels, and thus does not reduce the risk of harms associated with drinking alcohol.

Studies suggest that drinking caffeine and alcohol together may lead to hazardous and life-threatening behaviors. For example, serious concerns are raised about whether the combination of alcohol and caffeine is associated with an increased risk of alcohol-related consequences, including alcohol poisoning, sexual assault, and riding with a driver who is under the influence of alcohol.

Malt versions of premixed alcoholic beverages come in containers holding between 12 and 32 liquid ounces. Some may also contain stimulant ingredients in addition to caffeine. Their advertised alcohol-by-volume value is as high as 12 percent, compared to standard beer's usual value of 4 to 5 percent.

These alcoholic beverages are available in many states in convenience stores and other outlets. They often come in large, boldly colored cans comparable in size to "tall" cans of beer—or in containers resembling regular beer bottles.

Source: From "Serious Concerns Over Alcoholic Beverages with Added Caffeine," U.S. Food and Drug Administration (www.fda.gov), December 8, 2011.

Prevention Strategies

In 2008, thirteen State Attorneys General and the San Francisco, California, City Attorney initiated an investigation of CABs, which resulted in negotiated settlements with two CAB producers, who agreed to remove all stimulants from their products.

Because CABs may have higher alcohol content than beer, some states (for example, Montana) have classified CABs as liquor, thereby limiting the locations where these beverages can be sold.

States and communities are also developing educational strategies to alert consumers to the risks of mixing alcohol with energy drinks and CABs. One community has enacted an ordinance requiring retailers to post signs warning of the risks of CABs.

Additional Strategies Recommended By CDC

Effective population-based strategies for preventing excessive alcohol consumption and related harms should also be implemented, including increasing alcohol excise taxes, limiting alcohol outlet density, and maintaining existing restrictions on days of sale.

Youth exposure to alcohol marketing should also be reduced by lowering the voluntary industry standard governing the placement of alcohol advertising from the current 30% threshold to 15%, based on the proportion of the audience that is age 12–20 years.

Chapter 5

Binge Drinking

Binge Drinking Is A Nationwide Problem

New estimates show that binge drinking (which means men drinking five or more alcoholic drinks within a short period of time or women drinking four or more drinks within a short period of time) is a bigger problem than previously thought. More than 38 million U.S. adults binge drink, about four times a month, and the largest number of drinks per binge is on average eight. This behavior greatly increases the chances of getting hurt or hurting others due to car crashes, violence, and suicide. Drinking too much, including binge drinking, causes nearly 80,000 deaths in the United States each year. Binge drinking is a problem in all states, even in states with fewer binge drinkers, because they are bingeing more often and in larger amounts.

Problem

Binge drinking is a dangerous and costly public health problem:

- Binge drinking is about more than just the number of binge drinkers. The amount and number of times binge drinkers drink are also important to address.

- Age group with most binge drinkers: 18–34 years

- Age group that binge drinks most often: 65+ years

- Income group with most binge drinkers: more than $75,000

- Income group that binge drinks the most often and drinks most per binge: less than $25,000

About This Chapter: This chapter begins with excerpts from "Binge Drinking: Nationwide Problem, Local Solutions," *CDC VitalSigns*, Centers for Disease Control and Preventions (www.cdc.gov), January 2012. Additional information is from "Excessive Drinking Costs U.S. $223.5 Billion," CDC, October 17, 2011.

- Most alcohol-impaired drivers binge drink.

- Most people who binge drink are not alcohol dependent or alcoholics.

- More than half of the alcohol adults drink is while binge drinking.

- More than 90% of the alcohol youth drink is while binge drinking.

Binge Drinking Costs Everyone

- Drinking too much, including binge drinking, cost $746 per person, or $1.90 a drink, in the U.S. in 2006. These costs include health care expenses, crime, and lost productivity. See below for more information.

- Binge drinking cost federal, state, and local governments about 62 cents per drink in 2006, while federal and state income from taxes on alcohol totaled only about 12 cents per drink.

Facts About Binge Drinking

Binge drinking is associated with many health problems, including the following:

- Unintentional injuries (for example, car crashes, falls, burns, drowning)
- Intentional injuries (for example, firearm injuries, sexual assault, domestic violence)
- Alcohol poisoning
- Sexually transmitted diseases
- Unintended pregnancy
- Children born with fetal alcohol spectrum disorders
- High blood pressure, stroke, and other cardiovascular diseases
- Liver disease
- Neurological damage
- Sexual dysfunction
- Poor control of diabetes

Adult binge drinking also casts a shadow on future generations. "Binge drinking by adults has a huge public health impact, and influences the drinking behavior of underage youth by the example it sets," said Substance Abuse and Mental Health Services Administrator Pamela S. Hyde. "We need to reduce binge drinking by adults to prevent the immediate and long–term effects it has on the health of adults and youth."

Source: Excerpted from "Binge Drinking," a Centers for Disease Control and Prevention (CDC) Fact Sheet dated December 17, 2010; and "Binge Drinking Is Bigger Problem Than Previously Thought," a CDC press release dated January 10, 2012.

- Drinking too much contributes to more than 54 different injuries and diseases, including car crashes, violence, and sexually-transmitted diseases.

- The chance of getting sick and dying from alcohol problems increases significantly for those who binge drink more often and drink more when they do.

Percent Of Adults Who Binge Drink

Binge drinking varies from state to state, and estimates of adults who binge drink range from 10.9% in Utah to 25.6% in Wisconsin. Binge drinking is most common in the Midwest, New England, the District of Columbia, Alaska, and Hawaii.

The average largest number of drinks within a short period of time among binge drinkers ranged from six drinks in the District of Columbia to nine drinks in Wisconsin. The largest number of drinks consumed by binge drinkers is highest in the Midwest and southern Mountain states (Arizona, Nevada, New Mexico, and Utah), and some states such as Louisiana, Mississippi, and South Carolina where binge drinking is less common.

Everyone Can Help Prevent Binge Drinking

The U.S. government can collaborate with states and communities to support effective community strategies to prevent binge drinking strategies such as those recommended by the Community Guide (The Community Guide recommendations can be found at http://www .thecommunityguide.org/alcohol.) The U.S. government can also help states and communities in gather statistics, evaluate laws and regulations that control the marketing and sale of alcohol, and determine whether prevention strategies are working.

States and communities can implement effective community strategies to prevent binge drinking, gather statistics, and develop community coalitions that build partnerships among schools, community- and faith-based organizations, law enforcement, health care, and public health agencies to reduce binge drinking.

Doctors, nurses, and other healthcare providers can recognize that drinking too much causes 80,000 deaths in the U.S. each year and contributes to over 54 different injuries and diseases. They can also recognize that most binge drinkers are not alcohol dependent or alcoholics, support effective community strategies to prevent binge drinking, and screen patients for binge drinking and advise those who do to reduce their use.

People can choose not to binge drink themselves and help others not to do it. Adults can drink in moderation if they do drink. The U.S. dietary guidelines on alcohol consumption recommend no more than one drink per day for women and no more than two drinks per day for men. Pregnant women and underage youth should not drink alcohol. People can also support effective community strategies to prevent binge drinking, support local control of the marketing and sale of alcohol, and support the minimum legal drinking age of 21.

Excessive Drinking Costs U.S. $223.5 Billion

A new study finds that excessive alcohol consumption cost the United States $223.5 billion in 2006, or about $1.90 per drink. By implementing effective community-based prevention strategies, we can reduce excessive alcohol consumption and its costs.

Excessive alcohol consumption is known to kill about 79,000 people in the United States each year, but a new study released by the Centers for Disease Control and Prevention (CDC) and The Lewin Group shows that it also has a huge impact on our wallets as well.

The cost of excessive alcohol consumption in the United States reached $223.5 billion in 2006 or about $1.90 per drink. Almost three-quarters of these costs were due to binge drinking. Binge drinking is defined as consuming four or more alcoholic beverages per occasion for women or five or more drinks per occasion for men, and is the most common form of excessive alcohol consumption in the United States.

The researchers found that the cost of excessive drinking was quite far-reaching, reflecting the effect this dangerous behavior has on many aspects of the drinker's life and on the lives of those around them. The costs largely resulted from losses in workplace productivity (72% of the total cost), health care expenses for problems caused by excessive drinking (11% of total), law enforcement and other criminal justice expenses related to excessive alcohol consumption (9% of total), and motor vehicle crash costs from impaired driving (6% of the total).

The study analyzed national data from multiple sources to estimate the costs due to excessive drinking in 2006, the most recent year for which data were available. The study did not consider a number of other costs such as those because of pain and suffering among either the excessive drinker or others that were affected by their drinking, and thus may be an underestimate. Nevertheless, the researchers estimated that excessive drinking cost $746 for every man, woman, and child in the United States in 2006.

What You Need To Know About Binge Drinking

Binge drinking is reported by about 15% of U.S. adults. Binge drinking is most common among men, 18- to 34-year-olds, whites, and people with household incomes of $75,000 or more. Most binge drinkers are not alcohol dependent.

Preventing Excessive Alcohol Consumption And Reducing Its Economic Costs

There are many evidence-based strategies that communities can use to prevent excessive drinking, including increasing alcohol excise taxes, reducing alcohol outlet density, reducing the days and hours of alcohol sales, and holding alcohol retailers liable for injuries or damage done by their intoxicated or underage customers. By implementing these evidence-based strategies, we can reduce excessive alcohol consumption and the many health and social costs related to it.

Leprechauns, Shamrocks, And... Binge Drinking?

St. Patrick's Day, once a religious holiday that celebrated the patron saint of Ireland, has become a day for revelry and partying. In fact, it has become one of the biggest drinking days of the year.

Binge drinking—sucking down four or five drinks within about two hours—seems to be encouraged, with many bars hosting day-long parties and serving green beer and Irish whiskey.

What's The Harm?

While downing pints of green beer may be a St. Patrick's Day tradition for some, it's really not a good one for your brain. Research shows that binge drinking damages the brain, even if you do it only once in a while. Young people are at special risk, since their brains are still developing—growing and making new connections until their mid-20s.

Binge drinking can lead to alcohol poisoning and also affects the frontal cortex, an area involved with judgment, thinking, memory, and feeling.

Binge drinking also can have serious consequences after the party's over. If you're driving under the influence, or riding with someone who's drunk, you'll need a ton of "Irish luck" to get home safely. St. Patrick's Day is one of the deadliest on the road. More than one in three drivers involved in fatal crashes have a blood alcohol concentration over the legal limit—and of course, no amount of alcohol is legal for those under age 21.

In 2011, the National Highway Traffic Safety Administration started a program with the slogan, "Kiss Me, I'm Sober," to keep "buzzed" drivers off the road on St. Patrick's Day. The first and most important step is to choose a designated driver who will not drink alcohol during the festivities.

Be Green!

St. Patrick's Day is meant for light-hearted fun, and you don't have to drink alcohol to enjoy it.

Source: "St. Patrick's Day: Leprechauns, Shamrocks, and… Binge Drinking?" National Institute on Drug Abuse (teens .drugabuse.gov), March 15, 2012.

Chapter 6

Alcohol Poisoning

Excessive drinking can be hazardous to everyone's health. It can be particularly stressful if you are the sober one taking care of your drunken friend, who is vomiting while you are trying to do your homework or study for an exam.

Some people laugh at the behavior of others who are drunk. Some think it's even funnier when they pass out. But there is nothing funny about the aspiration of vomit leading to asphyxiation or the poisoning of the respiratory center in the brain, both of which can result in death.

Do you know about the dangers of alcohol poisoning? When should you seek professional help for a friend? Sadly enough, too many students say they wish they would have sought medical treatment for a friend. Many end up feeling responsible for alcohol-related tragedies that could have easily been prevented.

Common myths about sobering up include drinking black coffee, taking a cold bath or shower, sleeping it off, or walking it off. But these are just myths, and they don't work. The only thing that reverses the effects of alcohol is time—something you may not have if you are suffering from alcohol poisoning. And many different factors affect the level of intoxication of an individual, so it's difficult to gauge exactly how much is too much.

What happens to your body when you get alcohol poisoning?

Alcohol depresses nerves that control involuntary actions such as breathing and the gag reflex (which prevents choking). A fatal dose of alcohol will eventually stop these functions.

About This Chapter: From "Facts about Alcohol Poisoning," College Drinking—Changing the Future (www .collegedrinkingprevention.gov), a project of the National Institute on Drug Abuse, July 11, 2007. Reviewed by David A. Cooke, MD, FACP, December 2012.

It is common for someone who drank excessive alcohol to vomit since alcohol is an irritant to the stomach. There is then the danger of choking on vomit, which could cause death by asphyxiation in a person who is not conscious because of intoxication.

You should also know that a person's blood alcohol concentration (BAC) can continue to rise even while he or she is passed out. Even after a person stops drinking, alcohol in the stomach and intestine continues to enter the bloodstream and circulate throughout the body. It is dangerous to assume the person will be fine by sleeping it off.

What are critical signs and symptoms of alcohol poisoning?

- Mental confusion, stupor, coma, or person cannot be roused

- Vomiting

- Seizures

- Slow breathing (fewer than eight breaths per minute)

- Irregular breathing (10 seconds or more between breaths)

- Hypothermia (low body temperature), bluish skin color, paleness

About Alcohol Poisoning: A Summary

Alcohol depresses nerves that control involuntary actions such as breathing and the gag reflex, which prevents choking. Someone who drinks a fatal dose of alcohol will eventually stop breathing. Even if someone survives an alcohol overdose, he or she can suffer irreversible brain damage. Rapid binge drinking (which often happens on a bet or a dare) is especially dangerous because the victim can drink a fatal dose before losing consciousness.

A person's blood alcohol concentration can continue to rise even while he or she is passed out. Even after someone stops drinking, alcohol in the stomach and intestine continues to enter the blood-stream and circulate throughout the body. A person who appears to be sleeping it off may be in real danger.

Critical signs of alcohol poisoning include mental confusion, stupor, coma, or the person cannot be roused; vomiting; seizures; slow (fewer than eight breaths per minute) or irregular (10 seconds or more between breaths) breathing; and hypothermia (low body temperature), bluish skin color, and paleness.

Know the danger signals. If you suspect someone has alcohol poisoning, don't wait for all the critical signs to be present. If you suspect an alcohol overdose, call 911 immediately for help.

Source: "A Word About Alcohol Poisoning," National Institute on Alcohol Abuse and Alcoholism (www.niaaa.nih.gov), April 2012.

What should I do if I suspect someone has alcohol poisoning?

- Know the danger signals.

- Do not wait for all symptoms to be present.

- Be aware that a person who has passed out may die.

- If there is any suspicion of an alcohol overdose, call 911 for help. Don't try to guess the level of drunkenness.

What can happen to someone with alcohol poisoning that goes untreated?

- Victim chokes on his or her own vomit

- Breathing slows, becomes irregular, or stops

- Heart beats irregularly or stops

- Hypothermia (low body temperature)

- Hypoglycemia (too little blood sugar) leads to seizures

- Untreated severe dehydration from vomiting can cause seizures, permanent brain damage, or death

Even if the victim lives, an alcohol overdose can lead to irreversible brain damage. Rapid binge drinking (which often happens on a bet or a dare) is especially dangerous because the victim can ingest a fatal dose before becoming unconscious.

Don't be afraid to seek medical help for a friend who has had too much to drink. Don't worry that your friend may become angry or embarrassed-remember, you cared enough to help. Always be safe, not sorry.

Chapter 7

Alcohol Abuse And Alcoholism

When people drink too much, with time they risk becoming addicted to alcohol. This is called alcoholism, or alcohol dependence. It's a disease, and it can happen at any age. These are some of the common signs:

- **Craving:** A strong need or urge to drink

- **Loss Of Control:** Not being able to stop or cut down drinking

- **Not Feeling Well After Heavy Drinking:** Upset stomach, sweating, shakiness, or nervousness

- **A Need To Drink More:** To get the same effect as before

- **Neglecting Activities:** Giving up or cutting back on other activities

- **Continuing To Drink:** Even though alcohol is causing problems

It may be hard to imagine why people with alcoholism can't just "use a little willpower" to stop drinking. But the addiction creates an uncontrollable need for alcohol. It can be as strong as the need for food and water. People may want to stop because they know that drinking harms their health and their loved ones. But quitting is extremely difficult.

Although some people are able to recover from alcoholism without help, many need assistance. With treatment and support, many stop drinking and rebuild their lives.

About This Chapter: This chapter begins with text from "When Drinking Becomes A Disease," National Institute on Alcohol Abuse and Alcoholism (www.thecoolspot.gov), 2010. It continues with "FAQs on Alcohol Abuse and Alcoholism," College Drinking—Changing the Culture, a project of the National Institute on Drug Abuse, July 2007. Revised by David A. Cooke, MD, FACP, December 2012.

Frequently Asked Questions About Alcohol Abuse And Alcoholism

What is alcoholism?

Alcoholism, also known as alcohol dependence, is a disease that includes the following four symptoms:

- **Craving:** A strong need, or urge, to drink.

- **Loss Of Control:** Not being able to stop drinking once drinking has begun.

- **Physical Dependence:** Withdrawal symptoms, such as nausea, sweating, shakiness, and anxiety after stopping drinking.

- **Tolerance:** The need to drink greater amounts of alcohol to get "high."

For clinical and research purposes, formal diagnostic criteria for alcoholism also have been developed. Such criteria are included in the *Diagnostic and Statistical Manual of Mental Disorders* published by the American Psychiatric Association, as well as in the International Classification Diseases, published by the World Health Organization.

What are symptoms of an alcohol use disorder?

See if you recognize any of these symptoms in yourself. In the past year, have you...

- had times when you ended up drinking more, or longer, than you intended?
- more than once wanted to cut down or stop drinking, or tried to, but couldn't?
- more than once gotten into situations while or after drinking that increased your chances of getting hurt (such as driving, swimming, using machinery, walking in a dangerous area, or having unsafe sex)?
- had to drink much more than you once did to get the effect you want? or found that your usual number of drinks had much less effect than before?
- continued to drink even though it was making you feel depressed or anxious or adding to another health problem? or after having had a memory blackout?
- spent a lot of time drinking? or being sick or getting over other aftereffects?
- continued to drink even though it was causing trouble with your family or friends?
- found that drinking—or being sick from drinking—often interfered with taking care of your responsibilities? or caused school problems?

Is alcoholism a disease?

Yes, alcoholism is a disease. The craving that an alcoholic feels for alcohol can be as strong as the need for food or water. An alcoholic will continue to drink despite serious family, health, or legal problems.

Like many other diseases, alcoholism is chronic, meaning that it lasts a person's lifetime; it usually follows a predictable course; and it has symptoms. The risk for developing alcoholism is influenced both by a person's genes and by his or her lifestyle.

Is alcoholism inherited?

Research shows that the risk for developing alcoholism does indeed run in families. The genes a person inherits partially explain this pattern, but lifestyle is also a factor. Currently, researchers are working to discover the actual genes that put people at risk for alcoholism. Your friends, the amount of stress in your life, and how readily available alcohol is also are factors that may increase your risk for alcoholism.

But remember: Risk is not destiny. Just because alcoholism tends to run in families doesn't mean that a child of an alcoholic parent will automatically become an alcoholic too. Some people develop alcoholism even though no one in their family has a drinking problem. By

---

- given up or cut back on activities that were important or interesting to you, or gave you pleasure, in order to drink?
- more than once gotten arrested, been held at a police station, or had other legal problems because of your drinking?
- found that when the effects of alcohol were wearing off, you had withdrawal symptoms, such as trouble sleeping, shakiness, restlessness, nausea, sweating, a racing heart, or a seizure? or sensed things that were not there?

If you don't have symptoms, and if you're over the age of 21, then staying within low-risk drinking limits will reduce your chances of having problems in the future (for more information, see Chapter 3—Can Some People Consume Alcohol Safely?).

If you do have any symptoms, then alcohol may already be a cause for concern. The more symptoms you have, the more urgent the need for change. A health professional can look at the number, pattern, and severity of symptoms to see whether an alcohol use disorder is present and help you decide the best course of action.

Source: Excerpted from "Rethinking Drinking," National Institute on Alcohol Abuse and Alcoholism (www.niaaa.nih. gov), April 2010.

the same token, not all children of alcoholic families get into trouble with alcohol. Knowing you are at risk is important, though, because then you can take steps to protect yourself from developing problems with alcohol.

Can alcoholism be cured?

No, alcoholism cannot be cured at this time. Even if an alcoholic hasn't been drinking for a long time, he or she can still suffer a relapse. Not drinking is the safest course for most people with alcoholism.

Can alcoholism be treated?

Yes, alcoholism can be treated. Alcoholism treatment programs use both counseling and medications to help a person stop drinking. Treatment has helped many people stop drinking and rebuild their lives.

Which medications treat alcoholism?

Three oral medications—disulfiram (Antabuse), naltrexone (Depade, ReVia), and acamprosate (Campral)—are currently approved to treat alcohol dependence. In addition, an injectable, long-acting form of naltrexone (Vivitrol) is available. These medications have been shown to help people with dependence reduce their drinking, avoid relapse to heavy drinking, and achieve and maintain abstinence. Naltrexone acts in the brain to reduce craving for alcohol after someone has stopped drinking. Acamprosate is thought to work by reducing symptoms that follow lengthy abstinence, such as anxiety and insomnia. Disulfiram discourages drinking by making the person taking it feel sick after drinking alcohol.

Other types of drugs are available to help manage symptoms of withdrawal (such as shakiness, nausea, and sweating) if they occur after someone with alcohol dependence stops drinking.

Although medications are available to help treat alcoholism, there is no "magic bullet." In other words, no single medication is available that works in every case and/or in every person. Developing new and more effective medications to treat alcoholism remains a high priority for researchers.

Does alcoholism treatment work?

Alcoholism treatment works for many people. But like other chronic illnesses—such as diabetes, high blood pressure, and asthma—there are varying levels of success when it comes to treatment. Some people stop drinking and remain sober. Others have long periods of sobriety with bouts of relapse. And still others cannot stop drinking for any length of time. With treatment, one thing is clear, however: the longer a person abstains from alcohol, the more likely he or she will be able to stay sober.

Do you have to be an alcoholic to experience problems with alcohol?

No. Alcoholism is only one type of an alcohol problem. Alcohol abuse can be just as harmful. A person can abuse alcohol without actually being an alcoholic—that is, he or she may drink too much and too often but still not be dependent on alcohol. Some of the problems linked to alcohol abuse include not being able to meet work, school, or family responsibilities; drunk-driving arrests and car crashes; and drinking-related medical conditions. Under some circumstances, even social or moderate drinking is dangerous—for example, when driving, during pregnancy, or when taking certain medications.

Are specific groups of people more likely to have problems?

Alcohol abuse and alcoholism cut across gender, race, and nationality. In the United States, 17.6 million people—about one in every 12 adults—abuse alcohol or are alcohol dependent. In general, more men than women are alcohol dependent or have alcohol problems. And alcohol problems are highest among young adults ages 18–29 and lowest among adults ages 65 and older. We also know that people who start drinking at an early age—for example, at age 14 or younger—are at much higher risk of developing alcohol problems at some point in their lives compared to someone who starts drinking at age 21 or after.

How can you tell if someone has a problem?

Answering the following four questions can help you find out if you or a loved one has a drinking problem:

- Have you ever felt you should cut down on your drinking?
- Have people annoyed you by criticizing your drinking?
- Have you ever felt bad or guilty about your drinking?
- Have you ever had a drink first thing in the morning to steady your nerves or to get rid of a hangover?

One "yes" answer suggests a possible alcohol problem. More than one "yes" answer means it is highly likely that a problem exists. If you think that you or someone you know might have an alcohol problem, it is important to see a doctor or other health care provider right away. They can help you determine if a drinking problem exists and plan the best course of action.

Can a problem drinker simply cut down?

It depends. If that person has been diagnosed as an alcoholic, the answer is "no." Alcoholics who try to cut down on drinking rarely succeed. Cutting out alcohol—that is, abstaining—is usually the best course for recovery. People who are not alcohol dependent but who have experienced alcohol-related problems may be able to limit the amount they drink. If they can't stay within those limits, they need to stop drinking altogether.

If an alcoholic is unwilling to get help, what can you do about it?

This can be a challenge. An alcoholic can't be forced to get help except under certain circumstances, such as a traffic violation or arrest that results in court-ordered treatment. But you don't have to wait for someone to "hit rock bottom" to act. Many alcoholism treatment specialists suggest the following steps to help an alcoholic get treatment:

- **Stop all "cover ups."** Family members often make excuses to others or try to protect the alcoholic from the results of his or her drinking. It is important to stop covering for the alcoholic so that he or she experiences the full consequences of drinking.

- **Time your intervention.** The best time to talk to the drinker is shortly after an alcohol-related problem has occurred—like a serious family argument or an accident. Choose a time when he or she is sober, both of you are fairly calm, and you have a chance to talk in private.

- **Be specific.** Tell the family member that you are worried about his or her drinking. Use examples of the ways in which the drinking has caused problems, including the most recent incident.

- **State the results.** Explain to the drinker what you will do if he or she doesn't go for help—not to punish the drinker, but to protect yourself from his or her problems. What you say may range from refusing to go with the person to any social activity where alcohol will be served, to moving out of the house. Do not make any threats you are not prepared to carry out.

- **Get help.** Gather information in advance about treatment options in your community. If the person is willing to get help, call immediately for an appointment with a treatment counselor. Offer to go with the family member on the first visit to a treatment program and/or an Alcoholics Anonymous meeting.

- **Call on a friend.** If the family member still refuses to get help, ask a friend to talk with him or her using the steps just described. A friend who is a recovering alcoholic may be particularly persuasive, but any person who is caring and nonjudgmental may help. The intervention of more than one person, more than one time, is often necessary to coax an alcoholic to seek help.

- **Find strength in numbers.** With the help of a health care professional, some families join with other relatives and friends to confront an alcoholic as a group. This approach should only be tried under the guidance of a health care professional who is experienced in this kind of group intervention.

- **Get support.** It is important to remember that you are not alone. Support groups offered in most communities include Al-Anon, which holds regular meetings for spouses and other significant adults in an alcoholic's life, and Alateen, which is geared to children of alcoholics. These groups help family members understand that they are not responsible for an alcoholic's drinking and that they need to take steps to take care of themselves, regardless of whether the alcoholic family member chooses to get help.

You can call the National Drug and Alcohol Treatment Referral Routing Service (Center for Substance Abuse Treatment) at 800-662-HELP (4357) for information about treatment programs in your local community and to speak to someone about an alcohol problem.

What is a safe level of drinking?

For most adults, moderate alcohol use—up to two drinks per day for men and one drink per day for women and older people—causes few if any problems. (One drink equals one 12-ounce bottle of beer or wine cooler, one 5-ounce glass of wine, or 1.5 ounces of 80-proof distilled spirits.)

Certain people should not drink at all, however:

- Women who are pregnant or trying to become pregnant
- People who plan to drive or engage in other activities that require alertness and skill (such as driving a car)
- People taking certain over-the-counter or prescription medications
- People with medical conditions that can be made worse by drinking
- Recovering alcoholics
- People younger than age 21

Is it safe to drink during pregnancy?

No, alcohol can harm the baby of a mother who drinks during pregnancy. Although the highest risk is to babies whose mothers drink heavily, it is not clear yet whether there is any completely safe level of alcohol during pregnancy. For this reason, the U.S. Surgeon General released advisories in 1981 and again in 2005 urging women who are pregnant or may become pregnant to abstain from alcohol (http://www.lhvpn.net/hhspress.html). The damage caused by prenatal alcohol includes a range of physical, behavioral, and learning problems in babies. Babies most severely affected have what is called fetal alcohol syndrome (FAS). These babies may have abnormal facial features and severe learning disabilities. Babies can also be born with mild disabilities without the facial changes typical of FAS.

Does alcohol affect older people differently?

Alcohol's effects do vary with age. Slower reaction times, problems with hearing and seeing, and a lower tolerance to alcohol's effects put older people at higher risk for falls, car crashes, and other types of injuries that may result from drinking.

Older people also tend to take more medicines than younger people. Mixing alcohol with over-the-counter or prescription medications can be very dangerous, even fatal. In addition, alcohol can make many of the medical conditions common in older people, including high blood pressure and ulcers, more serious. Physical changes associated with aging can make older people feel "high" even after drinking only small amounts of alcohol. So even if there is no medical reason to avoid alcohol, older men and women should limit themselves to one drink per day.

How do you know if you have a problem?

Answering the following four questions can help you find out if you or someone close to you has a drinking problem.

- Have you ever felt you should cut down on your drinking?
- Have people annoyed you by criticizing your drinking?
- Have you ever felt bad or guilty about your drinking?
- Have you ever had a drink first thing in the morning to steady your nerves or to get rid of a hangover?

One "yes" answer suggests a possible alcohol problem. If you responded "yes" to more than one question, it is very likely that you have a problem with alcohol. In either case, it is important that you see your health care provider right away to discuss your responses to these questions.

Even if you answered "no" to all of the above questions, if you are having drinking-related problems with your job, relationships, health, or with the law, you should still seek help.

Source: Excerpted from "Alcoholism, Substance Abuse, and Addictive Behavior," Office on Women's Health (www.womens health.gov), March 29, 2010.

Does alcohol affect women differently?

Yes, alcohol affects women differently than men. Women become more impaired than men do after drinking the same amount of alcohol, even when differences in body weight are taken into account. There is some debate as to why this is true; it is suspected that differences in body composition or rate of alcohol metabolism are responsible. Regardless, women are more sensitive to alcohol, on average, and that is why the recommended drinking limit for women is lower than for men.

In addition, chronic alcohol abuse takes a heavier physical toll on women than on men. Alcohol dependence and related medical problems, such as brain, heart, and liver damage, develop and progress more rapidly in women than in men, and are seen at lower levels of alcohol intake.

Is alcohol good for your heart?

Studies have shown that moderate drinkers are less likely to die from one form of heart disease than are people who do not drink any alcohol or who drink more.

If you are a nondrinker, however, you should not start drinking solely to benefit your heart. You can guard against heart disease by exercising and eating foods that are low in fat. And if you are pregnant, planning to become pregnant, have been diagnosed as alcoholic, or have another medical condition that could make alcohol use harmful, or if you are younger than age 21, you should not drink.

If you can safely drink alcohol and you choose to drink, do so in moderation. Heavy drinking can actually increase the risk of heart failure, stroke, and high blood pressure, as well as cause many other medical problems, such as liver cirrhosis.

When taking medications, must people stop drinking?

Possibly. More than 150 medications interact harmfully with alcohol. These interactions may result in increased risk of illness, injury, and even death. Alcohol's effects are heightened by medicines that depress the central nervous system, such as sleeping pills, antihistamines, antidepressants, anti-anxiety drugs, and some painkillers. In addition, medicines for certain disorders, including diabetes, high blood pressure, and heart disease, can have harmful interactions with alcohol. If you are taking any over-the-counter or prescription medications, ask your doctor or pharmacist if you can safely drink alcohol.

How can a person get help for an alcohol problem?

There are many national and local resources that can help. The National Drug and Alcohol Treatment Referral Routing Service provides a toll-free telephone number, 800-662-HELP

(4357), offering various resource information. Through this service you can speak directly to a representative concerning substance abuse treatment, request printed material on alcohol or other drugs, or obtain local substance abuse treatment referral information in your state.

Many people also find support groups, such as Al-Anon/Alateen, Alcoholics Anonymous (AA), and National Association for Children of Alcoholics (NACOA), a helpful aid to recovery.

Why do some people become addicted, while others do not?

Nothing can predict whether or not a person will become addicted to alcohol or other drugs. But there are some risk factors for addiction. These risk factors include the following:

- **Biology:** Genes, gender, ethnicity, and the presence of other mental disorders may increase risk for alcohol or drug abuse and addiction.
- **Environment:** Peer pressure, physical and sexual abuse, stress, and family relationships can influence the course of substance abuse and addiction in a person's life.
- **Development:** Although drinking alcohol or taking drugs at any age can lead to addiction, the earlier that substance use begins, the more likely it is to progress to more serious abuse.

Source: Excerpted from "Alcoholism, Substance Abuse, and Addictive Behavior," Office on Women's Health (www.womenshealth.gov), March 29, 2010.

Chapter 8

The Stages Of Alcoholism

There are, and have been, many theories about alcoholism. The most prevailing theory, and now most commonly accepted, is called the "Disease Model." Its basic beliefs are that alcoholism is a disease with recognizable symptoms, causes, and methods of treatment. In addition, there are several stages of the disease which are often described as early, middle, and late. It is useful to understand these stages in terms of how the disease appears.

The Early Or Adaptive Stage

The early or adaptive stage of alcoholism is marked by increasing tolerance to alcohol and physical adaptations in the body which are largely unseen. This increased tolerance is marked by the alcoholic's ability to consume greater quantities of alcohol while appearing to suffer few effects and continuing to function. This tolerance is not created simply because the alcoholic drinks too much but rather because the alcoholic is able to drink increased quantities because of physical changes going on inside his or her body.

The early stage is difficult to detect. By appearances, an individual may be able to drink a great deal without becoming intoxicated, having hangovers, or suffering other apparent ill-effects from alcohol. An early stage alcoholic is often indistinguishable from a non-alcoholic who happens to be a fairly heavy drinker.

There is likely to be little or no obvious impact on the alcoholic's performance or conduct other than drinking. At this stage, the alcoholic is not likely to see any problem with his or her drinking and would scoff at any attempts to indicate that he or she might have a problem. The alcoholic is simply not aware of what is going on in his or her body.

About This Chapter: Excerpted from "Alcoholism," *Alcoholism in the Workplace: A Handbook for Supervisors*, Office of Personnel Management (www.omp.gov), 2006. Reviewed by David A. Cooke, MD, FACP, December 2012.

The Middle Stage

There is no clear line between the early and middle stages of alcoholism, but there are several characteristics that mark a new stage of the disease. Many of the pleasures the alcoholic obtained from drinking during the early stage are now being replaced by the destructive facets of alcohol abuse. The drinking that was done for the purpose of getting "high" is now being replaced by drinking to combat the pain and misery caused by prior drinking.

One basic characteristic of the middle stage is physical dependence. In the early stage, the alcoholic's tolerance to greater amounts of alcohol is increasing. Along with this, however, the body becomes used to these amounts of alcohol and now suffers from withdrawal when the alcohol is not present.

Another basic characteristic of the middle stage is craving. Alcoholics develop a very powerful urge to drink which they are eventually unable to control. As the alcoholic's tolerance increases along with the physical dependence, the alcoholic loses his or her ability to control drinking and craves alcohol.

The third characteristic of the middle stage is loss of control. The alcoholic simply loses his or her ability to limit his or her drinking to socially acceptable times, patterns, and places. This loss of control is due to a decrease in the alcoholic's tolerance and an increase in the withdrawal symptoms. The alcoholic cannot handle as much alcohol as they once could without getting drunk, yet needs increasing amounts to avoid withdrawal.

Another feature of middle stage alcoholics is blackouts. Contrary to what you might assume, the alcoholic does not actually pass out during these episodes. Instead, the alcoholic continues to function but is unable to remember what he or she has done or where he or she has been. Basically, the alcoholic simply can't remember these episodes because the brain has either stored these memories improperly or has not stored them at all. Blackouts may also occur in early stage alcoholics.

Impairment becomes evident during the middle stage. The alcoholic battles with loss of control, withdrawal symptoms, and cravings. This will become apparent in terms of any or all of the following: increased and unpredictable absences, poorly performed work assignments, behavior problems, inability to concentrate, accidents, increased days out sick, and possible deterioration in overall appearance and demeanor.

Late Stage

The late, or deteriorative stage, is best identified as the point at which the damage to the body from the toxic effects of alcohol is evident, and the alcoholic is suffering from a host of ailments.

An alcoholic in the final stages may be destitute, extremely ill, mentally confused, and drinking almost constantly. The alcoholic in this stage is suffering from many physical and psychological problems due to the damage to vital organs. His or her immunity to infections is lowered and mental condition is very unstable. Some of the very serious medical conditions the alcoholic faces at this point include heart failure, fatty liver, hepatitis, cirrhosis of the liver, malnutrition, pancreatitis, respiratory infections, and brain damage, some of which is reversible.

The Role Of Denial

Why does an alcoholic continue to drink despite the known facts about the disease and the obvious adverse consequences of continued drinking? The answer to this question is quite simple. In the early stage, the alcoholic does not consider himself or herself sick because his or her tolerance is increasing. In the middle stage, the alcoholic is unknowingly physically dependent on alcohol. He or she simply finds that continuing to use alcohol will prevent the problems of withdrawal. By the time an alcoholic is in the late stage, he or she is often irrational, deluded, and unable to understand what has happened.

In addition to the effects of these changes, the alcoholic is faced with one of the most powerful facets of addiction: denial. An alcoholic will deny that he or she has a problem. This denial is a very strong force. If an alcoholic did not deny the existence of a problem, he or she would most likely seek help when faced with the overwhelming problems caused by drinking. While denial is not a diagnosable physical symptom or psychiatric disorder, it is an accurate description of the state of the alcoholic's behavior and thinking and is very real.

Chapter 9

Concurrent Alcohol And Drug Use

Alcohol And Illicit Drug Use In Adolescence

It goes without saying that adolescents shouldn't use alcohol or illicit drugs. Both activities are illegal and dangerous to adolescents' health and safety. Still, by the time they reach their senior year of high school, 71 percent of adolescents have tried alcohol and nearly half have tried an illicit drug at least once. Although not all of the adolescents who try or use alcohol and drugs will develop an addiction, some will. In fact, more than one in 10 (12.5 percent) of youth ages 18 to 20 have an alcohol dependence, the highest rate of any age group.

Although strategies to prevent substance use work, treatment can help, and young people can and do recover, the best way for adolescents to avoid addiction is to never use alcohol or drugs. However, if an adolescent does develop an addiction, early intervention can help them to avoid carrying that problem into adulthood.

The most common and harmful form of alcohol use among all adolescents is *binge drinking* (having four or more drinks for women and five or more drinks for men within a couple of hours). Although the percentage of high school students who binge drink has declined in recent years, about one in four high school seniors surveyed in 2010 had binged within the past 30 days of the time the survey was taken.

In terms of illicit drug use, marijuana is the drug tried and used most often by adolescents, followed by prescription drugs without medical supervision, and then by inhalants and

About This Chapter: This chapter includes excerpts from "Alcohol and Illicit Drug Use in Adolescence," Office of Adolescent Health (www.hhs.gov/ash/oah), U.S. Department of Health and Human Services, September 2011; and Substance Abuse and Mental Health Services Administration, Office of Applied Studies. (March 19, 2009). *The NSDUH Report: Concurrent Illicit Drug and Alcohol Use*. Rockville, MD.

hallucinogens. After years of declining use, adolescents increased their use of marijuana between the mid-2000's and 2010.

Two federal initiatives have set goals and specific targets for preventing and reducing alcohol and illicit drug use in adolescence: the U.S. National Prevention Strategy (a comprehensive plan to increase the number of Americans who are healthy at every stage of life) and Healthy People 2020 (the federal government's 10-year health agenda). Specifically, efforts are focused on reducing the number of high school seniors who have engaged in binge drinking and on reducing the number of adolescents, ages 12 to 17, who have used an illicit drug in the last 30 days.

Several factors influence whether an adolescent will develop an addiction to alcohol or illicit drugs. These include genetics (for example, whether their parents had a substance abuse problem), as well as the age that they start using alcohol or illicit drugs (the earlier in life they use substances, the higher their chances are of addiction).

In a positive trend, the percentage of adolescents identified as having a substance dependency declined between 2002 and 2010. Still, in 2009 a substantial number (about eight percent) of all adolescents ages 12 to 17 required specialty treatment for problems with alcohol and illicit drugs. This includes 1.1 million adolescents suffering from alcohol dependency, and 1.2 million with an illicit drug problem. Of those youth in need, less than 10 percent received treatment. This low number is a result of a variety of reasons; however, the majority of adolescents with dependencies did not make an effort to get help, or did not think that they needed help.

Healthy People 2020 aims to increase access to services and increase the proportion of adolescents that receive treatment for dependency issues by 10 percent by 2020, in addition to improving prevention and screening activities for other adolescent substance abuse issues.

Concurrent Illicit Drug And Alcohol Use

Concurrent use of illicit drugs and alcohol is a serious public health concern because of the potential additive or interactive effects of multiple substance use, which may lead to more severe adverse consequences than use of a single substance. Little is known about the prevalence of illicit drug use at the same time or within a few hours of alcohol use. The National Survey on Drug Use and Health (NSDUH) can help to address the need for information in this area. This report examines this topic using annual averages based on combined 2006 and 2007 NSDUH data.

Illicit Drug Use Concurrent With Last Alcohol Use

Illicit drug use concurrent with the respondent's last alcohol use was reported by 5.6 percent of past month alcohol users aged 12 or older; this is equivalent to an estimated 7.1 million persons. The illicit drug most frequently used with alcohol was marijuana (4.8 percent), followed by cocaine and pain relievers (0.6 and 0.4 percent, respectively) (Figure 9.1).

Concurrent Illicit Drug And Alcohol Use, By Demographic Characteristics

Among past month alcohol users, males were nearly twice as likely as females to report illicit drug use concurrent with last alcohol use (7.1 vs. 3.9 percent). Rates were higher among adolescent and young adult past month drinkers than their older counterparts (14.2 percent among 12 to 17 year olds, 13.5 percent among 18 to 25 year olds, 7.7 percent among 26 to 34 year olds, 4.3 percent among 35 to 49 year olds, and 1.1 percent among those aged 50 or older) (Figure 9.2). American Indian or Alaska Native past month drinkers had the highest rate of illicit drug use concurrent with last alcohol use, and Asian drinkers had the lowest rate (11.7 and 2.1 percent, respectively) (Figure 9.3).

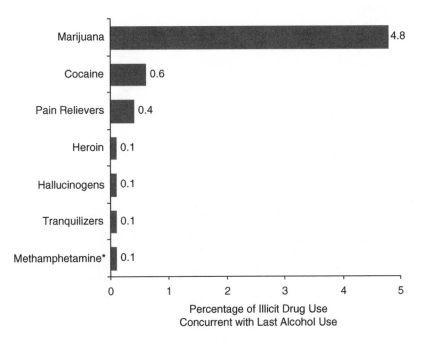

Figure 9.1. Illicit Drug Use Concurrent with Last Alcohol Use among Past Month Alcohol Users Aged 12 or Older, by Type of Illicit Drug: 2006 and 2007 (Source: 2006 and 2007 SAMHSA National Surveys on Drug Use and Health).

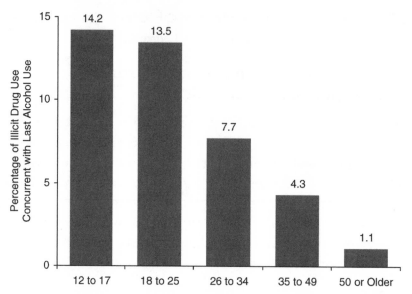

Figure 9.2. Concurrent Illicit Drug and Alcohol Use among Past Month Alcohol Users Aged 12 or Older, by Age Group: 2006 and 2007(Source: 2006 and 2007 SAMHSA National Surveys on Drug Use and Health).

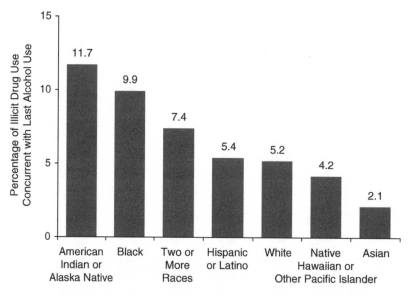

Figure 9.3. Concurrent Illicit Drug and Alcohol Use among Past Month Alcohol Users Aged 12 or Older, by Race/Ethnicity: 2006 and 2007 (Source: 2006 and 2007 SAMHSA National Surveys on Drug Use and Health).

Concurrent Illicit Drug Use And Level Of Alcohol Use

The likelihood of using illicit drugs concurrently with last alcohol use varied with the number of drinks consumed. Among past month alcohol users, those who binged on alcohol during their last occasion of use (that is, had five or more drinks within a couple of hours) were more likely than their counterparts who did not binge (that is, had four or fewer drinks) to have used illicit drugs concurrently with their last alcohol use (13.9 vs. 3.8 percent, respectively).

Discussion

Overall, about six percent of past month alcohol users used an illicit drug concurrently with their last alcohol use. However, this behavior was more prevalent among certain groups—namely, males, young people aged 12 to 25, and American Indians or Alaska Natives—perhaps reflecting differentials in rates of use of illicit drugs overall. Concurrent illicit drug use also was higher among those who engaged in binge drinking than those who drank less on their last occasion of alcohol use. Some of these differentials also may reflect lower awareness of the potential adverse health consequences of simultaneous alcohol and illicit drug use. Prevention and treatment providers should continue to emphasize the risks of using alcohol and illicit drugs together, with targeted messages for those groups at greatest risk for this behavior.

Chapter 10

Women And Alcohol: Increased Risks

Questions And Answers About Women And Alcohol

Women's drinking patterns are different from men's—especially when it comes to the type of beverage, amounts, and frequency. Women's bodies also react differently to alcohol than men's bodies. As a result, women face particular health risks and realities. Women should be aware of the health risks associated with drinking alcohol.

Why do women face higher risk?

Research shows that women start to have alcohol-related problems at lower drinking levels than men do. One reason is that, on average, women weigh less than men. In addition, alcohol disperses in body water, and pound for pound, women have less water in their bodies than men do. So after a man and woman of the same weight drink the same amount of alcohol, the woman's blood alcohol concentration will tend to be higher, putting her at greater risk for harm. Other biological differences, including hormones, may contribute, as well.

What are the health risks?

Liver Damage: Women who drink are more likely to develop alcoholic hepatitis (liver inflammation) than men who drink the same amount of alcohol. Alcoholic hepatitis can lead to cirrhosis.

About This Chapter: This chapter begins with information excerpted from "Women and Alcohol," National Institute on Alcohol Abuse and Alcoholism (www.niaaa.nih.gov), February 2011. It continues with text excerpted from "April Is Alcohol Awareness Month," Centers for Disease Control and Prevention (www.cdc.gov), April 6, 2011.

Heart Disease: Chronic heavy drinking is a leading cause of heart disease. Among heavy drinkers, women are more susceptible to alcohol-related heart disease than men, even though women drink less alcohol over a lifetime than men.

Breast Cancer: There is an association between drinking alcohol and developing breast cancer. Women who consume about one drink per day have a 10 percent higher chance of developing breast cancer than women who do not drink at all.

Pregnancy: Any drinking during pregnancy is risky. A pregnant woman who drinks heavily puts her fetus at risk for learning and behavioral problems and abnormal facial features. Even moderate drinking during pregnancy can cause problems. Drinking during pregnancy also may increase the risk for preterm labor.

How much is moderate drinking for adult women?

A standard drink is roughly 14 grams of pure alcohol, which is found in 12 ounces of beer, 5 ounces of wine, or 1.5 ounces of distilled spirits. The U.S. Department of Agriculture (USDA) defines moderate drinking as up to one drink per day for women (and up to two drinks per day for men).

What levels of alcohol consumption are related to alcohol problems?

Some women should never drink at all, including anyone under age 21, anyone who takes medications that can interact negatively with alcohol, and anyone who is pregnant or trying to conceive

Low risk drinking limits refer exclusively to adults (people 21 years of age and older), and they are different for men and women:

- **Adult Women:** No more than seven drinks per week and no more than three drinks on any single day

- **Adult Men:** No more than 14 drinks per week and no more than four drinks on any single day

To stay low risk, adults must keep within *both* the single-day and weekly limits. Low risk does not mean no risk. Even within these limits, people can have problems if they drink too quickly or have other health issues.

Adults who do drink can help minimize alcohol's effects by drinking slowly and making sure they eat enough while drinking. For more information please visit www.rethinking drinking.niaaa.nih.gov.

How often and how much do women drink?

These are selected consumption statistics for women and men (U.S. adults):

% who had at least one drink in the past year

- Women: 59.6
- Men: 71.8

% who had at least one drink in their lifetime, but not in the past year

- Women: 17.9
- Men: 16.6

% who had at least one drink in their lifetime

- Women: 77.5
- Men: 88.4

% total lifetime abstainers (not even one drink)

- Women: 22.5
- Men: 11.6

% of past-year drinkers, by usual number of drinks consumed per drinking day:

- Women who consume one drink per day: 48.2
- Men who consume one drink per day: 28.7
- Women who consume two drinks per day: 29.9
- Men who consume two drinks per day: 29.0
- Women who consume three or more drinks per day: 21.9
- Men who consume three or more drinks per day: 42.3

% of past-year drinkers who drank 4+(women)/5+(men) drinks on an occasion:

- Never in past year
  - Women: 71.2
  - Men: 56.9

- Ever in past year
  - Women: 28.8
  - Men: 43.1

- 1 to 11 times in past year (less than monthly)
  - Women: 14.2
  - Men: 15.3

- 12+ times in past year (monthly or more often)
  - Women: 14.6
  - Men: 27.8

% who drank 12+ drinks over the course of the past year

- Women: 42.1
- Men: 61.2

% who drank 12+ drinks over the course of some year, but not the past year

- Women: 13.4
- Men: 16.6

% who never drank 12+ drinks over the course of any year

- Women: 44.5
- Men: 22.2

Male And Female Drinkers Compared

Alcohol affects men and women differently. In general, men have more problems with alcohol compared with women. But women are often more sensitive than men to the effects of alcohol. Women tend to break alcohol down more slowly. Also, women have less water in their bodies than men, so alcohol becomes more concentrated. As a result, women may become more impaired than men after drinking the same amount. That is why the recommended drinking limit for women is lower than for men.

Source: Excerpted from "Alcohol Use and Older Adults," NIH SeniorHealth, National Institute on Aging (nihseniorhealth.gov), August 2010.

% of women who had a past-year pregnancy by drinking status:

- Did not drink at all in the past year: 41.0
- Drank during the past year, but not at all during pregnancy: 49.3
- Drank but in reduced quantities during pregnancy: 8.1
- Drank and did not reduce consumption during pregnancy: 1.5

Women And Alcohol Awareness

Gender Differences And Alcohol Consumption

Upon drinking equal amounts, women tend to absorb more alcohol when they drink, and take longer to break it down and remove it from their bodies compared to their male counterparts. These differences are caused by differences in body composition and chemistry between men and women. Even when they drink the same amount of alcohol, women tend to have higher levels of alcohol in their blood than men, and the immediate effects of impairment occur more quickly and last longer.

Alcohol tends to leave the body at a slower rate in women who take birth control pills compared with those who do not. The result can be greater alcohol impairment in women who take birth control pills.

Binge Drinking And The Risks To Women's Health

Binge drinking is defined as consuming four or more drinks per occasion for women and five or more drinks per occasion for men. It is a common and dangerous behavior that contributes to more than 11,500 deaths among women in the U.S. each year—approximately 32 deaths per day.

In 2009, more than one out of every ten women reported binge drinking during the past 30 days. On average, women who binge drink said they engaged in this risky behavior at least three times per month. Among women binge drinkers, they consume, on average, almost six drinks per drinking occasion, which exceeds the threshold for binge drinking.

Binge drinking usually leads to impairment, and women who binge drink with greater frequency and intensity put themselves and those around them at increased risk of experiencing alcohol-related harms, particularly if they are pregnant or may become pregnant.

Binge drinking increases the risk for breast cancer, heart disease, and stroke, all of which are leading causes of death in women.

Risk For Sexual Assault

Binge drinking is a risk factor for sexual assault, especially among young women in college settings. The risk for rape or sexual assault increases when both the perpetrator and victim have used alcohol before the attack.

Risk Of Sexually Transmitted Infections

Women who binge drink are more likely to have unprotected sex and multiple sex partners, which can increase their risk of acquiring the human immunodeficiency virus (HIV) and other sexually transmitted infections (STIs).

Alcohol Consumption And Pregnancy

No amount of alcohol is safe to drink while pregnant. There is also no safe time during pregnancy to drink, and no safe kind of alcohol.

Women who drink alcohol while pregnant increase their risk of having a baby with fetal alcohol spectrum disorders (FASDs). This group of conditions includes physical and intellectual disabilities, as well as problems with behavior and learning. Often, a person has a mix of these problems. FASDs are a leading known cause of intellectual disability and birth defects. FASDs are completely preventable if a woman does not drink while she is pregnant or may become pregnant.

Women should not drink alcohol if they are planning to become pregnant or are sexually active and do not use effective birth control because they could become pregnant and not know for several weeks.

National surveys show that about six out of every ten women of child-bearing age (18–44 years) use alcohol, and about one-third of women in this age group who drink alcohol binge drink.

Female binge drinkers are more likely to engage in unsafe sexual activities compared with women who are not binge drinkers. Binge drinking increases the risk for unintended pregnancy which may lead to a delay in recognizing pregnancy. If a woman does not recognize that she is pregnant and she continues drinking, she can expose her developing fetus to alcohol without realizing it.

Alcohol Consumption And Chronic Diseases

Women are often more vulnerable than men to the long-term effects of alcohol on their health. Over time, drinking too much alcohol can lead to these health consequences:

- **Cancer:** Alcohol consumption increases the risk for breast cancer and cancer of the mouth, throat, esophagus, liver, and colon.

- **Liver Disease:** The risk for cirrhosis and other alcohol-related liver diseases is higher for women than for men.

- **Heart Problems:** Studies have shown that women who drink excessively are at increased risk for damage to the heart muscle than men. Binge drinking can lead to high blood pressure and increase the risk for heart attack and stroke.

Preventing Alcohol-Related Problems

Prevention strategies require action at individual and population levels and must consider ways to create community environments that discourage binge drinking by women and their families.

These are some things all women can do:

- Avoid underage drinking.

- Avoid drinking alcohol if pregnant or planning to become pregnant. Fetal alcohol spectrum disorders are 100% preventable.

- Choose not to binge drink and help others not to do it. Binge drinking leads to many health and social problems for the drinkers, their families, and their communities. If adult women choose to drink alcoholic beverages, they should do so in moderation. Moderate drinking is defined as the consumption of up to one drink per day for women and up to two drinks per day for men.

- Seek care from a health care provider for excessive drinking.

Part Two
Underage Drinking

Chapter 11

Teens And Alcohol: A Dangerous Combination

Dangers Of Teen Drinking

Teens who drink don't just drink. They drink to excess. More than 7 percent of eighth graders, 16 percent of sophomores, and 23 percent of seniors report recent binge drinking (5+ drinks on the same occasion).

Statistics show that the majority of current teen drinkers got drunk in the previous month. That includes 50 percent of the high school sophomores who drink and 65 percent of the high school seniors who drink.

Underage drinking is linked to injury and risky behavior. According to the U.S. Surgeon General, about 5,000 kids under 21 die every year as a result of underage drinking—from crashes, homicides, and suicides. Teens who drink also are at risk for a long list of other injuries and potential life-long alcohol abuse. Reducing underage drinking can reduce drinking-related harm.

Brain Development And Alcohol Abuse

Research indicates that the human brain continues to develop into a person's early 20s, and that exposure of the developing brain to alcohol may have long-lasting effects on intellectual capabilities and may increase the likelihood of alcohol addiction.

The age when drinking starts affects future drinking problems. For each year that the start of drinking is delayed, the risk of later alcohol dependence is reduced by 14 percent.

About This Chapter: This chapter includes excerpts from "Dangers of Teen Drinking," "Alcohol Advertising," and "Answering Questions about Alcohol," produced by We Don't Serve Teens (www.dontserveteens.gov), a campaign of the Federal Trade Commission and most recently updated in 2011.

Drinking And Driving

Car crashes are the leading cause of death among people ages 15 to 20. About 1,900 people under 21 die every year from car crashes involving underage drinking.

Young people are more susceptible to alcohol-induced impairment of their driving skills. Drinking drivers aged 16 to 20 are twice as likely to be involved in a fatal crash as drinking drivers who are 21 or older.

Suicide

Alcohol use interacts with conditions like depression and stress, and contributes to an estimated 300 teen suicides a year. High school students who drink are twice as likely to have seriously considered attempting suicide, as compared to nondrinkers. High school students who binge drink are four times as likely to have attempted suicide, as compared to nondrinkers.

Sexual Behavior

Current teen drinkers are more than twice as likely to have had sexual intercourse within the past three months than teens who don't drink. Higher drinking levels increase the likelihood of sexual activity. Adolescents who drink are more likely to engage in risky sexual activities, like having sex with someone they don't know or failing to use birth control.

Other Risks

Teens who drink alcohol are more likely than nondrinkers to smoke marijuana, use inhalants, or carry a weapon. Binge drinking substantially increases the likelihood of these activities.

Academic Performance

A government study published in 2007 shows a relationship between binge drinking and grades. Approximately two-thirds of students with "mostly A's" are non-drinkers, while nearly half of the students with "mostly D's and F's" report binge drinking. It is not clear, however, whether academic failure leads to drinking, or vice versa.

Alcohol Advertising

Alcohol advertising and marketing is widespread. All of us encounter commercial messages from a myriad of sources every day. Learn how to tell the difference between the facts and the hype and to become a smarter, more responsible, and more confident consumer.

Warning Signs Of A Drinking Problem

Although the following signs may indicate a problem with alcohol or other drugs, some also reflect normal teenage growing pains. Experts believe that a drinking problem is more likely if several of these signs occur at the same time, if they occur suddenly, and if some of them are extreme in nature.

- **Mood Changes:** Flare-ups of temper, irritability, and defensiveness
- **School Problems:** Poor attendance, low grades, and/or recent disciplinary action
- **Rebellion:** Against family rules
- **Friend Changes:** Switching friends and a reluctance to have parents get to know the new friends
- **A "Nothing Matters" Attitude:** Sloppy appearance, a lack of involvement in former interests, and general low energy
- **Alcohol Presence:** In a child's room or backpack or on his or her breath
- **Physical Or Mental Problems:** Memory lapses, poor concentration, bloodshot eyes, lack of coordination, or slurred speech

Source: From "Warning Signs of a Drinking Problem," Substance Abuse and Mental Health Services Administration (www.toosmarttostart.samhsa.gov), July 2, 2012.

Alcohol Advertising Standards

Alcohol advertisers have pledged to comply with self-regulatory codes designed to limit targeting of teens. Among other provisions, these codes direct that no more than 30 percent of the audience for an ad may consist of people under 21 and that ad content should not appeal primarily to people under 21. The Federal Trade Commission, the nation's consumer protection agency, monitors compliance with the codes and has published the results of three major studies on alcohol advertising.

Let industry and the government know if you see an alcohol ad you think violates the standards. If you believe that an ad doesn't comply with the alcohol industry's self-regulatory codes, file a complaint in any of three ways: with the company, with one of the alcohol industry's self-regulatory agencies, or with the Federal Trade Commission (https://www.ftccomplaintassistant.gov). There are three organizations that serve the alcohol industry as self-regulatory organizations:

Distilled Spirits Council of the United States

1250 Eye Street, NW, Suite 400
Washington, DC 20005
http://www.discus.org

Beer Institute

122 C Street NW, Suite 350
Washington, DC 20001
http://www.beerinstitute.org

Wine Institute

425 Market Street Suite 1000
San Francisco, CA 94105
http://www.wineinstitute.org

Answering Questions About Alcohol

What can you say to people who think teen drinking is not a serious problem? Despite the statistics and the science, some people still think teen drinking is not a serious problem. Here are some of the more common questions neighbors and friends may ask about teen drinking—and the answers.

Wouldn't a lower drinking age allow parents to teach their kids to drink responsibly?

Parents don't have to drink with their children to teach them responsible drinking. Additionally, letting teens drink at home sends the wrong message about appropriate conduct away from home.

Don't kids binge because they haven't learned to drink when they're living at home?

This question assumes that binge drinking was less common when the legal drinking age was 18 or 19. That assumption is wrong—binge drinking by 12th graders has dropped by 15 percent since 21 was adopted as the national legal drinking age.

Kids are going to drink anyway. They always have. Isn't it better to host a party so my friends aren't out driving?

It's not your decision to make. Letting other teens drink in your house undermines other parents, and in many states, violates the law. Drunk driving isn't the only danger associated with teen drinking, and you can't guarantee that your teen guests won't drive after they leave your house. Offer non-alcoholic choices rather than another drinking venue.

The legal drinking age in Europe is younger than it is in the U.S. Why don't European kids have alcohol-related problems?

The concept that European teens start drinking at a young age without problems is a myth. A recent National Institutes of Health publication shows that European countries with lower drinking ages have the same teen drinking problems as the U.S., or worse.

My parents drank when they were kids, so what's the problem with letting teens drink now?

Good thing that they're okay, but many teens are not as lucky. On average, 6.4 American teens die each day from alcohol-related crashes. Teen drinking is associated with long-term alcohol dependence, increased sexual activity, unprotected sex, suicide, smoking, and carrying weapons; in addition, it imposes high financial costs on society.

I don't believe that the reduction in teen drinking and driving accidents since 1983 is entirely due to the minimum drinking age. There must be more to it.

Seat belt requirements, zero tolerance laws, increased enforcement, and frankly, increased public education and information on the dangers of teen drinking have contributed to the downturn in teen drinking and accidents. However, after careful study, the U.S. Department of Transportation concluded that the minimum drinking age law, by itself, has played an important role in reducing both teen drinking and driving after drinking.

Doesn't a "legal drinking age" just make alcohol "forbidden fruit" that teenagers try harder to get?

If this were true, teen drinking would have increased after adoption of the legal drinking age. It didn't. Having a legal drinking age has substantially reduced drinking by teens. In addition, the drinking habits of 18-year-olds have a big influence on younger teens, particularly those who are 15 to 17.

If kids can vote and join the military at 18, why do they have to wait until they're 21 to drink legally?

It's the law. In addition, ages of "initiation" vary. You can work at 14, vote at 18 and drink at 21, but you can't run for Congress until you're 25. Researchers who have evaluated the data say the minimum legal drinking age delays the onset of alcohol use. As a result, it reduces drinking-related injuries among teens and the risk of alcohol abuse and dependence later in life.

Chapter 12

The Teen Brain:
Still Under Construction

Introduction

One of the ways that scientists have searched for the causes of mental illness is by studying the development of the brain from birth to adulthood. Powerful new technologies have enabled them to track the growth of the brain and to investigate the connections between brain function, development, and behavior.

The research has turned up some surprises, among them the discovery of striking changes taking place during the teen years. These findings have altered long-held assumptions about the timing of brain maturation. In key ways, the brain doesn't look like that of an adult until the early 20s.

An understanding of how the brain of an adolescent is changing may help explain a puzzling contradiction of adolescence: young people at this age are close to a lifelong peak of physical health, strength, and mental capacity, and yet, for some, this can be a hazardous age. Mortality rates jump between early and late adolescence. Rates of death by injury between ages 15 to 19 are about six times that of the rate between ages 10 and 14. Crime rates are highest among young males and rates of alcohol abuse are high relative to other ages. Even though most adolescents come through this transitional age well, it's important to understand the risk factors for behavior that can have serious consequences. Genes, childhood experience, and the environment in which a young person reaches adolescence all shape behavior. Adding to this complex picture, research is revealing how all these factors act in the context of a brain that is changing, with its own impact on behavior.

About This Chapter: "The Teen Brain: Still Under Construction," National Institute of Mental Health (www.nimh .nih.gov), 2011.

The more we learn, the better we may be able to understand the abilities and vulnerabilities of teens, and the significance of this stage for life-long mental health.

The fact that so much change is taking place beneath the surface may be something to keep in mind during the ups and downs of adolescence.

The "Visible" Brain

A clue to the degree of change taking place in the teen brain came from studies in which scientists did brain scans of children as they grew from early childhood through age 20. The scans revealed unexpectedly late changes in the volume of gray matter, which forms the thin, folding outer layer or cortex of the brain. The cortex is where the processes of thought and memory are based. Over the course of childhood, the volume of gray matter in the cortex increases and then declines. A decline in volume is normal at this age and is in fact a necessary part of maturation.

Alcohol And The Developing Brain

Alcohol can cause alterations in the structure and function of the developing brain, which continues to mature into a person's mid 20s, and it may have consequences reaching far beyond adolescence.

In adolescence, brain development is characterized by dramatic changes to the brain's structure, neuron connectivity (that is, "wiring"), and physiology. These changes in the brain affect everything from emerging sexuality to emotionality and judgment.

Not all parts of the adolescent brain mature at the same time, which may put an adolescent at a disadvantage in certain situations. For example, the limbic areas of the brain mature earlier than the frontal lobes. The limbic areas regulate emotions and are associated with an adolescent's lowered sensitivity to risk. The frontal lobes are responsible for self-regulation, judgment, reasoning, problem-solving, and impulse control. Differences in maturation among parts of the brain can result in impulsive decisions or actions and a disregard for consequences. Furthermore, although alcohol is a central nervous system depressant, alcohol can appear to be a stimulant because, initially, it depresses the part of the brain that controls inhibitions.

Alcohol affects an adolescent's brain development in many ways. The effects of underage drinking on specific brain activities are explained below.

Cerebral Cortex: Alcohol slows down the cerebral cortex as it works with information from a person's senses.

Central Nervous System: When a person thinks of something he wants his body to do, the central nervous system—the brain and the spinal cord—sends a signal to that part of the body. Alcohol slows down the central nervous system, making the person think, speak, and move slower.

The assumption for many years had been that the volume of gray matter was highest in very early childhood, and gradually fell as a child grew. The more recent scans, however, revealed that the high point of the volume of gray matter occurs during early adolescence.

While the details behind the changes in volume on scans are not completely clear, the results push the timeline of brain maturation into adolescence and young adulthood. In terms of the volume of gray matter seen in brain images, the brain does not begin to resemble that of an adult until the early 20s.

The scans also suggest that different parts of the cortex mature at different rates. Areas involved in more basic functions mature first: those involved, for example, in the processing of information from the senses, and in controlling movement. The parts of the brain responsible for more top-down control, controlling impulses, and planning ahead—the hallmarks of adult behavior—are among the last to mature.

Frontal Lobes: The brain's frontal lobes are important for planning, forming ideas, making decisions, and using self-control. When alcohol affects the frontal lobes of the brain, a person may find it hard to control his or her emotions and urges. The person may act without thinking or may even become violent. Drinking alcohol over a long period of time can damage the frontal lobes forever.

Hippocampus: The hippocampus is the part of the brain where memories are made. When alcohol reaches the hippocampus, a person may have trouble remembering something he or she just learned, such as a name or a phone number. This can happen after just one or two drinks. Drinking a lot of alcohol quickly can cause a blackout—not being able to remember entire events, such as what he or she did last night. If alcohol damages the hippocampus, a person may find it hard to learn and to hold on to knowledge.

Cerebellum: The cerebellum is important for coordination, thoughts, and awareness. A person may have trouble with these skills when alcohol enters the cerebellum. After drinking alcohol, a person's hands may be so shaky that they can't touch or grab things normally, and they may lose their balance and fall.

Hypothalamus: The hypothalamus is a small part of the brain that does an amazing number of the body's housekeeping chores. Alcohol upsets the work of the hypothalamus. After a person drinks alcohol, blood pressure, hunger, thirst, and the urge to urinate increase while body temperature and heart rate decrease.

Medulla: The medulla controls the body's automatic actions, such as a person's heartbeat. It also keeps the body at the right temperature. Alcohol actually chills the body. Drinking a lot of alcohol outdoors in cold weather can cause a person's body temperature to fall below normal. This dangerous condition is called hypothermia.

Source: Excerpted from "Alcohol and the Developing Brain," Substance Abuse and Mental Health Services Administration (www.toosmarttostart.gov), May 14, 2012.

What's Gray Matter?

The details of what is behind the increase and decline in gray matter are still not completely clear. Gray matter is made up of the cell bodies of neurons, the nerve fibers that project from them, and support cells. One of the features of the brain's growth in early life is that there is an early blooming of synapses—the connections between brain cells or neurons—followed by pruning as the brain matures. Synapses are the relays over which neurons communicate with each other and are the basis of the working circuitry of the brain. Already more numerous than an adult's at birth, synapses multiply rapidly in the first months of life. A two-year-old has about half again as many synapses as an adult. (For an idea of the complexity of the brain: a cube of brain matter, 1 millimeter on each side, can contain between 35 and 70 million neurons and an estimated 500 billion synapses.)

Scientists believe that the loss of synapses as a child matures is part of the process by which the brain becomes more efficient. Although genes play a role in the decline in synapses, animal research has shown that experience also shapes the decline. Synapses exercised by experience survive and are strengthened, while others are pruned away. Scientists are working to determine to what extent the changes in gray matter on brain scans during the teen years reflect growth and pruning of synapses.

A Spectrum Of Change

Research using many different approaches is showing that more than gray matter is changing:

- Connections between different parts of the brain increase throughout childhood and well into adulthood. As the brain develops, the fibers connecting nerve cells are wrapped in a protein that greatly increases the speed with which they can transmit impulses from cell to cell. The resulting increase in connectivity—a little like providing a growing city with a fast, integrated communication system—shapes how well different parts of the brain work in tandem. Research is finding that the extent of connectivity is related to growth in intellectual capacities such as memory and reading ability.

- Several lines of evidence suggest that the brain circuitry involved in emotional responses is changing during the teen years. Functional brain imaging studies, for example, suggest that the responses of teens to emotionally loaded images and situations are heightened relative to younger children and adults. The brain changes underlying these patterns involve brain centers and signaling molecules that are part of the reward system with which the brain motivates behavior. These age-related changes shape how much different parts of the brain are activated in response to experience, and in terms of behavior, the urgency and intensity of emotional reactions.

- Enormous hormonal changes take place during adolescence. Reproductive hormones shape not only sex-related growth and behavior, but overall social behavior. Hormone systems involved in the brain's response to stress are also changing during the teens. As with reproductive hormones, stress hormones can have complex effects on the brain, and as a result, behavior.

- In terms of sheer intellectual power, the brain of an adolescent is a match for an adult's. The capacity of a person to learn will never be greater than during adolescence. At the same time, behavioral tests, sometimes combined with functional brain imaging, suggest differences in how adolescents and adults carry out mental tasks. Adolescents and adults seem to engage different parts of the brain to different extents during tests requiring calculation and impulse control, or in reaction to emotional content.

Young Drinkers Risk Slowing Down Brain Power

Drinking may harm adolescents' ability to concentrate and to understand spatial relationships. A recent study led by Susan Tapert at the University of California, San Diego compared the standardized test scores of 76 kids (ages 12 to 14 years old) with their scores after about three years. At the three-year follow-up, 36 of the kids had begun drinking at moderate to heavy levels and 40 continued not using alcohol or other drugs. The study defined moderate to heavy drinking as drinking at least monthly and having three or more drinks at a time, or drinking less frequently, but having four or more drinks at a time. The kids in this study were consuming an average of about eight drinks per month by the time they reached the follow-up.

During the study's three-year time period, the team discovered once teens began to drink, they performed more poorly on cognitive tests than before they began drinking. Interestingly, the kinds of skills affected varied between girls and boys.

The researchers found that girls' scores on tasks requiring them to visualize and reproduce a complicated line drawing decreased after they began drinking. The researchers also found that boys' scores on tests requiring sustained attention decreased after they began drinking.

Tapert's study suggests that these behavioral effects may point toward alcohol's underlying effect on brain structure. Brain scans demonstrate that adolescent drinking can reduce the health of white matter in the brain. White matter is where brain cells communicate with each other, so damage to this area can result in slower, less efficient thinking. Reduced white matter integrity may cause girls to have difficulty understanding spatial relationships. This damage may be long-lasting since the adolescent brain is still undergoing significant developmental changes, making it especially vulnerable to alcohol's toxic effects.

Source: Excerpted from "Research Highlights: Young Drinkers Risk Slowing Down Brain Power," National Institute on Alcohol Abuse and Alcoholism (www.niaaa.nih.gov), April 30, 2010.

- Research suggests that adolescence brings with it brain-based changes in the regulation of sleep that may contribute to teens' tendency to stay up late at night. Along with the obvious effects of sleep deprivation, such as fatigue and difficulty maintaining attention, inadequate sleep is a powerful contributor to irritability and depression. Studies of children and adolescents have found that sleep deprivation can increase impulsive behavior; some researchers report finding that it is a factor in delinquency. Adequate sleep is central to physical and emotional health.

The Changing Brain And Behavior In Teens

One interpretation of all these findings is that in teens, the parts of the brain involved in emotional responses are fully online, or even more active than in adults, while the parts of the brain involved in keeping emotional, impulsive responses in check are still reaching maturity. Such a changing balance might provide clues to a youthful appetite for novelty, and a tendency to act on impulse—without regard for risk.

While much is being learned about the teen brain, it is not yet possible to know to what extent a particular behavior or ability is the result of a feature of brain structure—or a change in brain structure. Changes in the brain take place in the context of many other factors, among them, inborn traits, personal history, family, friends, community, and culture.

Teens And The Brain: More Questions For Research

Scientists continue to investigate the development of the brain and the relationship between the changes taking place, behavior, and health. The following questions are among the important ones that are targets of research:

How do experience and environment interact with genetic preprogramming to shape the maturing brain, and as a result, future abilities and behavior? In other words, to what extent does what a teen does and learns shape his or her brain over the rest of a lifetime?

In what ways do features unique to the teen brain play a role in the high rates of illicit substance use and alcohol abuse in the late teen to young adult years? Does the adolescent capacity for learning make this a stage of particular vulnerability to addiction?

Why is it so often the case that, for many mental disorders, symptoms first emerge during adolescence and young adulthood?

This last question has been the central reason to study brain development from infancy to adulthood. Scientists increasingly view mental illnesses as developmental disorders that have their roots in the processes involved in how the brain matures. By studying how the circuitry of the brain develops, scientists hope to identify when and for what reasons development goes off track. Brain imaging studies have revealed distinctive variations in growth patterns of brain tissue in youth who show signs of conditions affecting mental health. Ongoing research is providing information on how genetic factors increase or reduce vulnerability to mental illness; and how experiences during infancy, childhood, and adolescence can increase the risk of mental illness or protect against it.

The Adolescent And Adult Brain

It is not surprising that the behavior of adolescents would be a study in change, since the brain itself is changing in such striking ways. Scientists emphasize that the fact that the teen brain is in transition doesn't mean it is somehow not up to par. It is different from both a child's and an adult's in ways that may equip youth to make the transition from dependence to independence. The capacity for learning at this age, an expanding social life, and a taste for exploration and limit testing may all, to some extent, be reflections of age-related biology.

Understanding the changes taking place in the brain at this age presents an opportunity to intervene early in mental illnesses that have their onset at this age. Research findings on the brain may also serve to help adults understand the importance of creating an environment in which teens can explore and experiment while helping them avoid behavior that is destructive to themselves and others.

Alcohol And The Teen Brain

Adults drink more frequently than teens, but when teens drink they tend to drink larger quantities than adults. There is evidence to suggest that the adolescent brain responds to alcohol differently than the adult brain, perhaps helping to explain the elevated risk of binge drinking in youth. Drinking in youth, and intense drinking are both risk factors for later alcohol dependence. Findings on the developing brain should help clarify the role of the changing brain in youthful drinking, and the relationship between youth drinking and the risk of addiction later in life.

Chapter 13

Alcohol, Peers, And Peer Pressure

Peer Pressure And Underage Drinking

What is peer pressure?

Your classmates keep asking you to have them over because you have a pool, everyone at school is wearing silly hats so you do too, and your best friend begs you to go running with her because you both need more exercise, so you go, too. These are all examples of peer pressure. Don't get it yet?

- *Pressure* is the feeling that you are being pushed toward making a certain choice—good or bad.

- A *peer* is someone in your own age group.

- *Peer pressure* is—you guessed it—the feeling that someone your own age is pushing you toward making a certain choice, good or bad.

What's so difficult about avoiding peer pressure?

Have you ever given in to pressure? Like when a friend begs to borrow something you don't want to give up or to do something your parents say is off limits? Chances are you probably have given into pressure at some time in your life.

About This Chapter: This chapter begins with information "Peer Pressure and Underage Drinking," National Institute on Alcohol Abuse and Alcoholism (www.thecoolspot.gov), 2010. It continues with "Need Advice?" from the Substance Abuse and Mental Health Services Administration (www.toosmarttostart.gov), July 2, 2012. Text under the heading "Factors That Influence When Teens Are More Or Less Likely To Drink" is excerpted from "How You Make a Difference," Office of Adolescent Health (http://www.hhs.gov/ash/oah), 2009.

If you did something you wish you hadn't, then most likely you didn't feel too good about it. You might have felt sad, anxious, guilty, like a wimp or pushover, or disappointed in yourself.

Everyone gives in to pressure at one time or another, but why do people sometimes do things that they really don't want to do? Here are a few reasons:

- They are afraid of being rejected by others

- They want to be liked and don't want to lose a friend

- They want to appear grown up

- They don't want to be made fun of

- They don't want to hurt someone's feelings

- They aren't sure of what they really want

- They don't know how to get out of the situation

Ways To Say "No" To Alcohol

It may seem like so many people drink. But lots of teenagers have figured out that they don't have to drink to have fun or feel comfortable at a party. Of course it can be tough to say "no" when other people are drinking. Lots of times, though, people respect you more when you stand up for what you think is right.

Here are some ways to say "no" to alcohol:

- I'd get kicked off the team if I was caught around booze.
- None for me. I'm driving. I'd like to keep my car in one piece.
- No, thanks. I'm not into that stuff.
- You know, I'm not going to drink anymore. It'd be great if you'd help me out.
- I've seen too many people throw up or get messed up. I'll pass.

Your best bet in dealing with alcohol may be to avoid it as much as possible. Consider these suggestions:

- Don't go to places where there will be drinking. See if your friends want to catch a movie, go out to dinner, go shopping, or go to a school play or sports event.
- Keep in mind that you don't have to do everything your friends do to stay close with them.
- If your friends seem to want to drink a lot, you might look for friends who have the same interests as you, like through a school club.

Source: Excerpted from "Ways to Say "No" to Alcohol," Office on Women's Health (www.girlshealth.gov), May 18, 2010.

When you face pressure you *can* stand your ground.

Almost everyone faces peer pressure once in a while. Friends have a big influence on our lives, but sometimes they push us to do things that we may not want to do. Unless you want to give in every time you face this, you're going to need to learn how to handle it.

The first step to standing up to peer pressure is to understand it. Learn to recognize the different things people do when they pressure others. Pay attention to the differences between spoken and unspoken pressures. The tricks include put-downs, rejections, and reasoning, as well as pressure without words, or unspoken pressure. Once you know about the peer pressure bag of tricks, you'll be able to spot peer pressure and deal with it.

Perhaps your friends have used these lines on you:

- Who needs you as a friend anyway?

- You're such a baby!

- It won't hurt you!

These are a few of the tactics in the peer pressure bag-of-tricks. Did you give in, even though you didn't want to? Learn to spot the tricks. Being aware of the pressure is the first step to resisting it.

Is peer pressure always bad?

Peer pressure isn't all bad. You and your friends can pressure each other into some things that will improve your health and social life and make you feel good about your decisions.

Think of a time when a friend pushed you to do something good for yourself or to avoid something that would've been bad. Here are some good things friends can pressure each other to do:

- Be honest

- Avoid Alcohol

- Avoid drugs

- Not smoke

- Be nice

- Respect others

- Work hard

- Exercise (together!)

You and your friends can also use good peer pressure to help each other resist bad peer pressure.

If you see a friend taking some heat, try some of these lines:

- We don't want to drink.

- We don't need to drink to have fun.

- Let's go and do something else.

- Leave her alone. She said she didn't want any.

A School's Scholastic Success Can Keep Kids From Drugs, Alcohol

For kids who are at risk for drinking, smoking, using drugs, and delinquent behavior, attending a higher-performing school may be protective. A study published in the March 2011 issue of *Prevention Science* evaluated the effect of school environment on kids in 61 public schools in urban, low-income, ethnic/minority areas in Chicago between 2002 and 2005. The study found that students at schools with *value-added education*, a measure showing higher than expected academic achievement and better attendance records given the profile of the student body, were much less likely than kids attending similar, but poorer-performing schools to drink, smoke, use illegal drugs, or have behavior problems.

The study measured value-added education based on the proportion of students in each school who meet or exceed the national standards for reading and math and who had better than anticipated attendance during the academic year. Of the 61 schools, seven were identified as value-added, and five were identified as *value-attenuated*, meaning they had lower than average performance. The schools in the middle were termed *normative*.

Students also answered two questions about alcohol use from the National Institute on Drug Abuse annual Monitoring the Future study. The questions were: "How many times did you drink in the past 30 days? and "How many times did you have five or more alcoholic beverages in the past two weeks?" Based on the researchers' analysis, value-added education was associated with much lower rates of alcohol use within two weeks as well as lower rates of cigarette and marijuana use, stealing, and fighting, when compared with the normative educational environments.

These findings suggest that school environment can serve as a protective factor against underage alcohol use.

Source: "A School's Scholastic Success Can Keep Kids From Drugs, Alcohol," *NIAAA Spectrum*, National Institute on Alcohol Abuse and Alcoholism, Vol. 3, Issue 2, June 2011.

Need Advice?

Is drinking no big deal?

Question: My friends say that drinking alcohol is no big deal. Everybody is doing it, and I should, too. What should I do?

Answer: First, be assured that the great majority (84.1 percent) of 12- to 17-year-old youth do not drink. Alcohol plays a significant role in risky behavior, various types of injuries, and suicide.

Remember, too, that underage drinking is illegal. If you are caught drinking, you could delay your chance of getting a driver's license or lose the one you already have. You could also be barred from playing on an athletic team.

What's right?

Question: People try to get me to drink at parties. I don't want to break the law or violate my parents' trust, but I don't want to be seen as a "square" who doesn't do what everyone else does. How can I do the right thing?

Answer: Make sure you know what the consequences will be if parents, police, and other adults find out that you have been drinking.

Will alcohol make me less shy?

Question: I'm shy and have a hard time making friends. The idea of going out on a date makes me break into a sweat. Someone told me that a drink or two would give me more confidence and lower my inhibitions. Is this true?

Answer: Some drinkers feel less shy and ill at ease with others temporarily. However, alcohol impairs judgment so that drinkers often do things they wouldn't consider doing if sober. Their behavior can lead to embarrassment, regret, serious trouble, even tragedy.

"Just about everybody feels shy sometimes," says Dr. Colleen Sherman in an article on shyness. Talk with a parent or another adult you trust about your feelings. School counselors and nurses know where you can find help. So do ministers, priests, rabbis, and other faith leaders.

Am I an alcoholic?

Question: I started drinking with my friends whenever we got together away from our parents. Now I want to drink even when I'm by myself. I wonder if I am turning into an alcoholic? How can I find out?

Answer: You're doing the smart thing by finding out now. People at any age may discover that what seemed like great fun isn't so much fun anymore, doesn't feel right, and might be turning into a problem.

The online test at www.checkyourself.com (click on the "Quizzes" tab) will help you recognize if you are on your way to having a serious problem with alcohol. If you score high enough when you submit your confidential quiz responses, you will go to another page that explains what you can do next.

I did something stupid. What now?

Question: I did something stupid when I was drinking with my friends recently. Now some of them treat me differently and aren't as friendly as they used to be. What should I do?

Answer: Perhaps you said or did something that was embarrassing or unkind or annoying. Friends will probably accept your apology and your sincere promise not to do anything like this again.

Maybe you broke something. You need to repair the damage, pay for someone else to fix it, or replace the item. And you should offer a sincere apology.

Doing "something stupid" under the influence of alcohol can also mean something much more serious, such as crime and violence, exposure to sexually transmitted diseases, driving under the influence, and other dangerous acts. Talk with your parent or another adult you trust and ask for help. Or, call the Substance Abuse and Mental Health Service Administration's 24-hour toll-free treatment referral helpline: 800-662-HELP (800-662-4357).

School Connectedness

School connectedness—the belief held by students that adults and peers in the school care about their learning as well as about them as individuals—is an important protective factor. Research has shown that young people who feel connected to their school are less likely to engage in many risk behaviors, including early sexual initiation, alcohol, tobacco, and other drug use, and violence and gang involvement.

Students who feel connected to their school are also more likely to have better academic achievement, including higher grades and test scores, have better school attendance, and stay in school longer.

Source: Excerpted from "School Connectedness," Centers for Disease Control and Prevention (www.cdc.gov), October 30, 2012.

How can I help my friends?

Question: Some friends of mine do things I know they don't mean to do whenever they drink. I don't want to get them in trouble or be a snitch. What can I do to help them?

Answer: It isn't snitching to get help for someone who may be in trouble because of drinking. About 5,000 underage drinkers die every year. A lot of them die in highway crashes. But many others die from alcohol poisoning or from trying to do something dangerous while they are impaired.

A friend with a drinking problem is in trouble already and needs help before the problem worsens or leads to tragedy. Visit The Cool Spot's list of resources (available online at (www .thecoolspot.gov/real_life2.asp) or the Help a Friend page on the Above the Influence website (www.abovetheinfluence.com/help/helpafriend) to make a difference in your friend's life.

Factors That Influence When Teens Are More Or Less Likely To Drink

Teens are more likely to drink when these conditions apply to their circumstances:

- Others close to them drink, including parents, brothers and sisters, and friends.

- Family history includes alcoholism, antisocial behavior, or depression.

- Parents encourage supervised drinking by teens, believing incorrectly that it will teach responsible alcohol use.

- They focus on perceived benefits of alcohol use.

- The child experienced maltreatment or neglect.

- The child's mother drank during pregnancy.

- They smoke or use other drugs.

- They have certain traits, such as impulsivity, risk taking, or a high tolerance for alcohol.

Teens are less likely to drink when these conditions apply to their circumstances:

- Their parents disapprove of underage drinking and actively discourage alcohol use by young people, particularly early use.

- They have a close relationship with their mothers and fathers.

- Their family is relatively free of conflict.

- They are raised by parents who offer a balance of discipline, boundaries, support, and appreciation.

- They do well in school and are involved in other positive, structured activities.

- They have good impulse control and can manage their own emotions and behaviors.

- They focus on the negative consequences of using alcohol.

Chapter 14

Underage Drinking Is A Serious Problem

Underage Drinking

Underage drinking is a serious public health problem in the United States. Alcohol is the most widely used substance of abuse among America's youth and drinking by young people poses enormous health and safety risks.

The consequences of underage drinking can affect everyone—regardless of age or drinking status. We all feel the effects of the aggressive behavior, property damage, injuries, violence, and deaths that can result from underage drinking. This is not simply a problem for some families—it is a nationwide concern.

Underage Drinking Statistics

Many young people drink alcohol:

- By age 15, more than 50 percent of teens have had at least one drink.

- By age 18, more than 70 percent of teens have had at least one drink.

- In 2009, 10.4 million young people ages 12–20 reported that they drank alcohol beyond "just a few sips" in the past month.

Youth Ages 12–20 Often Binge Drink: People ages 12 through 20 drink 11 percent of all alcohol consumed in the United States. Although youth drink less often than adults do, when

About This Chapter: This chapter includes information from "Underage Drinking," National Institute on Alcohol Abuse and Alcoholism (www.niaaa.nih.gov), March 2012; "Underage Drinking: One Step Forward, Many More to go," *NIAAA Spectrum*, Volume 4, Issue 2, June 2012; and "Age 21 Minimum Legal Drinking Age," Centers for Disease Control and Prevention (www.cdc.gov), July 20, 2010.

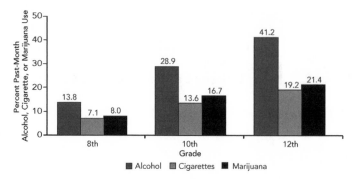

Figure 14.1. More adolescents use alcohol than cigarettes or marijuana. (Source of data: Johnston, L.D.; O'Malley, P.M.; Bachman, J.G.; and Schulenberg, J.E. Monitoring the Future National Survey Results on Drug Use, 1975–2009: Volume I: Secondary School Students, NIH Publication No. 10–7584. Bethesda, MD: National Institute on Drug Abuse, 2010.)

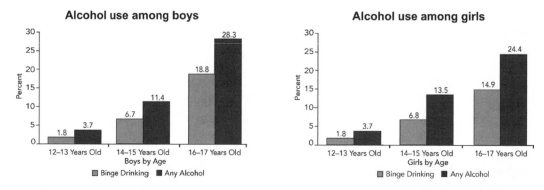

Figure 14.2. Drinking patterns vary by age and gender. (Source of data: Substance Abuse and Mental Health Services Administration. Results From the 2009 National Survey on Drug Use and Health: Volume I. Summary of National Findings (Office of Applied Studies, NSDUH Series H-38A, HHS Publication No. SMA 10–4586 Findings). Rockville, MD: Substance Abuse and Mental Health Services Administration, 2010.)

they do drink, they drink more. That is because young people consume more than 90 percent of their alcohol by binge drinking. Binge drinking is consuming many drinks on an occasion. (A standard drink is roughly 14 grams of pure alcohol, which is found in 12 ounces of beer, 5 ounces of wine, or 1.5 ounces of distilled spirits.) Drinking alcohol and binge drinking become more prevalent as young people get older.

- 6.9 million young people had five or more drinks on the same occasion, within a few hours, at least once in the past month.

- 2.1 million young people had five or more drinks on the same occasion on five or more days over the past month.

What is "binge drinking?" For adults, binge drinking means drinking so much within about two hours that blood alcohol concentration (BAC) levels reach 0.08g/dL, the legal limit of intoxication. For women, this usually takes about four drinks, and for men, about five. But, according to recent research estimates, it takes fewer drinks for children to reach these BAC levels.

Drinking Patterns Vary By Age And Gender: As adolescents get older, they tend to drink more, and boys generally drink more than girls.

Underage Drinking Is Dangerous

Underage drinking poses a range of risks and negative consequences. It is dangerous for these reasons:

- **It causes many deaths:** Every year in the United States, about 5,000 young people under age 21 die as a result of underage drinking. This includes 1,900 deaths from motor vehicle crashes; 1,600 from homicides; 1,200 from alcohol poisoning, falls, burns, and drowning; and 300 from suicides.

- **It causes many injuries:** In 2008 alone, about 190,000 people under age 21 visited an emergency room for alcohol-related injuries.

Young People And Drinking Patterns

Alcohol use starts young and increases with age. The percentages of 8th, 10th, and 12th graders who admitted drinking alcohol in the 30-day period prior to the 2010 Monitoring the Future survey were 14 percent, 29 percent, and 41 percent respectively.

Those who start drinking at a young age are more likely to have problems with alcohol as adults. Youth who drink before age 15 are five times more likely to develop alcohol dependence than those who start at 21.

Ninety percent of 12th graders say that it is fairly easy or very easy for them to get alcohol. In most cases, an adult is buying the alcohol for them, selling it to them, or condoning its use in some way. Teens say they rely on adults more than anyone else to help them make tough decisions and to provide good advice.

Source: Excerpted from "Did You Know?" from the Substance Abuse and Mental Health Services Administration (www.toosmarttostart.gov), September 9, 2011

- **It impairs judgment:** Drinking can lead to poor decisions about engaging in risky behavior, including drinking and driving, sexual activity (such as unprotected sex), and aggressive or violent behavior.

- **It increases the risk of physical and sexual assault:** Underage drinkers are more likely to carry out or be the victim of a physical or sexual assault after drinking than others their age who do not drink.

- **It can lead to other problems:** Drinking may cause youth to have trouble in school or with the law. Drinking alcohol also is associated with the use of other drugs.

- **It increases the risk of alcohol problems later in life:** Research shows that people who start drinking before the age of 15 are four times more likely to meet the criteria for alcohol dependence at some point in their lives.

- **It interferes with brain development:** Research shows that young people's brains keep developing well into their 20s. Alcohol can alter this development, affecting both brain structure and function. This may cause cognitive or learning problems and/or make the brain more prone to alcohol dependence. This is especially a risk when people start drinking young and drink heavily.

Why Do So Many Young People Drink?

As children mature, it is natural for them to assert their independence, seek new challenges, and try taking risks. Underage drinking is a risk that attracts many developing adolescents and teens. Many want to try alcohol, but often do not fully recognize its effects on their health and behavior. Some other reasons young people drink alcohol include peer pressure and stress.

In addition, many youth have easy access to alcohol. A recent study showed that 93.4 percent of adolescents ages 12 to 14 who drank alcohol in the past month got it for free. In many cases, adolescents have access to alcohol through family members, or find it at home.

Preventing Underage Drinking

Preventing underage drinking is a complex challenge. Any successful approach must consider many factors, including genetics, personality, rate of maturation and development, level of risk, social factors, and environmental factors. Several key approaches have been found to be successful:

- **Environmental Interventions:** This approach makes alcohol harder to get—for example, by raising the price of alcohol and keeping the minimum drinking age at 21. Enacting zero-tolerance laws that outlaw driving after any amount of drinking for people under 21 also can help prevent problems.

- **Individual-Level Interventions:** This approach seeks to change the way young people think about alcohol, so they are better able to resist pressures to drink.

- **School-Based Interventions:** These are programs that provide students with the knowledge, skills, motivation, and opportunities they need to remain alcohol free.

- **Family-Based Interventions:** These are efforts to empower parents to set and enforce clear rules against drinking, as well as improve communication between children and parents about alcohol.

Facts About Alcohol Consumption

- Alcohol use can make you act and look stupid. Alcohol can make you feel more social and daring, but it actually is a depressant that slows down parts of your brain. That's why people who have been drinking behave in ways they never would while sober.
- Underage drinking makes you accident prone. Alcohol interferes with your vision, coordination, and concentration by acting as a sedative on your central nervous system. Nearly 190,000 12-to 20-year-olds wind up in an emergency room each year for alcohol-related problems. (The majority of those who do are male.)
- Underage drinking can harm your brain The human brain is not fully developed until the mid-20s. Drinking alcohol, as with other drugs, can interfere with brain development.
- Underage drinking kills. Alcohol interferes with your vision, coordination, and concentration by acting as a sedative on your central nervous system. Each year, about 5,000 young people die from injuries caused by alcohol use.
- Alcohol use may cause depression or make it worse. Young people who feel depressed are more likely to drink alcohol, but alcohol is not a cure for depression. If you are depressed, ask an adult for help.
- Buying or possessing alcohol beverages is illegal for anyone under age 21 in all 50 states, the District of Columbia, and most U.S. territories.
- Alcohol is alcohol. A 12-ounce can of beer or 1.5 ounces of hard liquor contain the same amount of alcohol and have the same effects on your mind and body. There are no "safer" drinks.
- You can't make yourself sober after drinking. It takes an average of two to three hours for a single drink to leave a person system. Drinking coffee, taking a cold shower, or "walking it off" can't speed up this process.

Source: Excerpted from "Did You Know?" from the Substance Abuse and Mental Health Services Administration (www .toosmarttostart.gov), September 9, 2011

Warning Signs Of Underage Drinking

Adolescence is a time of change and growth, including behavior changes. These changes usually are a normal part of growing up but sometimes can point to an alcohol problem. The following warning signs may indicate underage drinking:

- Changes in mood, including anger and irritability
- Academic and/or behavioral problems in school
- Rebelliousness
- Changing groups of friends
- Low energy level
- Less interest in activities and/or care in appearance
- Finding alcohol among a young person's things
- Smelling alcohol on a young person's breath
- Problems concentrating and/or remembering
- Slurred speech
- Coordination problems

Treating Underage Drinking Problems

Some young people can experience serious problems as a result of drinking, including alcohol use disorders. These problems require intervention by trained professionals. Professional treatment options include seeing a counselor, psychologist, psychiatrist, or other trained professional and participating in outpatient or inpatient treatment at a substance abuse treatment facility or other licensed program.

Underage Drinking: One Step Forward, Many More To Go

In December 2011, an annual survey of drug use by American youth offered some promising news: Alcohol use by 8th, 10th, and 12th graders is at its lowest point since the survey began collecting data in 1975.

Monitoring the Future, one of three major surveys sponsored by the U.S. Department of Health and Human Services that provide data on substance abuse among youth, shows that

63.5 percent of 12th graders reported drinking alcohol last year, down from a high in 1997 of 74.8 percent. Of those who drank, 21.6 percent engaged in binge drinking, which means they had five or more drinks in a row during the preceding two weeks—down from 25.4 percent in 2006. These statistics are a sign of progress, but they nevertheless remain too high.

"On the one hand, we're encouraged by the findings—it shows we're on the right track. We've been on the case for a while now and we know more, so clearly it's paying off somehow," says Vivian Faden, Ph.D., associate director for Behavioral Research and director of the Office of Science Policy and Communications at NIAAA, and a leading expert on underage and college drinking.

"But alcohol is still the drug of choice among adolescents. We still have a lot of work to do to continue to better understand and address underage drinking; the problem is far from solved," Dr. Faden continued.

Dr. Faden and her colleagues believe that understanding underage drinking as a developmental issue holds a key to figuring out how to reduce it. As they move into adolescence and beyond, young people experience dramatic physical, emotional, and lifestyle changes, including important transitions such as starting high school or learning to drive. These changes can factor into an adolescent's decisions about drinking.

"By developmental, we mean that development affects the choices kids make to drink, and then, in turn, those choices affect their development," Dr. Faden explained. For example, research shows that the human brain actually continues to develop through adolescence and into our twenties. Different parts of the brain mature at different points in development; understanding this helps explain why adolescents are more likely to take risks, including experimenting with alcohol.

"Underage drinking is one way young people experiment in our culture. If alcohol wasn't available to them, they would still be taking risks, just not with alcohol," said Dr. Faden.

But the risks of underage drinking include a whole range of possible short- and long-term consequences that can change lives. Short-term problems include injuries and even deaths from accidents as well as from homicides and suicides. According to the Centers for Disease Control and Prevention, about 190,000 people under age 21 visited an emergency room for alcohol-related injuries in 2008 alone. Underage drinking can also interfere with school attendance, disrupt concentration, and impact academic performance. In addition, underage drinking can result in aggressive or violent behavior, as well as infections and pregnancies from unplanned and unprotected sex.

"Even the short-term problems can affect a teen's trajectory in life, whether it is having an arrest record or a driving accident or landing in the hospital. That could throw off someone's plans for academic success, or excelling on a sports team, or learning how to develop healthy relationships. You just don't know," said Dr. Faden.

The longer-term problems are also more intertwined with development. For some, starting to drink at an early age is associated with alcohol dependence later in life. This association can affect young drinkers across the board, regardless of whether they have a family history of alcohol problems. In addition, adolescents who drink often may not develop the skills necessary to socialize or deal with stress without drinking alcohol. These skills are a critical part of the maturation process.

There is also new research accumulating about the impact alcohol can have on the brain, including how it grows, develops, and functions. These problems may cause some youth to have difficulty performing tasks requiring memory performance and other critical cognitive skills in the short term and potentially in the long term, too.

"There is still a lot that we just do not know about how the brain responds to alcohol, and more research is needed," said Dr. Faden.

The National Institute on Alcohol Abuse and Alcoholism (NIAAA) is planning a large longitudinal study to investigate alcohol's effects on the developing brain by collecting baseline information on children before they begin drinking and then again afterward. It may also examine the extent to which changes in the brain caused by or associated with alcohol use may resolve if individuals stop or reduce their drinking. Even with this further research, though, it will still be hard to predict what consequences may affect an individual child.

"We can't really know what problems will affect a particular adolescent. But we do know that there are many adolescents out there who drink, and who drink a lot, and who are experiencing a whole range of these problems," said Dr. Faden.

Addressing underage drinking and the many problems associated with it requires identifying the adolescents who may be at risk as early as possible. To address this challenge, NIAAA recently released an alcohol screening guide for health care professionals who work with children. The guide helps practitioners screen their young patients for alcohol consumption and intervene with them based on their age and level of risk.

"We need to screen children and adolescents on a regular basis, so we can appropriately intervene with as many kids as we can," said Dr. Faden. "That will translate to our ultimate goal—which is to prevent the problems of underage drinking from hurting families, kids, and society as a whole."

Teen Brain, A Work In Progress

Have you ever wondered why you have to be 16 to get your driver's license or 18 to vote or 21 to legally drink alcohol?

It's partly because your brain is not ready to take on these responsibilities, since your brain is not fully developed when you're a teen.

During the teen years, essential parts of the brain are still forming—like the prefrontal cortex, which allows people to weigh the pros and cons of situations instead of acting on impulse. This is one reason why teens are generally more likely to take risks than adults.

For example, with alcohol, teens may be less able to judge when to stop drinking. The Centers for Disease Control and Prevention (CDC) tells us that each year, more than 4,600 alcohol-related deaths occur among those less than 21 years old—that is way too many.

Research shows that alcohol and other drugs change the brain's structure and how it works in the short and long term. In the short term, drugs affect your brain's judgment and decision-making abilities, while long-term use causes brain changes that can set people up for addiction and other problems. The brains of people who become addicted get altered so that drugs are now their top priority—and they will compulsively seek and use drugs even though doing so brings devastating consequences for their lives and for those who care about them.

Do yourself a favor and use your brain to make smart choices, reach your goals, and achieve your full potential in life.

Source: Excerpted from "The Teen Brain: A Work in Progress," National Institute on Drug Abuse (www.nida.nih.gov), September 1, 2011.

Age 21 Minimum Legal Drinking Age

Public Health Problem

- Excessive alcohol consumption contributes to more than 4,600 deaths among underage youth, that is, persons less than 21 years of age, in the United States each year.

- Underage drinking is strongly associated with many health and social problems among youth including alcohol-impaired driving, physical fighting, poor school performance, sexual activity, and smoking.

- Most underage youth who drink do so to the point of intoxication, that is, they binge drink (defined as having five or more drinks in a row), typically on multiple occasions.

- Current drinking during the previous month among persons aged 18 to 20 years declined significantly from 59% in 1985 to 40% in 1991, coincident with states' adopting an age 21 minimum legal drinking age, but increased to 47% by 1999.

- The prevalence of current drinking among persons aged 21 to 25 also declined significantly from 70% in 1985 to 56% in 1991, but increased to 60% by 1999.

Relationship Between Youth And Adult Drinking

- Binge drinking by adults is a strong predictor of binge drinking by college students living in the same state.

- There are approximately 1.5 billion episodes of binge drinking among persons aged 18 years or older in the United States annually, most of which involve adults age 26 years and older.

- More than half of all active duty military personnel report binge drinking in the past month, and young adult service members exposed to combat are at significantly greater risk of binge drinking than older service members.

- More than 90% of adult binge drinkers are not alcohol dependent.

Prevention Of Underage Drinking

- The Task Force on Community Preventive Services recommends implementing and maintaining an age 21 minimum legal drinking age (MLDA) based on strong evidence of effectiveness, including a median 16% decline in motor vehicle crashes among underage youth in states that increased the legal drinking age to 21 years.

- The Task Force on Community Preventive Services also recommends enhanced enforcement of laws prohibiting the sale of alcohol to minors to reduce such sales.

- Age 21 MLDA laws result in lower levels of alcohol consumption among young adults age 21 years and older as well as those less than age 21 years.

- States with more stringent alcohol control policies tend to have lower adult and college binge drinking rates.

- In addition to the age 21 MLDA, other effective strategies for preventing underage drinking include increasing alcohol excise taxes11 and limiting alcohol outlet density. Youth exposure to alcohol marketing should also be reduced.

Chapter 15

A Developmental Perspective On Underage Alcohol Use

Dramatic developmental changes unfold as individuals mature from birth to childhood, from childhood to adolescence, and from adolescence to early adulthood. These include physiological changes—such as physical growth, brain development, and puberty—as well as psychological and social changes—such as an evolving sense of self, forming more mature relationships with friends, and transitioning from middle school to high school.

Developmental changes factor into underage drinking. For example, as a high school student transitions to college, he or she may experience greater freedom and autonomy, creating more opportunities to use alcohol. Underage drinking also can influence development, potentially affecting the course of a person's life. For example, alcohol use can interfere with school performance and/or negatively affect peer relationships.

This text examines the complex relationship between underage drinking and development: how developmental factors influence drinking, the social and physical consequences of alcohol use, and how various developmental stages can be specifically targeted to design more effective measures for preventing or treating underage drinking.

Key Stages In Human Development

As children mature, they achieve key developmental milestones such as changing the way they relate to parents and peers, beginning school and moving through different grades and school settings, undergoing puberty, gaining greater independence, and taking on more

About This Chapter: Excerpted from "A Developmental Perspective on Underage Alcohol Use," *Alcohol Alert*, No. 78, National institute on Alcohol Abuse and Alcoholism (www.niaaa.nih.gov), July 2009. The complete text of this document, including references, can be found online at http://pubs.niaaa.nih.gov/publications/AA78/AA78.htm.

responsibilities. These milestones may come earlier for some individuals than others, depending on how quickly they mature, but tend to correspond, in general, to certain ages and developmental stages:

- Prenatal: Prior to birth

- Ages 0–10: childhood

- Ages 10–15: early to mid-adolescence

- Ages 16–20: late adolescence

- Ages 21–25: transition to early adulthood

Each stage in development carries risks for alcohol use and its consequences. Studies show that alcohol use typically begins in early adolescence (ages 12–14) and that between ages 12 and 21, rates of alcohol use and binge drinking increase sharply before leveling off in the twenties. (Binge drinking is defined as consuming five or more drinks in a row for men and four or more drinks in a row for women.)

How Developmental Factors Influence Drinking And Risk For Drinking

Researchers are investigating the complex relationship between developmental factors and alcohol use to better understand how the risks for drinking and alcohol-related problems emerge across development.

Personality And Behavior: Aspects of personality/temperament and certain behaviors that are evident early in life—often before children enter elementary school—such as antisocial behavior, poor self-regulation, poor self-control, anxiety, a tendency toward depression, and shyness may predict initiation of alcohol use in early adolescence, as well as future heavy use and alcohol use disorders (AUDs). Individuals with the most persistent personality and behavior problems are those most likely to experience more chronic and severe forms of AUDs in adulthood.

Family Dynamics: Family dynamics also factor into a child's risk for underage drinking. When parents respond well to their child's needs, that child is better able to regulate his or her emotions and behavior. The most effective family environments are characterized by greater warmth, moderate discipline, and limited stress. Conversely, parents who are depressed, antisocial, or aggressive toward their children or who create a family atmosphere marked by conflict may hinder their child's ability to regulate and control his or her own behavior. Problems with behavioral control, in turn, increase the risk for involvement with alcohol and other drugs

(AODs). Early exposure to AOD use by parents and siblings also increases the risk for underage alcohol use.

Peer Relationships And Culture: As they mature, adolescents place increased importance on peer relationships. Peers who drink may encourage experimentation with alcohol use. This experimentation can have potentially dangerous consequences. Yet, as researchers note, the increased risk-taking and experimentation that is characteristic of adolescence marks an important developmental progression, as individuals begin to form their own identities and to develop strong bonds with peers.

Gene–Environment Interaction: Research suggests that the interaction of inherited and environmental factors strongly influences drinking behavior and that their relative influence varies across adolescence. For example, the initiation of alcohol use is tied more to environmental than to genetic influences. In contrast, across mid- to late adolescence, the relative influence of genetic factors on underage drinking increases, although there are important individual differences. Some of the genetic factors that influence problem drinking are specific to alcohol, whereas others influence a range of behaviors that reflect a general lack of impulse control in late adolescence and early adulthood.

Adolescent Brain Development And Gaps In Maturity: All regions of the brain do not mature at the same time or at the same pace. For example, a region deep within the brain that governs emotions and mediates fear and anxiety (the limbic system) matures in early adolescence. Its development is believed to be triggered by the hormones that set puberty in motion. In contrast, the frontal cortex—the region responsible for self-regulation, decision-making, and behavioral control—develops more gradually, as a result of age and experience. This creates a period of time during adolescence in which emotions are heightened, but the ability to regulate these emotions and regulate one's behavior still is developing. Some researchers believe this differential maturation of brain regions may contribute to the increased risk-taking behavior common during adolescence.

Differences In Sensitivity To Alcohol: Research with animals suggests that compared with adults, adolescents are less sensitive to the negative effects of alcohol intoxication—such as sedation, hangover, and loss of coordination—but are more sensitive to the way alcohol eases social situations. Because human adolescents may be less sensitive than adults to certain aversive effects of alcohol, they may be at higher risk for consuming more drinks per drinking occasion. This developmental phenomenon may help explain why adolescents are able to drink larger amounts of alcohol (as in binge drinking) without experiencing the same levels of physiological effects (such as sleepiness and poor coordination) as adults.

How Drinking Can Influence Development

The immediate, short-term, and long-term effects of alcohol vary with developmental period.

Prenatal: The developing embryo and fetus are particularly vulnerable to the adverse effects of alcohol. Prenatal exposure to alcohol can result in a wide range of physical abnormalities, growth retardation, and nervous system impairments (collectively referred to as fetal alcohol spectrum disorder; the most severe form of this disorder is called fetal alcohol syndrome).

Childhood And Adolescence: Underage drinking can interfere with school attendance, disrupt concentration, damage relationships with parents and peers, and potentially alter brain function and/or other aspects of development, all of which have consequences for future success in such areas as work, adult relationships, health, and overall well-being. A person who begins drinking early in life also is more likely to become a heavy drinker during adolescence and to experience alcohol abuse or dependence on alcohol in adulthood.

In addition, chronic heavy drinking during adolescence has been linked to cognitive deficits and alterations in brain activity and structure. It is unclear, however, whether these deficits resulted from alcohol consumption itself or existed prior to the initiation of drinking and may in fact have contributed to that individual's alcohol use. It is also unknown if and to what extent these deficits will resolve with abstinence or decreased drinking. Human studies have shown, however, that adolescents are more vulnerable than adults to alcohol-related effects on memory. Additionally, evidence from rodent studies of binge-type drinking suggests that adolescent animals are more vulnerable than adults to brain damage.

Late Adolescence: Across multiple studies, there seems to be a strong relationship between drinking in later adolescence and in early adulthood. Research also shows that people who drink heavily in late adolescence are more likely than others to be diagnosed with an alcohol use disorder (AUD) later in life. In addition, alcohol use in late adolescence is associated with a number of other serious problems in adulthood, including drug dependence, antisocial behavior, and depression, although evidence of this latter association has been inconsistent.

Prevention

The harmful consequences of alcohol use underscore the importance of evidence-based preventive interventions and policy measures for preventing underage drinking. Preventive interventions may target every member of an eligible population or a particular subpopulation with a higher risk of problems, including AUDs. Findings from recent research studies are summarized below.

Family-Focused Interventions: These interventions typically address a range of risk and protective factors associated with life within a family. For instance, do parents carefully monitor the child's activities, are they "close" (that is, bonded) to the child, do they practice effective discipline, and are they involved in the child's home life and school? Many family-focused interventions have been aimed at families with preschool-aged children and have focused on improving parent-child relationships, decreasing aggressive behavior, and enhancing the children's social and psychological readiness to make the transition to school. Most studies evaluating these interventions have concentrated on the effectiveness of these measures in curbing aggressive behavior. Only one preschool program evaluated alcohol use later in life and showed reduced drinking by participants when they reached their teen years.

Few family-focused interventions for elementary school–aged children have been implemented and assessed, although interventions for this population often have family and school components. Several of these interventions have shown effectiveness in delaying the initiation of alcohol use and reducing drinking during the teenage years.

For adolescents aged 10–15, family-focused interventions have shown considerable promise. Interventions for this age-group can be either home based or administered in small groups, and analysis indicates that small-group interventions show relatively stronger evidence of effect than home-based interventions. Family-focused interventions have not shown this same degree of effectiveness for older adolescents who do not enter college, although studies focusing on college-bound adolescents have shown some success.

School-Based Interventions: Unlike family-based approaches, which tend to focus on strengthening parenting skills and parent-child relationships, school-based approaches focus on life skills, peer refusal skills, role-playing, strengthening positive peer relationships, and providing accurate information on how many children actually use alcohol. Such interventions have been shown to significantly reduce aggressive and disruptive behavior in younger children, as well as early initiation and progression of alcohol use in adolescents. However, many studies have important limitations, including not following children long enough to evaluate eventual alcohol use. Among the programs reviewed, there were no effective interventions with children in later elementary school years (grades 3 to 5) with respect to early alcohol use. Similarly, the researchers found only two promising school-based interventions targeted to high school students.

Multi-Domain Interventions: As the name implies, these interventions address several aspects of an adolescent's life (for example, the individual, family, school, and community/environment) and typically focus on younger adolescents. Research indicates that these interventions can be effective, but there is a need for further research to develop and assess such interventions for older adolescents. In addition, there are challenges to large-scale implementation of these programs, including the extensive resources required to sustain quality implementation.

Policy, Law, And Environmentally Focused Interventions. These types of interventions typically focus on older adolescents. The research considered here did not find any effective policy interventions aimed at adolescents younger than age 16, nor did it identify policy interventions that could be shown to delay initiation of alcohol use or reduce alcohol use among younger adolescents. For older adolescents, several interventions have shown promise, including those focused on reducing the sale of alcohol to minors, increasing identification checks ("carding") by vendors, and reducing the community's tolerance of the sale of alcohol to minors and of underage drinking in general. However, studies assessing the effectiveness of these measures often did not investigate alcohol use outcomes specifically, or they involved so few communities that it is impossible to say if these measures would be effective for all communities.

One policy that has been extensively studied is the effectiveness of laws raising the minimum legal drinking age from 18 to 21. Most studies have found a positive effect on health and safety when the minimum drinking age is increased to 21. Studies also have shown that changes in the drinking age laws can reduce the rates of underage drinking, single-vehicle nighttime car crashes (the most common crash associated with alcohol use), and vehicle fatalities. Other studies, however, found no changes in the rates of crashes and fatalities after the introduction of such laws.

Treatment

Researchers have developed a variety of treatment approaches for adolescents with alcohol and other drug (AOD) use disorders. Medications rarely are used in this age-group, although some studies have examined the effects of certain drugs aimed at treating coexisting psychiatric conditions, such as depression or anxiety, in this population. For example, in one study of adolescents with bipolar disorder and an AOD use disorder, those who received lithium treatment were less likely to screen positive for AOD use and exhibited greater clinical improvement than did adolescents in a placebo group. Findings from a recent review if research evaluating treatment in underage drinkers are summarized below.

Behavioral Therapy: This intervention attempts to identify the behaviors and situations in which AOD use occurs and then to disrupt those behaviors by equipping adolescents with skills to resist AOD use. It emphasizes stress management, assertiveness training, and self-control. One study of adolescents seeking treatment for AOD use disorders found that those receiving behavioral therapy reported less frequent drug use than adolescents in a comparison group. The treatment-seeking group also had improved school attendance and performance. Another study comparing behavioral therapy with supportive counseling in adolescents and adults found that those in the behavioral therapy group showed much greater reductions in AOD use than those in the supportive therapy group, both immediately after treatment and at a nine-month followup. The behavioral therapy group also showed greater improvements in other areas, including the number of days in school.

Cognitive-Behavioral Therapy (CBT): Built on basic behavioral therapy, CBT includes strategies to help the adolescent better understand the factors and situations that precede AOD use as well as the consequences of that use. A study compared CBT (presentations, modeling, role playing, and homework exercises) with traditional group therapy among adolescents who abused AODs in addition to having other psychiatric disorders. Adolescents in the CBT group achieved lower scores on the Teen Addiction Severity Index—a tool that assesses a variety of aspects (or domains) to determine the adolescent's need for treatment or counseling—than the comparison group.

Family-Based Interventions And Multisystemic Therapy (MST): These approaches use family therapy principles to improve adolescent health-risk behaviors. MST provides intensive, home-based treatment addressing the child's environment, including his or her family, peer groups, school, and community. Research using an MST approach with juvenile offenders (which focused on changing behavior by identifying the strengths and weaknesses of each participant and forming an individualized treatment plan) found positive effects on several high-risk behaviors. Study participants were less likely to use AODs, to be arrested for AOD-related offenses, and to be convicted for aggressive criminal behaviors than a similar group that did not receive the intervention.

When family therapy was combined with CBT, adolescents who received the family therapy/CBT intervention, on average, were less likely to use alcohol during the six-month follow-up period and reported lower marijuana use than did adolescents who received only a basic-information intervention.

Similarly, a study of 182 alcohol- and marijuana-abusing adolescents who received either multidimensional family therapy (designed to improve overall family functioning through multiple interventions in several key areas of life), adolescent group therapy, or a multifamily education intervention found that adolescents assigned to multidimensional family therapy showed the greatest improvement (compared with the other groups), with more than 40 percent of participants in this group reporting reduced AOD use, which persisted throughout the one-year follow-up period.

Motivational Enhancement Therapy: Also known as motivational interviewing (MI), motivational enhancement therapy is designed to enhance a person's motivation to make changes regarding AOD use and to recognize and cope with those life situations that may trigger or sustain AOD use. MI is particularly appealing for treating AOD-abusing adolescents, who often do not seek treatment on their own and need to be motivated to do so and to change their behaviors. In one study, researchers found that students receiving a single, brief MI session during their freshman year in college significantly reduced their drinking and had fewer alcohol-related consequences at six-month and two-year followups than did students who did not receive the intervention. In another MI study, one session significantly reduced adolescents' nicotine, alcohol, and marijuana use at the three-month followup, relative to those who received only basic AOD education.

Conclusion

The developmental pathway from childhood to adulthood is marked by significant change. Studies examining the complex relationship between development and alcohol use help illustrate how a person's risk for drinking and alcohol-related problems emerges across childhood, adolescence, and early adulthood. The consequences of drinking alcohol also vary with developmental period. These effects can be far-reaching, ranging from altered brain function, reduced academic and work performance, and increased risk of problems with alcohol and other psychiatric problems during adulthood, to increased risk for injury or death (for example, from alcohol-related falls or traffic crashes).

Understanding the interaction between alcohol and development enables scientists to design better-targeted and more effective approaches for preventing underage alcohol use. Some of these approaches, which act at the level of the family, school, or multiple domains simultaneously, have been shown to be effective at least for certain age-groups in delaying the initiation of drinking and reducing the amount of alcohol consumed. Still, not all developmental stages have been equally explored, and population subgroups, such as certain rural, cultural, or ethnic populations, may not respond as well to existing interventions. More research is needed to determine what works and what doesn't in different settings.

Equally important, knowledge of the interrelationship between developmental stage and drinking behavior will help researchers and clinicians design more effective treatment programs for adolescents with AUDs that can effectively reduce alcohol consumption and its associated consequences.

Chapter 16

Abusive And Underage College Drinking

College Drinking

Abusive and underage college drinking are significant public health problems, and they exact an enormous toll on the intellectual and social lives of students on campuses across the United States.

Drinking at college has become a ritual that students often see as an integral part of their higher-education experience. Many students come to college with established drinking habits, and the college environment can exacerbate the problem. Research shows that more than 80 percent of college students drink alcohol, and almost half report binge drinking in the past two weeks.

Virtually all college students experience the effects of college drinking—whether they drink or not.

Binge Drinking

Many college alcohol problems are related to binge drinking. Binge drinking is a pattern of drinking that brings blood alcohol concentration (BAC) levels to 0.08 g/dL. This usually occurs after four drinks for women and five drinks for men—in about two hours.

Drinking this way can pose serious health and safety risks, including car crashes, drunk-driving arrests, sexual assaults, and injuries. Over the long term, frequent binge drinking can damage the liver and other organs.

About This Chapter: The main text in this chapter includes excerpts from "College Drinking," National Institute on Alcohol Abuse and Alcoholism (www.nih.niaaa.gov), April 2012; text from "Secondary Effects of Alcohol Abuse," U.S. Department of Education (http://www.higheredcenter.org), 2008; and, "Addressing Alcohol Use on Campus," U.S. Department of Education, 2008. Reviewed by David A. Cooke, MD, FACP, December 2012.

Annual College Drinking Consequences

The consequences of excessive and underage drinking affect virtually all college campuses, college communities, and college students, whether they choose to drink or not. The following statistics report estimates for the number of college students affected by drinking-related consequences every year:

- **Death:** 1,825 college students between the ages of 18 and 24 die from alcohol-related unintentional injuries, including motor vehicle crashes.

- **Injury:** 599,000 students between the ages of 18 and 24 are unintentionally injured under the influence of alcohol.

- **Assault:** 696,000 students between the ages of 18 and 24 are assaulted by another student who has been drinking.

- **Sexual Abuse:** 97,000 students between the ages of 18 and 24 are victims of alcohol-related sexual assault or date rape.

- **Unsafe Sex:** 400,000 students between the ages of 18 and 24 had unprotected sex and more than 100,000 students between the ages of 18 and 24 report having been too intoxicated to know if they consented to having sex.

- **Academic Problems:** About 25 percent of college students report academic consequences of their drinking including missing class, falling behind, doing poorly on exams or papers, and receiving lower grades overall.

- **Health Problems/Suicide Attempts:** More than 150,000 students develop an alcohol-related health problem, and between 1.2 and 1.5 percent of students indicate that they tried to commit suicide within the past year due to drinking or drug use.

- **Drunk Driving:** 3,360,000 students between the ages of 18 and 24 drive under the influence of alcohol.

- **Vandalism:** About 11 percent of college student drinkers report that they have damaged property while under the influence of alcohol.

- **Property Damage:** More than 25 percent of administrators from schools with relatively low drinking levels and over 50 percent from schools with high drinking levels say their campuses have a "moderate" or "major" problem with alcohol-related property damage.

- **Police Involvement:** About 5 percent of four-year college students are involved with the police or campus security as a result of their drinking, and 110,000 students between the ages of 18 and 24 are arrested for an alcohol-related violation such as public drunkenness or driving under the influence.

- **Alcohol Abuse And Dependence:** 31 percent of college students met criteria for a diagnosis of alcohol abuse and 6 percent for a diagnosis of alcohol dependence in the past 12 months, according to questionnaire-based self-reports about their drinking.

Source: From "A Snapshot of Annual High-Risk College Drinking Consequences," National Institute on Alcohol Abuse and Alcoholism, July 2010. The complete text of this document, including references for the statistics, can be found online at http://www.collegedrinkingprevention.gov/statssummaries/snapshot.aspx.

To avoid binge drinking and its consequences, college students (and all drinkers who are old enough to drink; underage minors should not drink at all) are advised to track the number of drinks they consume over a given period of time. That is why it is important to know exactly what counts as a drink.

In the United States, a standard drink is one that contains about 14 grams of "pure" alcohol. This is the amount of alcohol found in 12 ounces of beer (which is usually about 5% alcohol), 5 ounces of wine (which is typically about 12% alcohol), or 1.5 ounces of distilled spirits (which is about 40% alcohol). Unfortunately, although the standard drink amounts are helpful for following health guidelines, they often do not reflect customary serving sizes, particularly in a college environment. A large cup of beer, an over-poured glass of wine, or a single mixed drink could contain much more alcohol than a standard drink.

Alcohol Poisoning

Thousands of college students are transported to the emergency room each year for alcohol poisoning, which occurs when high levels of alcohol suppress the nervous and respiratory systems and the body struggles to rid itself of toxins produced from the breakdown of alcohol. Signs of this dangerous condition can include the following:

- Mental confusion, stupor, coma, or the person cannot be roused

- Vomiting

- Slow or irregular breathing

- Hypothermia (low body temperature), bluish or pale skin

Alcohol poisoning can lead to permanent brain damage or death, so a person showing any of these signs requires immediate medical attention. Don't wait. Call 911 if you suspect alcohol poisoning.

Factors Affecting Student Drinking

Although the majority of students come to college already having some experience with alcohol, certain aspects of college life, such as unstructured time, the widespread availability of alcohol, inconsistent enforcement of underage drinking laws, and limited interactions with parents and other adults, can intensify the problem. In fact, college students have higher binge-drinking rates and a higher incidence of drunk driving than their non-college peers.

The first six weeks of freshman year is an especially vulnerable time for heavy drinking and alcohol-related consequences because of student expectations and social pressures at the start of the academic year.

Factors related to specific college environments also are significant. Students attending schools with strong Greek systems and with prominent athletic programs tend to drink more than students at other types of schools. In terms of living arrangements, alcohol consumption is highest among students living in fraternities and sororities and lowest among commuting students who live with their families.

An often overlooked preventive factor involves the continuing influence of parents. Research shows that students who choose not to drink often do so because their parents discussed alcohol use and its adverse consequences with them.

Addressing College Drinking

Ongoing research continues to improve our understanding of how to address this persistent and costly problem. Successful efforts typically involve a mix of prevention, intervention, and treatment strategies that target individual students, the student body as a whole, and the broader college community.

Strategies Targeting Individual Students: Strategies that target individual students, including those at risk for alcohol problems, are effective, particularly alcohol screening and brief intervention programs conducted in campus health centers. These programs evaluate students' alcohol use and provide feedback about the risks of drinking, how these risks interfere with meeting their goals, how to monitor and reduce drinking, and how to handle high-risk situations.

A focus on individual intervention and treatment is significant, as research shows that 19 percent of college students between the ages of 18 and 24 meet the criteria for alcohol abuse and dependence, but only 5 percent of them seek treatment assistance.

Strategies Targeting The Campus And Surrounding Community: In combination with individually oriented interventions, strategies that focus on the college environment are another key component of a comprehensive program. These prevention efforts target the entire student body as well as the broader college community and include strategies that provide alcohol education, limit alcohol availability and enforce underage-drinking laws, provide alcohol-free campus activities, notify parents of alcohol-related infractions, and adjust academic schedules to include more Friday classes and reduce the number of long weekends during the semester.

Social-norms approaches, which focus on correcting student misperceptions about how much their peers drink, have been widely implemented. However, new research shows that these approaches may work best in individual and online applications, in which students receive personalized feedback, but they are much less effective as part of campus-wide campaigns.

Accumulating research shows that campus-community partnerships can be effective. With the involvement of campus administrators, local law enforcement, merchants, residents, and local leaders, these partnerships address college drinking through the application and consistent enforcement of community policies. Effective campus-community partnership strategies can include publicizing and enforcing underage-drinking and zero-tolerance laws for drivers under age 21, establishing partnerships between the college and the local residential and business communities to reduce access to alcohol and to address violations, and increasing the price of alcohol, such as the elimination of low-cost drink specials in bars near college campuses, because research shows that when alcohol is more expensive people drink less and have fewer alcohol-related problems.

Strong leadership from a concerned college president in combination with an involved campus community and a comprehensive program of evidence-based strategies can help address harmful student drinking.

Secondary Effects Of Alcohol Abuse

Students who are not heavy drinkers or who abstain from drinking altogether still suffer negative consequences from other students' alcohol abuse, called secondary effects. Additionally, the campus as a whole suffers as the academic mission of a college or university is compromised by students who abuse alcohol. Finally, the secondary effects of high-risk drinking can reach as far as neighboring communities.

Secondary Effects On Campus

The majority of college and university students are not heavy drinkers, with 22.8 percent abstaining altogether from all alcohol use. However, even students who don't abuse alcohol can be affected by others' heavy drinking. In fact, according to the Harvard School of Public Health's College Alcohol Study (CAS), over three-quarters of students who live in campus housing report experiencing one or more secondary effects of alcohol:

- 60 percent had interrupted study or sleep
- 48 percent took care of a drunk fellow student
- 29 percent were insulted or humiliated
- 20 percent (females) experienced an unwanted sexual advance
- 19 percent had a serious argument or quarrel
- 15 percent had property damaged

- 9 percent had been pushed, hit, or assaulted

- 1 percent (females) were sexually assaulted or victims of acquaintance rape

Moreover, entire campuses suffer the secondary effects of vandalism, riots, hazing, and other forms of violence committed by intoxicated students.

Secondary Effects In The Community

College drinking can negatively affect the quality of life of individuals and families who live in local communities. People who live within one mile of a campus are more likely to experience excessive noise, public drunkenness, litter, vandalism, and public urination and vomiting on their property than those who live farther away.

Effective Prevention

An environmental management approach to prevention influences behavior change on multiple levels and can have a large-scale effect on reducing the secondary effects of alcohol abuse on campus and in the community.

Getting community leaders on board with the planning and implementation of these alcohol prevention efforts can help ensure that local citizens' viewpoints are considered and their problems addressed.

Academic Performance

Poor academic performance among college students is associated with alcohol consumption. Alcohol abuse contributes to students missing class, failing tests, dropping out due to do poor grades, and compromising the academic mission of colleges and universities.

One of the most common consequences of alcohol abuse by students is difficulty keeping up with academic responsibilities. The number of drinks a student consumes is directly associated with the student's grades. Core Institute research shows the following correlation between grades and alcoholic drink consumption:

- Students with B averages consume 1.1 more drinks per week than A students.

- Students with C averages consume 2.7 more drinks per week than A students.

- Students with D and F averages consume 6.4 more drinks per week than A students.

Source: Excerpted from "Academic Performance," U.S. Department of Education (http://www.higheredcenter.org), 2008. Reviewed by David A. Cooke, MD, FACP, December 2012.

Addressing Alcohol Use On Campus

Traditional Prevention Approaches

Historically, institutions of higher education have addressed the issues of student alcohol use by focusing on education and intervention strategies that target students individually. Many of the typical education and awareness programs offered on campuses are based on the idea that students simply don't have enough information on the dangers of alcohol use: teach them, and their behavior will change.

These kinds of programs are offered during freshman orientation, in conjunction with an Alcohol Awareness Week, or through peer education programs. On some campuses, lessons about the dangers of alcohol use are integrated into course work, a strategy known as curriculum infusion. Evaluation data from typical education and awareness programs demonstrate that while such programs may be a necessary and productive component of a more comprehensive alcohol prevention strategy, they are ineffective when used as stand-alone programs.

A Comprehensive Approach

Drawing on more than two decades of prevention research, the Higher Education Center developed a comprehensive approach to student alcohol use, which addresses the issues not only through educational channels but also by bringing about change at the institutional, community, and public policy level. This approach is grounded in the principle that people's attitudes, decisions, and behavior—and in this case, those that relate to alcohol use—are shaped by the physical, social, economic, and legal environment. The many aspects of this environment can be shaped by prevention advocates, campus officials, government officials, and others. This model, termed environmental management, has since been supported by scientific research for its effectiveness in bringing about lasting and positive change on a college campus.

Environmental Management

Environmental management addresses several factors that, though they may vary in the degree to which they exist on a college campus, have significant effects on students' decisions regarding alcohol use:

- Students lack (or lack awareness of) adequate social, recreational, and extracurricular options to deter them from drinking.
- Students perceive a strong normative pressure to drink in college.

- College students are often the targets of aggressive marketing and promotion tactics by the alcohol industry.

- Alcohol is often abundantly available in and around college campuses.

- Campus and local laws and policies on alcohol can be vague or nonexistent and are not always consistently or adequately enforced.

Accordingly, the environmental management approach employs five strategies to target these factors:

- Offer and promote social, recreational, extracurricular, and public service alcohol-free options.

- Create a social, academic, and residential environment that supports health-promoting norms.

- Restrict marketing and promotion of alcoholic beverages both on and off campus.

- Limit alcohol availability both on and off campus.

- Develop campus policies and enforce laws at the campus, local, state, and federal levels.

For a campus to succeed in its efforts to address student alcohol use, campus officials not only have to measure the extent and nature of the problem but also the variety of factors that are driving the problem. Then a campus can engage in a strategic planning process by which it maps out a plan for addressing the most critical factors that underlie the campus alcohol problem. In developing this framework for effective alcohol prevention, the Higher Education Center also acknowledges that alcohol use is both a campus and community problem, and campuses and community collaboration is necessary to address it.

Chapter 17

Emergency Department Visits Involving Underage Alcohol Use

Despite laws in all 50 states and the District of Columbia that prohibit underage drinking, consumption of alcohol by adolescents and young adults younger than 21 remains a significant public health concern. More adolescents and young adults younger than 21 use alcohol than tobacco or illicit drugs, making it the most widely abused substance by this age group. The 2008 National Survey on Drug Use and Health (NSDUH) shows that 26.4 percent of persons aged 12 to 20 had consumed alcohol in the past month and 17.4 percent were binge drinkers (that is, drank five or more drinks on the same occasion on at least one day in the 30 days prior to the survey). NSDUH data also show that adolescents and young adults who consumed alcohol in the past month drank more alcoholic drinks per occasion, on average, than persons over the legal drinking age (4.9 *vs.* 2.8 drinks).

In recognition of the scope of the underage drinking problem, in 2007 the Surgeon General issued the *Call to Action to Prevent and Reduce Underage Drinking*. The report noted the association between underage drinking and a host of negative consequences, including risky sexual behavior, violence, illicit drug use, injury, damage to the developing brain, and death. Adolescents and young adults that experience medical emergencies severe enough to require treatment in an emergency department (ED) may be at higher risk for such negative consequences. ED visits involving underage drinking therefore provide a unique opportunity to identify these high-risk adolescents and young adults.

About This Chapter: This chapter includes text excerpted from: Substance Abuse and Mental Health Services Administration, Office of Applied Studies. (July 29, 2010). *The DAWN Report: Emergency Department Visits Involving Underage Alcohol Use: 2008*. Rockville, MD. The complete text of this document, including references, is available online at http://www.oas.samhsa.gov/2k10/DAWN005/UnderageDrinkingHTML.pdf.

The Drug Abuse Warning Network (DAWN) is a public health surveillance system that monitors drug-related ED visits in the United States. To be a DAWN case, an ED visit must have involved a drug, either as the direct cause of the visit or as a contributing factor. DAWN includes ED visits for underage persons involving alcohol only or in combination with other drug(s) and can, therefore, be used to examine underage alcohol use that results in ED visits. Using 2008 data, this text focuses on alcohol-related ED visits among adolescents and young adults aged 12 to 20 and provides an update to a similar report [published in June 2009].

Overview

In 2008, an estimated 575,092 drug-related ED visits were made by patients aged 12 to 20. About one third of these visits (32.9 percent, or 188,981 visits) involved alcohol. Of all alcohol-related ED visits made by patients aged 12 to 20, 70.0 percent involved alcohol only, and 30.0 percent involved alcohol in combination with other drugs.

Of the 56,727 alcohol-related ED visits by patients aged 12 to 20 in which alcohol was combined with another drug, 57.3 percent involved marijuana. Anti-anxiety drugs, narcotic pain relievers, and cocaine were indicated in 17.8, 15.3, and 13.3 percent of these visits, respectively.

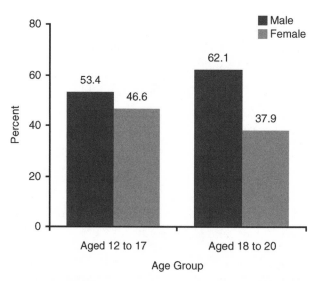

Figure 17.1. Alcohol-Related Emergency Department (ED) Visits by Patients Aged 12 to 20, by Age Group and Gender: 2008 (Source: 2008 [08/2009 update] SAMHSA Drug Abuse Warning Network.)

Risky Behavior: The Road To The Emergency Department

When you ask friends what they're going to do for homecoming or the prom or graduation, spending the night in the local emergency department probably isn't on their list. Unfortunately, for many young people, alcohol may change their plans. According to a study by the Substance Abuse and Mental Health Services Administration (SAMHSA), emergency departments get 546 underage drinking-related emergency department visits every day—many more on special celebration days.

Emergency department visits can cost $1,000 or more—not including the cost of an ambulance or a hospital stay if you have to be admitted to the hospital. If a drinker in the ER is under 18, the hospital has to call their parents or guardians. To make matters worse, minors can also get into legal trouble since underage drinking is against the law.

Not to pile on, BUT people who drink before their 21st birthday are more likely to use drugs, get bad grades, become a victim of a violent or sexual crime, and get addicted to alcohol. In fact, More than four in ten people who begin drinking before age 15 eventually become alcoholic.

Better to celebrate special events in a way you'll be glad to remember the next morning!

Source: "Risky Behavior Leads to Emergency Rooms," National Institute on Drug Abuse (www.nida.nih.gov), April 21, 2011.

Gender And Age

The majority (58.6 percent) of alcohol-related ED visits made by patients aged 12 to 20 were made by males. Patients aged 18 to 20 accounted for about six in ten (60.3 percent) alcohol-related ED visits made by adolescents and young adults. Of ED visits made by underage drinkers, 62.1 percent of patients aged 18 to 20 were male compared with 53.4 percent of patients aged 12 to 17 (see Figure 17.1).

Discharge Of Underage Drinkers From The ED

Follow-up care in DAWN is defined as admission to an inpatient unit in the hospital, transfer to another health care facility, or referral to a detoxification program or substance abuse treatment. About one in five (19.1 percent) alcohol-related ED visits made by patients aged 12 to 20 had evidence of follow-up care (see Table 17.1). Most patients were treated and released to home (72.3 percent).

Evidence of follow-up care for patients from EDs was related to whether visits involved alcohol only or alcohol in combination with other drugs. When ED visits involved alcohol only, 12.0 percent had evidence of follow-up care. However, when visits involved alcohol in combination with other drugs, 35.5 percent had evidence of follow-up care. This pattern held for both age groups and genders (see Figures 17.2 and 17.3).

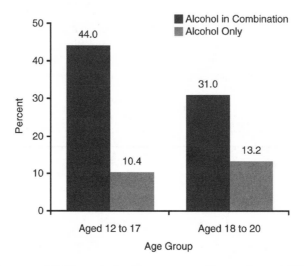

Figure 17.2. Evidence of Follow-up for Emergency Department (ED) Visits Involving Alcohol Only and Visits Involving Alcohol in Combination with Other Drugs by Patients Aged 12 to 20, by Age Group: 2008 (Source: 2008 [08/2009 update] SAMHSA Drug Abuse Warning Network.)

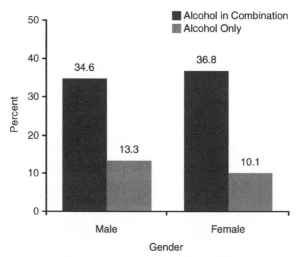

Figure 17.3. Evidence of Follow-up for Emergency Department (ED) Visits Involving Alcohol Only and Visits Involving Alcohol in Combination with Other Drugs by Patients Aged 12 to 20, by Gender: 2008 (Source: 2008 [08/2009 update] SAMHSA Drug Abuse Warning Network.)

Discussion

DAWN data show the extent of the underage drinking problem through the lens of alcohol-related ED visits made by patients aged 12 to 20. The findings in this report point to underage drinking as a costly public health concern and suggest the need for continued efforts to prevent and reduce underage drinking.

The ED offers a unique opportunity to identify and intervene with underage drinkers, particularly those at greatest risk for severe and negative long-term consequences of alcohol abuse. In this report, most alcohol-related ED visits involving adolescents and young adults resulted in a discharge home without any evidence of follow-up care. Adolescents and young adults who experience alcohol-related episodes severe enough to require ED treatment likely require a substance abuse assessment at a minimum. Health professionals in the ED are well

Table 17.1. Follow-Up Status And Disposition Of Alcohol-Related Emergency Department (ED) Visits By Patients Aged 12 To 20: 2008 (Source of data: 2008 [08/2009 update] SAMHSA Drug Abuse Warning Network.)

Follow-up And Disposition	Estimated Number of ED Visits	Percent of Visits
Total	**188,981**	**100.0**
No Follow-up	**152,921**	**80.9**
Released to home	136,548	72.3
Released to police/jail	11,437	6.1
Left against medical advice	1,939	1.0
Other*	2,998	1.6
Follow-up	**36,060**	**19.1**
Admitted to same hospital	18,018	9.5
Intensive care unit/critical care unit	4,546	2.4
Psychiatric unit	4,346	2.3
Chemical dependency/detoxification unit	1,959	1.0
Other inpatient unit	7,166	3.8
Transferred to another hospital or health care facility	12,868	6.8
Referred to detoxification or substance use treatment facility	5,174	2.7

* "Other" includes Other, Died, and Unknown.

placed to provide referrals for assessment and treatment, as well as brief interventions for these adolescents and young adults. Brief interventions in the ED, particularly brief motivational interventions, have been found to be effective in reducing alcohol use among adolescents and young adults as well. The use of a brief intervention in EDs may be particularly important in reducing future alcohol use and abuse and improving the long-term health and well-being of adolescents and young adults prone to alcohol misuse.

Drinking Can Put A Chill On Your Summer Fun

Summer is a wonderful time for outdoor activities with family and friends. For many people, a day at the beach, on the boat, or at a backyard barbecue will include drinking alcoholic beverages. But excessive drinking by adults (or any drinking by minors) and summer activities don't mix. Drinking impairs both physical and mental abilities, and it also decreases inhibitions—which can lead to tragic consequences on the water, on the road, and in the great outdoors. In fact, research shows that half of all water recreation deaths of teens and adults involve the use of alcohol.

Swimmers can get in over their heads.

Alcohol impairs judgment and increases risk-taking, a dangerous combination for swimmers. Even experienced swimmers may venture out farther than they should and not be able to make it back to shore, or they may not notice how chilled they're getting and develop hypothermia. Surfers could become over-confident and try to ride a wave beyond their abilities. Even around a pool, too much alcohol can have deadly consequences. Inebriated divers may collide with the diving board or dive where the water is too shallow.

Boaters can lose their bearings.

According to research funded by the National Institute on Alcohol Abuse and Alcoholism, alcohol may be involved in 60 percent of boating fatalities, including falling overboard. And a boat operator with a blood alcohol concentration (BAC) over 0.1 percent is 16 times more likely to be killed in a boating accident than an operator with zero BAC. According to the U.S. Coast Guard and the National Association of State Boating Law Administrators, alcohol can impair a boater's judgment, balance, vision, and reaction time. It can also increase fatigue and susceptibility to the effects of cold-water immersion. And if problems arise, intoxicated boaters are ill equipped to find solutions. For passengers, intoxication can lead to slips on deck, falls overboard, or accidents at the dock.

Source: Excerpted from "Risky Drinking Can Put a Chill on Your Summer Fun," National Institute on Alcohol Abuse and Alcoholism (www.niaaa.nih.gov), July 2011.

Part Three
Alcohol's Physical Effects

Chapter 18

Understanding Alcohol's Impact On Your Health

Beyond Hangovers

A brightly colored cosmopolitan is the drink of choice for the glamorous characters in *Sex and the City*. James Bond depends on his famous martini—shaken, not stirred—to unwind with after confounding a villain. And what wedding concludes without a champagne toast?

Alcohol is part of our culture—it helps us celebrate and socialize, and it enhances our religious ceremonies. But drinking too much (on a single occasion or over time) or too soon (before age 21) can have serious consequences for your health. Most Americans recognize that drinking too much can lead to accidents and dependence. But that's only part of the story. In addition to these serious problems, alcohol abuse can damage organs, weaken the immune system, and contribute to cancers. Plus, much like smoking, alcohol affects different people differently. Genes, environment, and even diet can play a role in whether you develop an alcohol-related disease. Sound complicated? It sure can be. To stay healthy, and to decide what role alcohol should play in your life, you need accurate, up-to-date information.

This chapter is designed to offer you guidance based on the latest research on alcohol's effect on health. Information about alcohol *use* that is not considered *abuse* refers to consumption only by adults. Alcohol consumption by people under the age of 21 carries increased health-related risks, and it is illegal in all 50 states of the United States.

About This Chapter: From "Beyond Hangovers: Understanding Alcohol's Impact on Your Health," National Institute on Alcohol Abuse and Alcoholism (www.niaaa.nih.gov), September 2010.

A Little Goes A Long Way

Knowing how much alcohol constitutes a *standard* drink can help you determine how much you are drinking and understand the risks. One standard drink contains about 0.6 fluid ounces or 14 grams of pure alcohol. In more familiar terms, the following amounts constitute one standard drink:

- 12 fluid ounces of beer (about 5% alcohol)

- 8 to 9 fluid ounces of malt liquor (about 7% alcohol)

- 5 fluid ounces of table wine (about 12% alcohol)

- 1.5 fluid ounces of hard liquor (about 40% alcohol)

Research demonstrates low-risk drinking levels for adult men are no more than four drinks on any single day AND no more than 14 drinks per week. For adult women, low-risk drinking levels are no more than three drinks on any single day AND no more than seven drinks per week. To stay low-risk, adults must keep within *both* the single-day and weekly limits. There is no amount of consumption that is considered low-risk for people under the age of 21; any underage alcohol consumption is high risk.

Even within low-risk limits, people can have problems if they drink too quickly, have health conditions, or are over age 65. Adults who are older than 65 should have no more than three drinks on any day and no more than seven drinks per week.

Based on their health and how alcohol affects them, some people may need to drink less or not at all. People who should abstain from alcohol completely include those who fall into these categories:

- Plan to drive a vehicle or operate machinery

- Are pregnant or trying to become pregnant

- Take medications that interact with alcohol

- Have a medical condition that alcohol can aggravate

Effects On The Brain

You're chatting with friends at a party and a waitress comes around with glasses of champagne. You drink one, then another, maybe even a few more. Before you realize it, you are laughing more loudly than usual and swaying as you walk. By the end of the evening, you are too slow to move out of the way of a waiter with a dessert tray and have trouble speaking clearly. The next morning, you wake up feeling dizzy and your head hurts. You may have a hard time remembering everything you did the night before.

These reactions illustrate how quickly and dramatically alcohol affects the brain. The brain is an intricate maze of connections that keeps our physical and psychological processes running smoothly. Disruption of any of these connections can affect how the brain works. Alcohol also can have longer-lasting consequences for the brain—changing the way it looks and works and resulting in a range of problems.

Most people do not realize how extensively alcohol can affect the brain. But recognizing these potential consequences will help you make better decisions about what amount of alcohol is appropriate for you.

Immediate Health Risks Associated With Alcohol Consumption

Excessive alcohol use has immediate effects that increase the risk of many harmful health conditions. These immediate effects are most often the result of binge drinking and include the following:

- Unintentional injuries, including traffic injuries, falls, drownings, burns, and unintentional firearm injuries.
- Violence, including intimate partner violence and child maltreatment. About 35% of victims report that offenders are under the influence of alcohol. Alcohol use is also associated with two out of three incidents of intimate partner violence. Studies have also shown that alcohol is a leading factor in child maltreatment and neglect cases, and is the most frequent substance abused among these parents.
- Risky sexual behaviors, including unprotected sex, sex with multiple partners, and increased risk of sexual assault. These behaviors can result in unintended pregnancy or sexually transmitted diseases.
- Miscarriage and stillbirth among pregnant women, and a combination of physical and mental birth defects among children that last throughout life.
- Alcohol poisoning, a medical emergency that results from high blood alcohol levels that suppress the central nervous system and can cause loss of consciousness, low blood pressure and body temperature, coma, respiratory depression, or death.

Source: Excerpted from "Alcohol Use and Health," Centers for Disease Control and Prevention (www.cdc.gov), October 28, 2011.

Inside The Brain

The brain's structure is complex. It includes multiple systems that interact to support all of your body's functions—from thinking to breathing to moving.

These multiple brain systems communicate with each other through about a trillion tiny nerve cells called neurons. Neurons in the brain translate information into electrical and chemical signals the brain can understand. They also send messages from the brain to the rest of the body.

Chemicals called neurotransmitters carry messages between the neurons. Neurotransmitters can be very powerful. Depending on the type and the amount of neurotransmitter, these chemicals can either intensify or minimize your body's responses, your feelings, and your mood. The brain works to balance the neurotransmitters that speed things up with the ones that slow things down to keep your body operating at the right pace.

Alcohol can slow the pace of communication between neurotransmitters in the brain.

Discovering The Brain Changes

There still is much we do not understand about how the brain works and how alcohol affects it. Researchers are constantly discovering more about how alcohol interrupts communication pathways in the brain and changes brain structure, and the resulting effects on behavior and functioning. A variety of research methods broaden our understanding in different ways:

Brain Imaging: Various imaging tools, including structural magnetic resonance imaging (MRI), functional magnetic resonance imaging (fMRI), diffusion tensor imaging (DTI), and positron emission tomography (PET), are used to create pictures of the brain. MRI and DTI create images of brain structure, or what the brain looks like. fMRI looks at brain function, or what the brain is doing. It can detect changes in brain activity. PET scans look at changes in neurotransmitter function. All of these imaging techniques are useful to track changes in the alcoholic brain. For example, they can show how an alcoholic brain changes immediately after drinking stops, and again after a long period of sobriety, to check for possible relapses.

Psychological Tests: Researchers also use psychological tests to evaluate how alcohol-related brain changes affect mental functioning. These tests demonstrate how alcohol affects emotions and personality, as well as how it compromises learning and memory skills.

Animal Studies: Testing the effect of alcohol on animals' brains helps researchers better understand how alcohol injures the human brain, and how abstinence can reverse this damage.

Defining The Brain Changes

Using brain imaging and psychological tests, researchers have identified the regions of the brain most vulnerable to alcohol's effects:

Cerebellum: This area controls motor coordination. Damage to the cerebellum results in a loss of balance and stumbling, and also may affect cognitive functions such as memory and emotional response.

Limbic System: This complex brain system monitors a variety of tasks including memory and emotion. Damage to this area impairs each of these functions.

Cerebral Cortex: Our abilities to think, plan, behave intelligently, and interact socially stem from this brain region. In addition, this area connects the brain to the rest of the nervous system. Changes and damage to this area impair the ability to solve problems, remember, and learn.

Alcohol Shrinks And Disturbs Brain Tissue

Heavy alcohol consumption—even on a single occasion—can throw the delicate balance of neurotransmitters off course. Alcohol can cause your neurotransmitters to relay information too slowly, so you feel extremely drowsy. Alcohol-related disruptions to the neurotransmitter balance also can trigger mood and behavioral changes, including depression, agitation, memory loss, and even seizures.

Long-term, heavy drinking causes alterations in the neurons, such as reductions in the size of brain cells. As a result of these and other changes, brain mass shrinks and the brain's inner cavity grows bigger. These changes may affect a wide range of abilities, including motor coordination; temperature regulation; sleep; mood; and various cognitive functions, including learning and memory.

One neurotransmitter particularly susceptible to even small amounts of alcohol is called glutamate. Among other things, glutamate affects memory. Researchers believe that alcohol interferes with glutamate action, and this may be what causes some people to temporarily "black out," or forget much of what happened during a night of heavy drinking.

Alcohol also causes an increased release of serotonin, another neurotransmitter, which helps regulate emotional expression, and endorphins, which are natural substances that may spark feelings of relaxation and euphoria as intoxication sets in. Researchers now understand that the brain tries to compensate for these disruptions. Neurotransmitters adapt to create balance in the brain despite the presence of alcohol. But making these adaptations can have negative results, including building alcohol tolerance, developing alcohol dependence, and experiencing alcohol withdrawal symptoms.

Factors That Make A Difference

Different people react differently to alcohol. That is because a variety of factors can influence your brain's response to alcohol. These factors include the following:

- **How Much And How Often You Drink:** The more you drink, the more vulnerable your brain is.

- **Your Genetic Background And Family History:** Certain ethnic populations can have stronger reactions to alcohol, and children of alcoholics are more likely to become alcoholics themselves.

- **Your Physical Health:** If you have liver or nutrition problems, the effects of alcohol will take longer to wear off.

Are Brain Problems Reversible?

Abstaining from alcohol over several months to a year may allow structural brain changes to partially correct. Abstinence also can help reverse negative effects on thinking skills, including problem-solving, memory, and attention.

Long-Term Health Risks Associated With Alcohol Consumption

Over time, excessive alcohol use can lead to the development of chronic diseases, neurological impairments and social problems. These include but are not limited to the following:

- Neurological problems, including dementia, stroke, and neuropathy.
- Cardiovascular problems, including myocardial infarction, cardiomyopathy, atrial fibrillation, and hypertension.
- Psychiatric problems, including depression, anxiety, and suicide.
- Social problems, including unemployment, lost productivity, and family problems.
- Cancer of the mouth, throat, esophagus, liver, colon, and breast. In general, the risk of cancer increases with increasing amounts of alcohol.
- Liver diseases, including alcoholic hepatitis and cirrhosis, which is among the 15 leading causes of all deaths in the United States.
- Among persons with hepatitis C virus, worsening of liver function and interference with medications used to treat this condition.
- Other gastrointestinal problems, including pancreatitis and gastritis.

Source: Excerpted from "Alcohol Use and Health," Centers for Disease Control and Prevention (www.cdc.gov), October 28, 2011.

Liver Damage That Affects The Brain

Not only does alcoholic liver disease affect liver function itself, it also damages the brain. The liver breaks down alcohol—and the toxins it releases. During this process, alcohol's by-products damage liver cells. These damaged liver cells no longer function as well as they should and allow too much of these toxic substances, ammonia and manganese in particular, to travel to the brain. These substances proceed to damage brain cells, causing a serious and potentially fatal brain disorder known as hepatic encephalopathy.

Hepatic encephalopathy causes a range of problems, from less severe to fatal. These problems can include sleep disturbances; mood and personality changes; anxiety; depression; shortened attention span; coordination problems, including asterixis, which results in hand shaking or flapping; coma; and death.

Doctors can help treat hepatic encephalopathy with compounds that lower blood ammonia concentrations and with devices that help remove harmful toxins from the blood. In some cases, people suffering from hepatic encephalopathy require a liver transplant, which generally helps improve brain function.

Fetal Alcohol Spectrum Disorders

Alcohol can affect the brain at any stage of development—even before birth. Fetal alcohol spectrum disorders are the full range of physical, learning, and behavioral problems, and other birth defects that result from prenatal alcohol exposure. The most serious of these disorders, fetal alcohol syndrome (FAS), is characterized by abnormal facial features and is usually associated with severe reductions in brain function and overall growth. FAS is the leading preventable birth defect associated with mental and behavioral impairment in the United States today. The brains of children with FAS are smaller than normal and contain fewer cells, including neurons. These deficiencies result in life-long learning and behavioral problems. Current research is investigating whether the brain function of children and adults with FAS can be improved with complex rehabilitative training, dietary supplements, or medications.

Effects On The Heart

Americans know how prevalent heart disease is—about one in 12 of us suffer from it. What we don't always recognize are the connections heart disease shares with alcohol. On the one hand, researchers have known for centuries that excessive alcohol consumption can damage the heart. Drinking a lot over a long period of time or drinking too much on a single occasion can put your heart—and your life—at risk. On the other hand, researchers now understand that drinking moderate amounts of alcohol can protect the hearts of some adults from the risks of coronary artery disease.

For adults, deciding how much, if any, alcohol is right can be complicated. To make the best decision, adults need to know the facts and then consult their health care providers.

Know The Function

Your cardiovascular system consists of your heart, blood vessels, and blood. This system works constantly—every second of your life—delivering oxygen and nutrients to your cells, and carrying away carbon dioxide and other unnecessary material.

Your heart drives this process. It is a muscle that contracts and relaxes over and over again, moving the blood along the necessary path. Your heart beats about 100,000 times each day, pumping the equivalent of 2,000 gallons of blood throughout your body.

The two sides, or chambers, of the heart receive blood and pump it back into the body. The right ventricle of the heart pumps blood into the lungs to exchange carbon dioxide from the cells for oxygen. The heart relaxes to allow this blood back into its left chamber. It then pumps the oxygen-rich blood to tissues and organs. Blood passing through the kidneys allows the body to get rid of waste products. Electrical signals keep the heart pumping continuously and at the appropriate rate to propel this routine.

Alcoholic Cardiomyopathy

Long-term heavy drinking weakens the heart muscle, causing a condition called alcoholic cardiomyopathy. A weakened heart droops and stretches and cannot contract effectively. As a result, it cannot pump enough blood to sufficiently nourish the organs. In some cases, this blood flow shortage causes severe damage to organs and tissues. Symptoms of cardiomyopathy include shortness of breath and other breathing difficulties, fatigue, swollen legs and feet, and irregular heartbeat. It can even lead to heart failure.

Arrhythmias

Binge drinking and long-term drinking can affect how quickly a heart beats. The heart depends on an internal pacemaker system to keep it pumping consistently and at the right speed. Alcohol disturbs this pacemaker system and causes the heart to beat too rapidly, or irregularly. These heart rate abnormalities are called arrhythmias. Two types of alcohol induced arrhythmias are atrial fibrillation and ventricular tachycardia:

Atrial Fibrillation: In this form of arrhythmia, the heart's upper, or atrial, chambers shudder weakly but do not contract. Blood can collect and even clot in these upper chambers. If a blood clot travels from the heart to the brain, a stroke can occur; if it travels to other organs such as the lungs, an embolism, or blood vessel blockage, occurs.

Ventricular Tachycardia: This form of arrhythmia occurs in the heart's lower (ventricular) chambers. Electrical signals travel throughout the heart's muscles, triggering contractions that keep blood flowing at the right pace. Alcohol-induced damage to heart muscle cells can cause these electrical impulses to circle through the ventricle too many times, causing too many contractions. The heart beats too quickly, and so does not fill up with enough blood between each beat. As a result, the rest of the body does not get enough blood. Ventricular tachycardia causes dizziness, lightheadedness, unconsciousness, cardiac arrest, and even sudden death. Drinking to excess on a particular occasion, especially when you generally don't drink, can trigger either of these irregularities. In these cases, the problem is nicknamed "holiday heart syndrome," because people who don't usually drink may consume too much alcohol at parties during the holiday season. Over the long-term, chronic drinking changes the course of electrical impulses that drive the heart's beating, which creates arrhythmia.

Strokes

A stroke occurs when blood cannot reach the brain. In about 80 percent of strokes, a blood clot prevents blood flow to the brain. These are called ischemic strokes. Sometimes, blood accumulates in the brain, or in the spaces surrounding it. This causes hemorrhagic strokes.

Both binge drinking and long-term heavy drinking can lead to strokes even in people without coronary heart disease. Recent studies show that people who binge drink are about 56 percent more likely than people who never binge drink to suffer an ischemic stroke over 10 years. Binge drinkers also are about 39 percent more likely to suffer any type of stroke than people who never binge drink.

In addition, alcohol exacerbates the problems that often lead to strokes, including hypertension, arrhythmias, and cardiomyopathy.

Hypertension

Chronic alcohol use, as well as binge drinking, can cause high blood pressure, or hypertension. Your blood pressure is a measurement of the pressure your heart creates as it beats, and the pressure inside your veins and arteries. Healthy blood vessels stretch like elastic as the heart pumps blood through them. Hypertension develops when the blood vessels stiffen, making them less flexible. Heavy alcohol consumption triggers the release of certain stress hormones that in turn constrict blood vessels. This elevates blood pressure. In addition, alcohol may affect the function of the muscles within the blood vessels, causing them to constrict and elevate blood pressure.

Cardiac Benefits Of Alcohol Consumption?

Research shows that healthy people who drink moderate amounts of alcohol may have a lower risk of developing coronary heart disease than nondrinkers. Moderate drinking is usually defined as no more than two drinks in a given day for adult men and one drink per day for adult women who are not pregnant or trying to conceive.

A variety of factors, including diet, genetics, high blood pressure, and age, can cause fat to build up in your arteries, resulting in coronary heart disease. An excess of fat narrows the coronary arteries, which are the blood vessels that supply blood directly to the heart. Clogged arteries reduce blood supply to the heart muscle, and make it easier for blood clots to form. Blood clots can lead to both heart attacks and strokes.

According to recent studies, drinking moderately can help protect adults from these conditions. Moderate drinking helps inhibit and reduce the build-up of fat in the arteries. It can raise the levels of HDL—high density lipoprotein, or "good" cholesterol—in the blood, which

---

Excessive Alcohol Use And Risks To Men's Health

Men are more likely than women to drink excessively. Excessive drinking is associated with significant increases in short-term risks to health and safety, and the risk increases as the amount of drinking increases. Men are also more likely than women to take other risks (for example, drive fast or without a safety belt), when combined with excessive drinking, further increasing their risk of injury or death.

Drinking Levels For Men

- Approximately 62% of adult men reported drinking alcohol in the last 30 days and were more likely to binge drink than women (47%) during the same time period.
- Men average about 12.5 binge drinking episodes per person per year, while women average about 2.7 binge drinking episodes per year.
- Most people who binge drink are not alcoholics or alcohol dependent.
- It is estimated that about 17% of men and about 8% of women will meet criteria for alcohol dependence at some point in their lives.

Injuries And Deaths As A Result Of Excessive Alcohol Use

- Men consistently have higher rates of alcohol-related deaths and hospitalizations than women.
- Among drivers in fatal motor-vehicle traffic crashes, men are almost twice as likely as women to have been intoxicated (a blood alcohol concentration of 0.08% or greater).

wards off heart disease. It can help guard against heart attack and stroke by preventing blood clots from forming and by dissolving blood clots that do develop. Drinking moderately also may help keep blood pressure levels in check.

These benefits may not apply to people with existing medical conditions, or who regularly take certain medications. In addition, researchers discourage people from beginning to drink just for the health benefits. Rather, you can use this research to help you spark a conversation with your medical professional about the best path for you.

Effects On The Liver

Liver disease is one of the leading causes of illness and death in the United States. More than two million Americans suffer from liver disease caused by alcohol. In general, liver disease strikes people who drink heavily over many years.

- Excessive alcohol consumption increases aggression and, as a result, can increase the risk of physically assaulting another person.
- Men are more likely than women to commit suicide and more likely to have been drinking prior to committing suicide.

Reproductive Health And Sexual Function

- Excessive alcohol use can interfere with testicular function and male hormone production resulting in impotence, infertility, and reduction of male secondary sex characteristics such as facial and chest hair.
- Excessive alcohol use is commonly involved in sexual assault. Impaired judgment caused by alcohol may worsen the tendency of some men to mistake a women's friendly behavior for sexual interest and misjudge their use of force. Also, alcohol use by men increases the chances of engaging in risky sexual activity including unprotected sex, sex with multiple partners, or sex with a partner at risk for sexually transmitted diseases.

Cancer

- Alcohol consumption increases the risk of cancer of the mouth, throat, esophagus, liver, and colon in men.

Source: From "Excessive Alcohol Use and Risks to Men's Health," Centers for Disease Control and Prevention (www.cdc.gov), June 20, 2010.

While many of us recognize that excessive alcohol consumption can lead to liver disease, we might not know why. Understanding the connections between alcohol and the liver can help you make smarter decisions about drinking and take better control of your health.

Know The Function

Your liver works hard to keep your body productive and healthy. It stores energy and nutrients. It generates proteins and enzymes your body uses to function and ward off disease. It also rids your body of substances that can be dangerous—including alcohol.

The liver breaks down most of the alcohol a person consumes. But the process of breaking alcohol down generates toxins even more harmful than alcohol itself. These by-products damage liver cells, promote inflammation, and weaken the body's natural defenses. Eventually, these problems can disrupt the body's metabolism and impair the function of other organs.

Because the liver plays such a vital role in alcohol detoxification, it is especially vulnerable to damage from excessive alcohol.

Know The Consequences

Heavy drinking—even for just a few days at a time—can cause fat to build up in the liver. This condition, called steatosis, or fatty liver, is the earliest stage of alcoholic liver disease and the most common alcohol-induced liver disorder. The excessive fat makes it more difficult for the liver to operate and leaves it open to developing dangerous inflammations, like alcoholic hepatitis.

For some, alcoholic hepatitis does not present obvious symptoms. For others, though, alcoholic hepatitis can cause fever, nausea, appetite loss, abdominal pain, and even mental confusion. As it increases in severity, alcoholic hepatitis dangerously enlarges the liver, and causes jaundice, excessive bleeding, and clotting difficulties.

Another liver condition associated with heavy drinking is fibrosis, which causes scar tissue to build up in the liver. Alcohol alters the chemicals in the liver needed to break down and remove this scar tissue. As a result, liver function suffers.

If you continue to drink, this excessive scar tissue builds up and creates a condition called cirrhosis, which is a slow deterioration of the liver. Cirrhosis prevents the liver from performing critical functions, including managing infections, removing harmful substances from the blood, and absorbing nutrients.

A variety of complications, including jaundice, insulin resistance and type 2 diabetes, and even liver cancer, can result as cirrhosis weakens liver function.

Risk factors ranging from genetics and gender, to alcohol accessibility, social customs around drinking, and even diet can affect a person's individual susceptibility to alcoholic liver disease. Statistics show that about one in five heavy drinkers will develop alcoholic hepatitis, while one in four will develop cirrhosis.

There's A Bright Side

The good news is that a variety of lifestyle changes can help treat alcoholic liver disease. The most critical lifestyle change is abstinence from alcohol. Quitting drinking will help prevent further injury to your liver. Cigarette smoking, obesity, and poor nutrition all contribute to alcoholic liver disease. It is important to stop smoking and improve your eating habits to keep liver disease in check. But when conditions like cirrhosis become severe, a liver transplant may be the primary treatment option.

Effects On The Pancreas

Each year, acute pancreatitis sends more than 200,000 Americans to the hospital. Many of those who suffer from pancreatic problems are also heavy drinkers. Habitual and excessive drinking damages the pancreas, and commonly causes pancreatitis.

Learning more about the links between alcohol and pancreatic problems can help you make better decisions to protect your health.

Know The Function

The pancreas plays an important role in food digestion and its conversion into fuel to power your body. It sends enzymes into the small intestine to digest carbohydrates, proteins, and fat. It also secretes insulin and glucagon, hormones that regulate the process of utilizing glucose, the body's main source of energy. Insulin and glucagon control glucose levels, which helps all cells use the energy glucose provides. Insulin also ensures that extra glucose gets stored away as either glycogen or fat.

When you drink, alcohol damages pancreatic cells and influences metabolic processes involving insulin. This process leaves the pancreas open to dangerous inflammations.

Know The Risks

A pancreas unaffected by alcohol sends enzymes out to the small intestine to metabolize food. Alcohol jumbles this process. It causes the pancreas to secrete its digestive juices internally, rather than sending the enzymes to the small intestine. These enzymes, as well as acetaldehyde—a substance produced from metabolizing, or breaking down the alcohol—are harmful to the pancreas. If you consume alcohol excessively over a long time, this continued process can cause inflammation, as well as swelling of tissues and blood vessels.

This inflammation is called pancreatitis, and it prevents the pancreas from working properly. Pancreatitis occurs as a sudden attack, called acute pancreatitis. As excessive drinking continues, the inflammation can become constant. This condition is known as chronic pancreatitis.

Pancreatitis is also a risk factor for the development of pancreatic cancer.

A heavy drinker may not be able to detect the build-up of pancreatic damage until the problems set off an attack. An acute pancreatic attack causes symptoms including abdominal pain, which may radiate up the back; nausea and vomiting; fever; rapid heart rate; diarrhea; and sweating.

Chronic pancreatitis causes these symptoms as well as severe abdominal pain, significant reduction in pancreatic function and digestion, and blood sugar problems. Chronic pancreatitis can slowly destroy the pancreas and lead to diabetes or even death.

While a single drinking binge will not automatically lead to pancreatitis, the risk of developing the disease increases as excessive drinking continues over time.

These risks apply to all heavy drinkers, but only about five percent of people with alcohol dependence develop pancreatitis. Some people are more susceptible to the disease than others, but researchers have not yet identified exactly what environmental and genetic factors play the biggest role.

Treatment Helps But Does Not Cure

Abstinence from alcohol can slow the progression of pancreatitis and reduce its painful symptoms. A low-fat diet also may help. It is also critical to guard against infections and to get supportive treatment. Treatment options, including enzyme-replacement therapy or insulin, can improve pancreatic function. In some cases, surgery is necessary to relieve pain, clear blockages, and reduce attacks.

The effects of alcoholic pancreatitis can be managed, but not easily reversed.

Cancer

Genetics, environment, and lifestyle habits can all heighten your risk of getting cancer. We can't do anything to change our genes, and we often can't do much to change our environment. But lifestyle habits are a different story.

Drinking too much alcohol is one lifestyle habit that can increase your risk of developing certain cancers. This does not mean that anyone who drinks too much will develop cancer. But numerous studies do show the more you drink, the more you increase your chances of developing certain types of cancer.

For example, a group of Italy-based scientists reviewed more than 200 studies examining alcohol's impact on cancer risk. The collective results of these studies clearly demonstrate that the more you drink, the higher your risk for developing a variety of cancers. The National Cancer Institute identifies alcohol as a risk factor for the following types of cancer:

- Mouth
- Esophagus
- Pharynx
- Larynx
- Liver
- Breast

At least seven out of ten people with mouth cancer drink heavily. Drinking five or more drinks per day can also increase your risk of developing other types of cancers, including colon or rectal cancer. In fact, summary estimates from the recent World Cancer Research Fund report indicate that women who drink five standard alcohol drinks each day have about 1.2 times the risk of developing colon or rectal cancer than women who do not drink at all.

People who drink are also more likely to smoke, and the combination increases the risk significantly. Smoking alone is a known risk factor for some cancers. But smoking and drinking together intensifies the cancer-causing properties of each substance. The overall effect poses an even greater risk.

The risk of throat and mouth cancers is especially high because alcohol and tobacco both come in direct contact with those areas. Overall, people who drink and smoke are 15 times more likely to develop cancers of the mouth and throat than nondrinkers and nonsmokers. In addition, recent studies estimate that alcohol and tobacco together are responsible for significant numbers of many different cancers:

- 80 percent of throat and mouth cancer in men
- 65 percent of throat and mouth cancer in women
- 80 percent of esophageal squamous cell carcinoma, a type of esophagus cancer
- 25 to 30 percent of all liver cancers

Women And Cancer

One recent, groundbreaking study followed the drinking habits of 1.2 million middle-aged women over seven years. The study found that alcohol increases women's chances of developing cancers of the breast, mouth, throat, rectum, liver, and esophagus. The researchers link alcohol to about 13 percent of these cancer cases.

In addition, the study concluded that cancer risk increases no matter how little or what kind of alcohol a woman drinks. Even one drink a day can raise risk, and it continues to rise with each additional drink. While men did not participate in this study, the researchers believe this risk is likely similar for men.

This study also attributes about 11 percent of all breast cancer cases to alcohol. That means that of the 250,000 breast cancer cases diagnosed in the United States in 2008, about 27,000 may stem from alcohol.

Know The Reasons

Scientists are still trying to figure out exactly how and why alcohol can promote cancer. There are a variety of possible explanations.

One explanation is that alcohol itself is not the primary trigger for cancer. We know that metabolizing, or breaking down, alcohol results in harmful toxins in the body. One of these toxins is called acetaldehyde. Acetaldehyde damages the genetic material in cells—and renders the cells incapable of repairing the damage. It also causes cells to grow too quickly, which makes conditions ripe for genetic changes and mistakes. Cancer can develop more easily in cells with damaged genetic material.

In addition, recent animal studies have shown that as cells try to break down alcohol, they cause the body to produce additional amounts of a protein called vascular endothelial growth factor (VEGF). VEGF promotes the growth of blood vessels and organ tissue. But, the flip side of having too much VEGF is that it allows blood vessels to grow in cancer cells that would die on their own. This allows the cancer cells to develop into tumors.

We also know that alcohol can damage the liver, causing cirrhosis. Cirrhosis results when too much scar tissue builds up within the liver and leaves it unable to perform its vital functions. One of the many complications that can result from cirrhosis is liver cancer.

Hormones may be the link between alcohol and breast cancer. Alcohol can increase the amounts of some hormones in the body, including estrogen. An excess of estrogen may lead to breast cancer.

Finally, genetics may play a role in preventing some heavy drinkers from developing cancer. A European research team examined 9,000 people with similar lifestyle habits to determine why some of them developed mouth and throat cancers, and some did not. Of the participants who were heavy drinkers, those who did not develop cancers had a particular genetic alteration that enabled them to break down alcohol about 100 times faster than in those without it. The study suggested that this gene is the reason why some people are less likely to develop cancer in response to heavy drinking.

There's A Bright Side

Fortunately, studies show that you can reduce your risk for cancer by drinking less. A recent Canadian report analyzed studies from 1966 through 2006 and concluded that risk reduction is possible, specifically for head and neck cancers. The study found that as people abstained from drinking, their risk for developing cancer plunged. After 20 years of abstinence, former drinkers had the same risk for head and neck cancers as people who never drank.

Effects On The Immune System

Germs and bacteria surround us everywhere. Luckily, our immune system is designed to protect our bodies from the scores of foreign substances that can make us sick. Drinking too much alcohol weakens the immune system, making your body a much easier target for disease. Understanding the effect alcohol can have on your immune system can inform the decisions you make about drinking alcohol.

Know The Facts

Your immune system is often compared to an army. This army defends your body from infection and disease. Your skin and the mucous that lines your respiratory and gastrointestinal tracts help block bacteria from entering or staying in your body. If foreign substances somehow make it through these barriers, your immune system kicks into gear with two defensive systems: innate and adaptive.

The innate system exists in your body before you are exposed to foreign substances like bacteria, viruses, fungi, or parasites. These substances, which are called antigens, can invade your body and make you sick. The components of the innate system include different kinds of cells and chemical messengers:

- **White Blood Cells:** White blood cells form your first line of defense against infection. They surround and swallow foreign bodies quickly.

Excessive Alcohol Use And Risks To Women's Health

Although men are more likely to drink alcohol and drink in larger amounts, gender differences in body structure and chemistry cause women to absorb more alcohol, and take longer to break it down and remove it from their bodies (to metabolize it). In other words, upon drinking equal amounts, women have higher alcohol levels in their blood than men, and the immediate effects occur more quickly and last longer. These differences also make women more vulnerable to alcohol's long-term effects on their health.

Reproductive Health

- National surveys show that about six out of every ten women of child-bearing age (aged 18–44 years) use alcohol, and slightly less than one-third of women who drink alcohol in this age group binge drink.

- In 2008, about 7.2% of pregnant women used alcohol.

- Excessive drinking may disrupt menstrual cycling and increase the risk of infertility, miscarriage, stillbirth, and premature delivery.

- Women who binge drink are more likely to have unprotected sex and multiple sex partners. These activities increase the risks of unintended pregnancy and sexually transmitted diseases.

Alcohol And Pregnancy

- Women who drink alcohol while pregnant increase their risk of having a baby with fetal alcohol spectrum disorders (FASD). The most severe form is fetal alcohol syndrome (FAS), which causes mental retardation and birth defects.

- FASD are completely preventable if a woman does not drink while pregnant or while she may become pregnant.

- Studies have shown that about one of 20 pregnant women drank excessively before finding out they were pregnant. No amount of alcohol is safe to drink during pregnancy. For

- **Natural Killer (NK) Cells:** Natural killers are special white blood cells that detect and destroy cells infected with cancer or viruses.

- **Cytokines:** White blood cells send out these chemical messengers directly to an infected site. Cytokines trigger inflammatory responses, like dilating blood vessels and increasing blood flow to the affected area. They also call on more white blood cells to swarm an infected area.

women who drink during pregnancy, stopping as soon as possible may lower the risk of having a child with physical, mental, or emotional problems.

- Research suggests that women who drink alcohol while pregnant are more likely to have a baby die from sudden infant death syndrome (SIDS). This risk substantially increases if a woman binge drinks during her first trimester of pregnancy.
- The risk of miscarriage is also increased if a woman drinks excessively during her first trimester of pregnancy.

Other Health Concerns

- **Liver Disease:** The risk of cirrhosis and other alcohol-related liver diseases is higher for women than for men.
- **Impact On The Brain:** Excessive drinking may result in memory loss and shrinkage of the brain. Research suggests that women are more vulnerable than men to the brain damaging effects of excessive alcohol use, and the damage tends to appear with shorter periods of excessive drinking for women than for men.
- **Impact On The Heart:** Studies have shown that women who drink excessively are at increased risk for damage to the heart muscle than men even for women drinking at lower levels.
- **Cancer:** Alcohol consumption increases the risk of cancer of the mouth, throat, esophagus, liver, colon, and breast among women. The risk of breast cancer increases as alcohol use increases.
- **Sexual Assault:** Binge drinking is a risk factor for sexual assault, especially among young women in college settings. Each year, about one in 20 college women are sexually assaulted. Research suggests that there is an increase in the risk of rape or sexual assault when both the attacker and victim have used alcohol prior to the attack.

Source: From "Excessive Alcohol Use and Risks to Women's Health," Centers for Disease Control and Prevention (www.cdc.gov), June 20, 2010.

The adaptive system kicks in after you are exposed to an infection for the first time. The next time you encounter the same infection, your adaptive system fights it off even faster and more efficiently than the first time. These are components of the adaptive system:

- **T-Lymphocyte Cells:** T-cells reinforce the work of white blood cells by targeting individual foreign substances. T-cells can identify and destroy a vast array of bacteria and viruses. They can also kill infected cells and secrete cytokines.

- **B-Lymphocyte Cells:** B-cells produce antibodies that fight off harmful substances by sticking to them and making them stand out to other immune cells.

- **Antibodies:** After B-cells encounter antigens, they produce antibodies. These are proteins that target specific antigens and then remember how to combat the antigen.

Know The Risks

Alcohol suppresses both the innate and the adaptive immune systems. Chronic alcohol use reduces the ability of white blood cells to effectively engulf and swallow harmful bacteria. Excessive drinking also disrupts the production of cytokines, causing your body to either produce too much or not enough of these chemical messengers. An abundance of cytokines can damage your tissues, whereas a lack of cytokines leaves you open to infection.

Chronic alcohol use also suppresses the development of T-cells and may impair the ability of NK cells to attack tumor cells. This reduced function makes you more vulnerable to bacteria and viruses and less capable of destroying cancerous cells.

With a compromised immune system, chronic drinkers are more liable to contract diseases like pneumonia and tuberculosis than people who do not drink too much. There is also data linking alcohol's damage to the immune system with an increased susceptibility to contracting infection with the human immunodeficiency virus. HIV develops faster in chronic drinkers who already have the virus.

Drinking a lot on a single occasion also can compromise your immune system. Drinking to intoxication can slow your body's ability to produce cytokines that ward off infections by causing inflammations. Without these inflammatory responses, your body's ability to defend itself against bacteria is significantly reduced. A recent study shows that slower inflammatory cytokine production can reduce your ability to fight off infections for up to 24 hours after getting drunk.

Still Looking For The Bright Side

At this point, scientists do not know whether abstinence, reduced drinking, or other measures will help reverse the effects of alcohol on the immune system. Nevertheless, it is important to keep in mind that avoiding drinking helps minimize the burden on your immune system, particularly if you are fighting a viral or bacterial infection.

Chapter 19

Blood Alcohol Concentration, Hangovers, And Memory Lapses

Blood Alcohol Concentration

Blood alcohol concentration (BAC) refers to the percentage of alcohol found in a person's blood.[1] Drinking alcohol at a rate that is faster than the body can process it will increase blood alcohol concentration. This amount influences a person's perceptions and emotions and the way the body and brain work.

Reading BAC And Legal Consequences

A BAC level can be discovered in a variety of different ways. Blood tests, urine analysis, and breath analysis (also known as Breathalyzer tests) can all be used to determine blood alcohol concentration. The most common of these tests, especially in cases of drunk driving, is breath analysis. Police who have pulled over an individual suspected of drunk driving administer this test because the results are shown almost immediately. Blood and urine tests cannot be accomplished by the roadside, and in the time it takes to get a sample, a person's BAC may change.[2]

Worldwide, most countries have established maximum legal BAC limits for drivers designed to deter people from driving while intoxicated. Some countries, such as Hungry and the Czech Republic, have a *zero-tolerance policy*, which means it is illegal to have any BAC level whatsoever. In the United States, the legal BAC level for a person over 21 is 0.08, but for those not yet of legal age it is illegal to drink any amount of alcohol. This means that a zero tolerance policy is applied for drivers under 21. If caught driving over the legal limit, offenders can have their driving licenses suspended or revoked. In some cases, cars will be equipped with a breath

---

About This Chapter: "Blood Alcohol Concentration, Hangovers, and Memory Lapses," by Zachary Klimecki, reviewed by David A. Cooke, M.D., F.A.C.P. December 2012. © 2013 Omnigraphics, Inc.

analysis device that will disable the ignition if the driver has had anything to drink. Offenders can also face heavy fines and jail time.[2,3]

Absorption Of Alcohol By The Body

When a person drinks an alcoholic beverage, most of it is pulled into the bloodstream from the small intestine and stomach. From there, alcohol travels to the liver where it is broken down and processed. The liver can only process so much at a time, so any excess alcohol circulates through the body until the liver has the ability to process the rest. It can take about one hour for the liver to process one alcoholic beverage.[4]

The amount of alcohol in the blood depends on how fast alcohol is emptied from the stomach and how much can be digested on the first pass through the stomach and liver. The rate at which alcohol is processed can vary depending on how often a person drinks, what they eat, how old they are, how much they weigh, whether they are male or female, and what time of day it is. Other factors can include how much alcohol a person drinks in a given time frame, if they have eaten recently or still have food in the stomach, and the type of alcoholic beverage they have consumed. Genetic factors can also influence how a person processes alcohol.[1]

Effects Of BAC

Measuring the amount of alcohol content in the blood can help determine the expected effects certain amounts of alcohol in a person's system can have on their brain and other organs. Table 19.1 lists the predicted effects of different BAC levels on body and brain function. Note that these values apply to people who do not have alcohol tolerance. People who are accustomed to regular, substantial alcohol intake may have fewer symptoms at a given level of intoxication that this table would suggest. It is not clear that habitual drinkers are better able to drive safely at higher alcohol levels, and the law does not make any distinctions.

Alcohol-Related Memory Lapses

A blackout can occur when the amount of alcohol in a person's system damages the ability to form new memories. Those who experience a blackout will have no recall or only partial knowledge of what happened while they were drinking. Binge drinking is commonly associated with blackouts. A person who has experienced an alcohol-related memory lapse may have engaged in risky behavior during the blackout, including unsafe sexual activity and getting into fights.[7]

Table 19.1. Effect on the Body and Mind at Different Blood Alcohol Concentration Levels.[5,6]

Blood Alcohol Concentration	Average Physical and Mental Effects
0.02	Change in mood Relaxation Slight body warmth Decline in visual function Decline in ability to multitask
0.05	Good feelings Exaggerated behavior Trouble focusing Lowered alertness Impaired judgment Reduced inhibition Reduced coordination
0.08	Poor muscle coordination Detecting danger becomes more difficult Short-term memory loss Impaired judgment, self-control, and reasoning Impaired concentration Impaired perception Reduced ability to process information
0.10	Slurred speech Slowed thinking Impaired reaction time Impaired reflexes Impaired vision
0.15	Far less muscle control than normal Mood swings Overexcitement Vomiting Major loss of balance
0.21–0.29	Stupor Severely impaired motor skills Loss of understanding Loss of consciousness Impaired sensations Blackouts
>0.30	Reduced bladder control Breathing trouble Slowed heart rate Unconsciousness Possible death

What Causes A Blackout?

Alcohol carried through the bloodstream to the brain impairs how the brain functions. Although blackouts usually happen after an individual has been drinking excessive amounts of alcohol, they are not necessarily related to how much a person drinks. They are more directly associated with a dramatic rise in blood alcohol concentration. Drinking on an empty stomach or chugging drinks, for example, can cause a rapid rise in BAC, which could make a person more prone to a blackout.

Alcohol affects the ability to transfer short-term memory to long-term memory while simultaneously impairing an individual's perception of incidents as they occur. Large quantities of alcohol can prevent specific parts of the brain from functioning normally, limiting the creation of new long-term memories. The hippocampus, the part of the brain largely responsible for creating memories, is particularly affected.

Dramatic and emotional events can be just as susceptible to memory loss as events that are boring and ordinary. Two primary types of alcohol-related memory lapses can occur, fragmentary blackouts and en bloc blackouts.[7]

En Bloc Blackouts

En bloc blackouts refer to situations when a person loses complete memory of the events that took place during a time of intoxication. This loss of memory persists even if the person is reminded of what happened. Individuals experiencing an en bloc blackout are able to retain some information in their short-term memory and may be able to engage in conversation or even relatively complicated tasks; however, they will forget events that just happened only minutes beforehand. En bloc blackouts are less common than fragmentary blackouts.[7]

Fragmentary Blackouts

Fragmentary blackouts describe when an individual can partially recall events that occurred while they were intoxicated, but not completely. Usually, people who experience a fragmentary blackout are unaware that they are missing any pieces of memory until someone else prompts them. When reminded, it is possible for the person to recover some of the memories they could not recall previously.[7]

Likelihood Of Experiencing A Blackout

The quantity of alcohol a person drinks and the rate at which their BAC rises have the most direct effect on the likelihood of a blackout.

Studies have also found that individuals who have experienced blackouts before are more likely to experience them again in the future when compared to those who do not have a history of blackouts. Researchers offer different theories to explain this observation. One theory suggests it is possible that someone who has consumed enough alcohol to blackout in the past is more susceptible to blackout in the future because the previous blackout damaged the brain in a way that makes the person more susceptible.[7] Another explanation is that some individuals are simply more vulnerable to blackouts. This can mean that certain people have a genetic disposition to getting blackouts.[8] Mothers who drink alcohol while pregnant may affect the way their children react to alcohol as adults. Individuals who were prenatally exposed to alcohol are associated with higher rates of alcohol-related problems, such as blackouts.[9]

Hangovers

The term *hangover* describes a variety of undesirable after-effects of drinking alcohol. Symptoms are typically experienced at the most increased levels of intensity when the blood alcohol concentration is reduced back to zero. Once they occur, the symptoms can persist for up to 24 hours.

The symptoms of a hangover are similar to mild alcohol withdrawal, although less intense and shorter in duration. Aside from causing bodily discomfort, research suggests that having a hangover does not necessarily impair a person's ability to perform simple or complex tasks. Common hangover symptoms include the following:

- Headache
- Muscle aches
- Fatigue
- Weakness
- Redness of the eyes
- Thirst
- Nausea
- Vomiting
- Stomach pain
- Decreased sleep
- Decreased REM

- Increased slow-wave sleep

- Dizziness

- Vertigo

- Sensitivity to light and sound

- Decreased attention and concentration

- Depression

- Anxiety

- Irritability

- Tremors

- Sweating

- Increased pulse and systolic blood pressure

Hangover Causes

Hangovers can be linked to several causes, such as the following:

- The effect of alcohol on the brain

- How the body metabolizes alcohol

- How organs react when exposed to alcohol

- Chemicals found inside an alcoholic beverage

- Behavior while drinking

- Personal character

Several other factors are proposed as contributors to hangover symptoms. These include an imbalance of bodily fluids, irritation of stomach and intestines, low blood sugar, sleep and body temperature disturbances, and alcohol withdrawal. Some factors can affect the symptoms experienced in a hangover but are not influenced by the alcohol itself. These include compounds other than alcohol in beverages, use of other drugs (especially nicotine), personality type, and a family history for alcoholism.

Treating And Preventing Hangovers

Many folk hangover cures have been proposed and sold throughout the years, but very few of them have been scientifically tested. Because of this, the effectiveness of any homebrew remedy or product marketed as a hangover cure is questionable. Non-steroidal anti-inflammatory medications, like Tylenol or Advil, can be used to relieve some of the symptoms associated with hangovers but must be used cautiously because they can further irritate the digestive system. In addition, the U.S. Food and Drug Administration reports that taking products containing acetaminophen (such a Tylenol) in conjunction with alcohol use increases the risk of serious liver injury.

It is never recommended to drink more alcohol in order to "cure" a hangover. Putting more alcohol into the body can potentially cause a worse hangover and lead to other alcohol-related problems in the long run. The most effective way to "cure" a hangover is to wait it out. Hangovers generally last about 8 to 24 hours.

Preventing a hangover from occurring in the first place is much more easily done. People who drink can help avoid hangovers by drinking in moderation, not getting intoxicated, and by paying attention to the total amount of alcohol they consume. Drinking alcohol with fewer impurities is also associated with fewer occurrences of hangovers. Although people who drink alcohol can take these measures to lessen the risk of experiencing a hangover, the only sure way to not get a hangover is by not drinking alcohol.[10] Additionally, people under the legal drinking age of 21 should avoid drinking alcohol irrespective of their perceived risk of hangover.

Notes

1. Zakhari, Samir Ph.D. Overview: How Is Alcohol Metabolized by the Body? *Alcohol Research & Health*. Vol. 29, No. 4. 2006. http://pubs.niaaa.nih.gov/publications/arh294/245-255.pdf

2. International Center for Alcohol Policies. "Module 16: Blood Alcohol Concentration Limits" in *ICAP Blue Book* (Washington: ICAP, 1995–2012). http://www.icap.org/policytools/icapbluebook/bluebookmodules/16bloodalcoholconcentrationlimits/tabid/176/default.aspx.

3. Highway Safety Research Center. Blood Alcohol Concentration (BAC) (Chapel Hill: University of North Carolina, nd) accessed October 2012, http://www.hsrc.unc.edu/safety_info/alcohol/blood_alcohol_concentration.cfm.

4. Centers for Disease Control and Prevention. Alcohol and Public Health, Frequently Asked Questions (Atlanta: CDC, October 15, 2012). http://www.cdc.gov/alcohol/faqs.htm#getDrunk.

5. Centers for Disease Control and Prevention. Effects of Blood Alcohol Concentration (BAC) (Atlanta: CDC, February 11, 2011). http://www.cdc.gov/Motorvehiclesafety/Impaired_Driving/bac.html.

6. Virginia Polytechnic Institute and State University. Alcohol's Effects (Blacksburg: Virginia Tech, 2012). http://www.alcohol.vt.edu/Students/alcoholEffects/index.htm.

7. White, Aaron M. What Happened? Alcohol, Memory Blackouts, and the Brain. *Alcohol Research & Health*. Vol. 27, No. 2. 2003. http://pubs.niaaa.nih.gov/publications/arh27-2/186-196.htm.

8. Nelson, Elliot C., et al. Genetic Epidemiology of Alcohol-Induced Blackouts. *Arch Gen Psychiatry*, Vol. 61. No. 3. 2004. doi:10.1001/archpsyc.61.3.257.

9. Baer, John S. PhD, et al. A 21-Year Longitudinal Analysis of the Effects of Prenatal Alcohol Exposure on Young Adult Drinking. *Arch Gen Psychiatry*, Vol. 60, No. 4. 2003. doi:10.1001/archpsyc.60.4.377.

10. Swift, Robert, et al. Alcohol Hangover: Mechanisms and Mediators. *Alcohol Research & Health*. Vol. 22, No. 1. 1998. http://pubs.niaaa.nih.gov/publications/arh22-1/54-60.pdf.

Chapter 20

Alcohol And The Liver

Understanding The Liver

Overview Of The Liver

Your liver is one of the largest and most important organs in your body. You only have one liver. It is the size of a football and weighs about three pounds in the average-size person. It is reddish-brown. Your liver is located on the right side of your abdomen behind your lower ribs, and your ribs help to protect your liver.

Your liver has many important jobs. One of the jobs that the liver does is to act as a "filter" for your body. The liver filters or detoxifies the blood.

Almost all the blood in your body passes through the liver. As blood passes through the liver, it breaks down substances, such as prescription or over-the-counter drugs, street drugs, alcohol, and caffeine.

Our bodies naturally produce some harmful (toxic) chemicals or poisons, and those are also broken down by the liver. In this way the liver acts as a filter to clean your blood.

The liver is also a "chemical factory." It performs more than 500 chemical functions in your body! The liver takes certain materials in your body and turns them into something else. For example, your liver turns proteins and sugars into things that your body needs. The liver

About This Chapter: This chapter begins with information from "Understanding the Liver: Entire Lesson," U.S. Department of Veterans Affairs (www.hepatitis.va.gov), July 3, 2012. Text under the heading "Questions and Answers about Cirrhosis" is excerpted from "What I Need to Know about Cirrhosis," National Institute of Diabetes and Digestive and Kidney Diseases (www.niddk.nih.gov), April 30, 2012.

produces blood-clotting factors that are needed to help you heal after an injury. It also stores vitamins, hormones, cholesterol, and minerals. Your liver lets go of these chemicals and nutrients when your body needs them, and they flow into your bloodstream.

The liver also produces a greenish fluid called bile. Tubes, called "bile ducts," connect the liver and another organ, the gallbladder, to the small intestine. The bile that is made by the liver helps to digest fats in the small intestine.

Here is a summary of the things the liver does:

- Filters your blood

- Makes proteins, including blood-clotting factors (needed to help you heal)

- Stores vitamins, sugars, fats, and other nutrients

- Helps regulate hormones

- Releases chemicals and nutrients into the body when needed

- Makes bile needed for digesting fats

- And much more

Important Definitions You Should Know

Advanced Liver Disease: Symptoms of advanced liver disease include: fatigue, difficulty concentrating, yellow jaundice, fluid in the abdomen, bleeding, and poor blood clotting.

Chronic Hepatitis C: Disease of the liver that remains throughout the course of the individual's life.

Cirrhosis: The end result of damage to the cells in the liver. Cirrhosis can be caused by many things, including viral hepatitis or alcohol, or both.

Fibrosis: Mild to moderate scarring of the liver.

Liver Biopsy: A procedure in which a small piece of liver is removed with a needle and examined to find out exactly how much liver damage is present. The biopsy is rated on a scale from 0 (normal liver) to 4 (cirrhosis).

Liver Cancer: A type of cancer, known as hepatocellular carcinoma, that develops in the liver as a result of viral hepatitis, cirrhosis, or alcohol.

Source: Excerpted from "Hepatitis C and Alcohol," U.S. Department of Veterans Affairs, available online at http://www .hepatitis.va.gov/pdf/alcohol-brochure.pdf; accessed June 25, 2012.

Liver Disease And Other Complications

Liver disease is caused by damage to the liver. Liver damage can be caused by many things, including viruses (such as the hepatitis viruses), drinking alcohol heavily, or being very overweight. Certain medications—for example, acetaminophen (Tylenol)—can cause severe liver damage in people who also have heavy alcohol use. In addition, exposure to industrial chemicals, including cleaning solvents, aerosolized paints, and paint thinners can damage the liver.

Liver damage can lead to livers that are swollen, shrunken, hard, or scarred. Such livers do not work well, and you can get very sick, or even die, if your liver stops working altogether.

Symptoms Of Acute Liver Disease

If something happens to the liver suddenly, it is *acute*. Some acute liver problems will cause symptoms suddenly as well. These are some of the symptoms of acute liver disease:

- Tiredness or weakness
- Jaundice (yellowing of the eyes and skin)
- Fever
- Nausea and vomiting
- Dark urine or very pale colored stools
- Pain under the ribs on the right side

Up to half of all people with acute liver disease have no symptoms at all. Some types of acute liver disease get better without treatment, and the liver heals itself entirely. On rare occasions an acute liver injury can require hospitalization and even liver transplant right away.

Symptoms Of Chronic Liver Disease

If something is continuing to affect the liver over time, after six months it is *chronic*. Many people with chronic liver problems will have no symptoms at all and may not even know they have a liver problem. Sometimes they develop symptoms only when the liver has been damaged for many years.

Hepatitis

The word *hepatitis* means inflammation or swelling of the liver. Many things can trigger this (for example, the hepatitis C virus). Medications, alcohol, and even some genetic diseases can cause inflammation. Genetic diseases are ones that are passed down from your biological parents.

Sometimes liver inflammation gets better on its own, but sometimes, as in the case of chronic hepatitis C, treatment with medications is required to stop the inflammation.

If you have hepatitis, you need to be very careful not to do things that might irritate your liver even more. Alcohol irritates the liver, even in someone who doesn't have any other liver problems.

To summarize: Hepatitis means inflammation of the liver. It can be caused by genetic diseases; medications (including over-the-counter drugs); alcohol; or viral hepatitis (such as hepatitis A, hepatitis B, and hepatitis C).

Fibrosis And Cirrhosis

Anything that damages the liver over many years can lead the liver to form scar tissue. Fibrosis is the first stage of liver scarring.

When scar tissue builds up and takes over most of the liver, this is a more serious problem called cirrhosis (pronounced "sir-o-sis"). Scar tissue cannot perform any of the jobs of normal liver cells, and this causes a person with cirrhosis to slowly become ill.

Not everyone with hepatitis or a chronic liver problem will develop cirrhosis. Cirrhosis does not happen overnight. In the early years of having cirrhosis, many people will have no obvious signs or be ill and many may not even be aware they have cirrhosis at all.

Cirrhosis can be caused by anything that damages the liver after years of irritation, not just alcohol. However, heavy alcohol use and having the hepatitis C virus for a long time (such as 20 to 30 years) increases your risk.

Over time, cirrhosis can lead a person to become ill. Symptoms can include fatigue, difficulty thinking clearly, fluid in the abdomen, bleeding in the intestines, and poor blood clotting. Anyone who has cirrhosis, with or without symptoms, needs very close medical attention.

Alcoholic Liver Disease

Alcoholic liver disease is a common form of liver disease in the United States. People get alcoholic liver disease by drinking large amounts of alcohol for many years. It doesn't matter whether the alcohol comes from hard liquor, beer, or wine. Any type of alcohol can cause liver damage.

One unit of an alcoholic beverage contains 10 grams of alcohol. A unit is roughly equivalent to one 12-ounce bottle of beer (5% alcohol); one 4-ounce glass of wine (12% alcohol); or one 1-ounce shot of hard liquor (40% alcohol).

So how much alcohol is too much? For people under age 21 any amount is too much. For adults, it depends on whether you're a man or a woman. Studies have shown that women experience liver disease at lower levels of alcohol intake than men.

Many liver specialists would agree that liver disease is likely at these levels:

- **For women:** Four or more units of alcohol daily for at least a year
- **For men:** Six or more units of alcohol daily for at least a year

Some people will experience liver damage even if they drink much less. The good news is that the livers of heavy drinkers can improve if they stop drinking entirely.

Fatty Liver

Fatty liver is the buildup of fat in liver cells. It is probably the most common type of liver disease in the United States. Fatty liver by itself rarely leads to severe liver damage.

Fatty liver can result from drinking too much alcohol. It can also happen in people who rarely drink. In this case, it is called "nonalcoholic fatty liver disease" or "nonalcoholic steato-hepatitis," or NASH. ("Steato-" means fat.) With NASH, a patient's liver shows some inflammation that in some cases can lead to liver damage and cirrhosis (scarring of the liver tissue).

It is not clear why fat builds up in the liver, but people are more likely to develop the condition if they have diabetes, are overweight, or have high levels of cholesterol or blood fats (called *triglycerides*). The amount of fat in the liver may decrease when overweight people lose weight, when diabetics have well-controlled blood sugars, and when cholesterol and triglyceride levels are lowered.

Liver Cancer

Like all other body organs, your liver can get cancer. Liver cancer is a disease in which some of the cells in your liver begin to reproduce faster than they should. This can lead to liver tumors, which are generally diagnosed by taking pictures of the liver with ultrasound, computerized tomography (CT) scan, or magnetic resonance imaging (MRI).

Having hepatitis B or hepatitis C can increase your chances of getting liver cancer, called hepatocellular carcinoma (HCC).

Most people with liver cancer do not have any symptoms from it early on. Those who do have symptoms often have some pain in the area of their liver (right side of the abdomen, under the ribs), or they may have a build-up of fluid in their abdomen (called *ascites*).

Liver cancer is very serious and can be deadly. If you find out that you have liver cancer, you need to get treated as soon as possible.

Other Liver Diseases

Some genetic disorders cause the liver to build up toxic substances. These include hemo-chromatosis (too much iron) and Wilson disease (too much copper). Other less common liver diseases include the following:

- Autoimmune hepatitis (the body attacks its own liver cells)
- Primary sclerosing cholangitis (the liver's large bile ducts become blocked, leading to infection, jaundice, and eventual cirrhosis)
- Primary biliary cirrhosis (liver's small bile ducts become inflamed and bile backs up, leading to itchy skin, jaundice, and eventual cirrhosis)

Liver Transplants

Liver transplants are considered only when a patient might die from liver disease. This is sometimes the case when a patient has liver cancer or when someone has advanced liver disease and the liver has stopped functioning properly. Being considered for a liver transplant does not mean that a patient is in danger of dying right away.

Liver transplantation is a long process that involves a lot of medical care. After a transplant, a patient needs lifelong drugs to keep the body from rejecting the new liver, and lifelong follow-up care from a specialist. Survival rates after a transplant are higher than 90% at one year, and patients usually have a good quality of life after their recovery.

Tests For Liver Damage

Most people with chronic liver disease will have no ongoing symptoms, and the damage will be detected only by blood tests. The tests (called a *liver panel*) measure these blood components:

- Your level of liver enzymes
- Your level of bilirubin (pronounced "billy-roo-bin"), which rises when the liver is not working well
- A protein called albumin (pronounced "al-byoo-min"), whose levels go down when the liver is damaged

Doctors can run more blood tests if they need to in order to find out what is causing the damage to your liver.

Ultrasound, CAT scans, and MRI are the three main methods of taking pictures of the liver. They can often show if the liver injury has become serious. A liver biopsy, in which a needle is used to take a sample of the liver itself, can tell even more about the liver's health.

Some people with liver problems can have a swollen liver. Others may have severe scarring or a shrunken liver. During an examination, a doctor can feel the liver to find out if it is shrunken, hard, or swollen.

Liver Enzymes

Enzymes are proteins found in your body that speed up certain chemical reactions. Liver enzymes perform these jobs within the liver. Two of the common ones are known as AST (aspartate aminotransferase) and ALT (alanine aminotransferase).

If the liver is damaged, AST and ALT pass into the bloodstream. When your doctor looks at the results from your blood tests, AST and ALT values are higher than normal if your liver is damaged.

The damage to the liver can come from viruses, such as the hepatitis C virus, over-the-counter drugs, and prescription and street drugs. If your doctor starts you on a certain medication, he or she may need to monitor your blood chemistries to make sure the medication is not causing further harm to your liver.

Test Results Summary

- A low level of liver enzymes in blood usually means the liver is healthy. However, a patient may have normal liver enzymes levels but still have liver damage.

- A higher than normal level of liver enzymes in blood can mean the liver is unhealthy. Patients also can have higher than normal liver enzyme levels related to problems in other organs, such as their bile ducts.

Reversing Liver Damage

The liver is one of the only organs in the body that is able to replace damaged tissue with new cells rather than scar tissue. For example, an overdose of acetaminophen (Tylenol) can destroy half of a person's liver cells in less than a week. Barring complications, the liver can repair itself completely and, within a month, the patient will show no signs of damage.

However, sometimes the liver gets overwhelmed and can't repair itself completely, especially if it's still under attack from a virus, drug, or alcohol. Scar tissue develops, which becomes difficult to reverse, and can lead to cirrhosis.

Keeping Your Liver Healthy

Here are some things to remember about keeping your liver healthy:

- Don't have unsafe sex (always use condoms).

- Don't inject drugs like heroin or cocaine.

- Don't drink alcohol. Alcohol is a poison to the liver and also can make liver diseases such as hepatitis much worse. Adults who do drink, should drink lightly.

- Don't share any personal items such as razors or toothbrushes that might have blood on them.

- Ask your doctor about getting vaccinated against hepatitis A and B. There is currently no vaccine against the hepatitis C virus.

- Follow strict food safety guidelines. Make sure that the water you drink and the food you eat are clean, especially when traveling to other countries. Most cases of infection with hepatitis A result from poor cleanliness during food preparation.

- If you take any medications, make sure your doctor knows about them. Also tell your doctor about any over-the-counter medicines, supplements, and natural or herbal remedies that you use. Certain medicines taken at the same time can cause damage to your liver, even if you can buy them without a prescription.

Alcohol, Hepatitis C, And Cirrhosis

Cirrhosis is severe scarring of the liver and is the end result of damage to liver cells. Cirrhosis can be caused by many things, including viral hepatitis or alcohol, or both.

How does alcohol affect cirrhosis?

Alcohol increases the damage done to the liver and speeds up the development of cirrhosis. Light drinkers or non-drinkers with hepatitis C (on average) have only moderate liver scarring, even up to 40 years after infection. Heavy drinkers—those who drink five or more drinks per day—develop scar tissue in their liver much more quickly. After about 25 years of hepatitis C infection, heavy drinkers show more than twice the scarring of light drinkers or non-drinkers. After 40 years of infection and heavy drinking, most heavy drinkers have developed cirrhosis.

What are the chances of getting cirrhosis?

In general, someone with hepatitis C has around a 20% chance of the fibrosis progressing all the way to development of cirrhosis. Alcohol use increases this chance severely. A heavy drinker with hepatitis C has 16 times the risk of cirrhosis that a non-drinker with hepatitis C has. Alcohol and hepatitis C both damage the liver, so together, the risk of serious liver damage (cirrhosis) is much higher than with either alone.

Source: "Alcohol and Cirrhosis," U.S. Department of Veterans Affairs (www.hepatitis.va.gov), July 3, 2012.

- Maintain a healthy body weight.

- Control blood sugars if you have diabetes.

- Keep cholesterol and blood fats within the recommended range. Ask your health care provider for advice on doing this.

Questions And Answers About Cirrhosis

What is cirrhosis?

Cirrhosis is scarring of the liver. Scar tissue forms because of injury or long-term disease. Scar tissue replaces healthy liver tissue and blocks the normal flow of blood through the liver. A healthy liver makes proteins, helps fight infections, cleans the blood, helps digest food, and stores a form of sugar that your body uses for energy.

Cirrhosis is scarring of the liver. A liver with too much scar tissue cannot work properly. You cannot live without a liver that works, but early treatment can control symptoms and keep cirrhosis from getting worse.

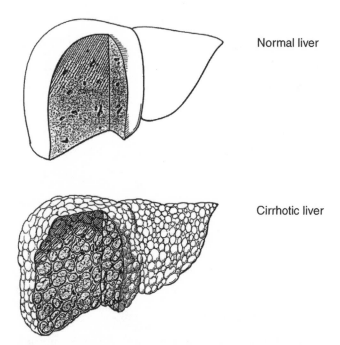

Normal liver

Cirrhotic liver

Figure 20.1. A liver with too much scar tissue cannot work properly (Source: NIDDK, 2012).

What causes cirrhosis?

Causes of cirrhosis include heavy alcohol use; some drugs, medicines, and harmful chemicals; infections; and chronic hepatitis B, C, or D—viral infections that attack the liver. Other causes include autoimmune hepatitis, which causes the body's immune system to destroy liver cells, nonalcoholic fatty liver disease, which is often caused by obesity, and diseases that damage or destroy bile ducts—tubes that carry bile from the liver.

Cirrhosis can sometimes be caused by certain inherited diseases—diseases that are passed from parent to child. These include hemochromatosis (a disease that causes iron to collect in the liver), Wilson disease (a condition that causes copper to build up in the liver), and porphyria (a disorder that affects the skin, bone marrow, and liver).

What are the symptoms of cirrhosis?

You may have no symptoms in the early stages of cirrhosis. As cirrhosis gets worse you may feel tired or weak; lose your appetite; feel sick to your stomach; lose weight; or notice red, spider-shaped blood vessels under your skin.

Cirrhosis can lead to other serious problems:

- You may bruise or bleed easily, or have nosebleeds.

- Bloating or swelling may occur as fluid builds up in your legs or abdomen—the area between your chest and hips. Fluid buildup in your legs is called edema; buildup in your abdomen is called ascites.

- Medicines, including those you can buy over the counter such as vitamins and herbal supplements, may have a stronger effect on you. Your liver does not break medicines down as quickly as a healthy liver would.

- Waste materials from food may build up in your blood or brain and cause confusion or difficulty thinking.

- Blood pressure may increase in the vein entering your liver, a condition called portal hypertension.

- Enlarged veins, called varices, may develop in your esophagus and stomach. Varices can bleed suddenly, causing you to throw up blood or pass blood in a bowel movement.

- Your kidneys may not work properly or may fail.

- Your skin and the whites of your eyes may turn yellow, a condition called jaundice.

- You may develop severe itching.

- You may develop gallstones.

- In the early stages, cirrhosis causes your liver to swell. Then, as more scar tissue replaces healthy tissue, your liver shrinks.

- A small number of people with cirrhosis also get liver cancer.

How is cirrhosis diagnosed?

Your doctor will examine you and may perform blood tests to see whether your liver is working properly or order imaging tests, which may show the size of your liver and show swelling or shrinkage. A liver biopsy, in which a doctor uses a needle to take a small piece of liver tissue to view with a microscope to look for scar tissue, may also be performed. In a liver biopsy, a doctor uses a needle to take a small piece of liver tissue to view with a microscope.

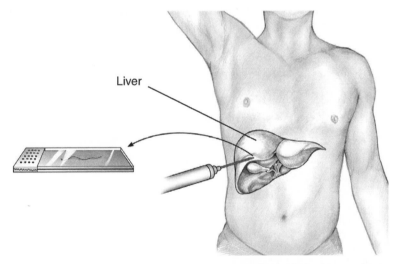

Liver

Figure 20.2. In a liver biopsy, a doctor uses a needle to take a small piece of liver tissue to view with a microscope (Source: NIDDK, 2012).

How is cirrhosis treated?

Once you have cirrhosis, nothing can make all the scar tissue go away. But treating the cause will keep cirrhosis from getting worse. For example, if cirrhosis is from heavy alcohol use, the treatment is to completely stop drinking alcohol. If cirrhosis is caused by hepatitis C, then the hepatitis C virus is treated with medicine.

159

Your doctor will suggest treatment based on the cause of your cirrhosis and your symptoms. Being diagnosed early and carefully following a treatment plan can help many people with cirrhosis. In the late stages of cirrhosis, certain treatments may not be effective. In that case, your doctor will work with you to prevent or manage the problems that cirrhosis can cause.

What if the cirrhosis treatment doesn't work?

If too much scar tissue forms, your liver could fail. Then you will need a liver transplant. A liver transplant can return you to good health.

How can I prevent cirrhosis if I already have liver disease?

To prevent cirrhosis, see your doctor for treatment of your liver disease. Many of the causes of cirrhosis are treatable. Early treatment may prevent cirrhosis.

Try to keep your weight in the normal range. Being overweight can make several liver diseases worse.

Do not drink any alcohol. Alcohol can harm liver cells. Drinking large amounts of alcohol over many years is one of the major causes of cirrhosis.

Do not use illegal drugs, which can increase your chances of getting hepatitis B or hepatitis C. See your doctor if you have hepatitis. Treatments for hepatitis B, C, and D are available. If you are on treatment, carefully follow your treatment directions. If you have autoimmune hepatitis, take your medicines and have regular checkups as recommended by your doctor or a liver specialist.

Points To Remember

- Cirrhosis is scarring of the liver. Scar tissue replaces healthy liver tissue.
- Some common causes of cirrhosis include heavy alcohol use, hepatitis infections, and nonalcoholic fatty liver disease.
- In the early stages of cirrhosis, you may have no symptoms. As the disease gets worse, cirrhosis can cause serious problems.
- Once you have cirrhosis, nothing can make all the scar tissue go away. But treatment can prevent cirrhosis from getting worse.
- If too much scar tissue forms and your liver fails, you will need a liver transplant.
- You can take steps to prevent cirrhosis or keep it from getting worse.

Source: NIDDK, 2012.

What can I do to keep cirrhosis from getting worse?

To keep cirrhosis from getting worse, do not drink any alcohol. Talk with your doctor before taking any medicines, including those you can buy over the counter such as vitamins and herbal supplements. Cirrhosis makes your liver sensitive to certain medicines.

Get vaccinated against hepatitis A and hepatitis B. Although hepatitis A does not cause cirrhosis, it can damage your liver.

Ask your doctor about getting a flu shot and being vaccinated against pneumonia.

Avoid eating raw oysters or other raw shellfish. Raw shellfish can have bacteria that cause severe infections in people with cirrhosis.

Chapter 21

Alcohol And The Pancreas

Heavy alcohol consumption can lead to a condition called pancreatitis.

What is pancreatitis?

Pancreatitis is inflammation of the pancreas. The pancreas is a large gland behind the stomach and close to the duodenum—the first part of the small intestine. The pancreas secretes digestive juices, or enzymes, into the duodenum through a tube called the pancreatic duct. Pancreatic enzymes join with bile—a liquid produced in the liver and stored in the gallbladder—to digest food. The pancreas also releases the hormones insulin and glucagon into the bloodstream. These hormones help the body regulate the glucose it takes from food for energy.

Normally, digestive enzymes secreted by the pancreas do not become active until they reach the small intestine. But when the pancreas is inflamed, the enzymes inside it attack and damage the tissues that produce them.

Pancreatitis can be acute or chronic. Either form is serious and can lead to complications. In severe cases, bleeding, infection, and permanent tissue damage may occur.

The gallbladder and the ducts that carry bile and other digestive enzymes from the liver, gallbladder, and pancreas to the small intestine are called the biliary system.

Both forms of pancreatitis occur more often in men than women.

About This Chapter: From "Pancreatitis," National institute of Diabetes and Digestive and Kidney Diseases (www .niddk.nih.gov), August 16, 2012.

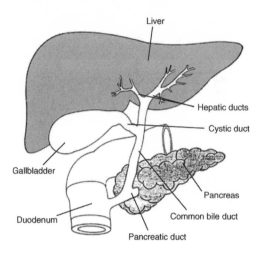

Figure 21.1. The gallbladder and the ducts that carry bile and other digestive enzymes from the liver, gallbladder, and pancreas to the small intestine are called the biliary system (Source: NIDDK, 2012).

What is acute pancreatitis?

Acute pancreatitis is inflammation of the pancreas that occurs suddenly and usually resolves in a few days with treatment. Acute pancreatitis can be a life-threatening illness with severe complications. Each year, about 210,000 people in the United States are admitted to the hospital with acute pancreatitis. The most common cause of acute pancreatitis is the presence of gallstones—small, pebble-like substances made of hardened bile—that cause inflammation in the pancreas as they pass through the common bile duct.

Chronic, heavy alcohol use is also a common cause. Acute pancreatitis can occur within hours or as long as two days after consuming alcohol. Other causes of acute pancreatitis include abdominal trauma, medications, infections, tumors, and genetic abnormalities of the pancreas.

Acute pancreatitis usually begins with gradual or sudden pain in the upper abdomen that sometimes extends through the back. The pain may be mild at first and feel worse after eating. But the pain is often severe and may become constant and last for several days. A person with acute pancreatitis usually looks and feels very ill and needs immediate medical attention. Other symptoms may include a swollen and tender abdomen, nausea and vomiting, fever, and a rapid pulse.

Severe acute pancreatitis may cause dehydration and low blood pressure. The heart, lungs, or kidneys can fail. If bleeding occurs in the pancreas, shock and even death may follow.

How is acute pancreatitis diagnosed?

While asking about a person's medical history and conducting a thorough physical examination, the doctor will order a blood test to assist in the diagnosis. During acute pancreatitis, the blood contains at least three times the normal amount of amylase and lipase, digestive enzymes formed in the pancreas. Changes may also occur in other body chemicals such as glucose, calcium, magnesium, sodium, potassium, and bicarbonate. After the person's condition improves, the levels usually return to normal.

Diagnosing acute pancreatitis is often difficult because of the deep location of the pancreas. The doctor will likely order one or more of the following tests:

Abdominal Ultrasound: Sound waves are sent toward the pancreas through a handheld device that a technician glides over the abdomen. The sound waves bounce off the pancreas, gallbladder, liver, and other organs, and their echoes make electrical impulses that create a picture—called a sonogram—on a video monitor. If gallstones are causing inflammation, the sound waves will also bounce off them, showing their location.

Computerized Tomography (CT) Scan: The CT scan is a noninvasive x ray that produces three-dimensional pictures of parts of the body. The person lies on a table that slides into a donut-shaped machine. The test may show gallstones and the extent of damage to the pancreas.

Endoscopic Ultrasound (EUS): After spraying a solution to numb the patient's throat, the doctor inserts an endoscope—a thin, flexible, lighted tube—down the throat, through the stomach, and into the small intestine. The doctor turns on an ultrasound attachment to the scope that produces sound waves to create visual images of the pancreas and bile ducts.

Magnetic Resonance Cholangiopancreatography (MRCP): MRCP uses magnetic resonance imaging, a noninvasive test that produces cross-section images of parts of the body. After being lightly sedated, the patient lies in a cylinder-like tube for the test. The technician injects dye into the patient's veins that helps show the pancreas, gallbladder, and pancreatic and bile ducts.

How is acute pancreatitis treated?

Treatment for acute pancreatitis requires a few days' stay in the hospital for intravenous (IV) fluids, antibiotics, and medication to relieve pain. The person cannot eat or drink so the pancreas can rest. If vomiting occurs, a tube may be placed through the nose and into the stomach to remove fluid and air.

Unless complications arise, acute pancreatitis usually resolves in a few days. In severe cases, the person may require nasogastric feeding—a special liquid given in a long, thin tube inserted through the nose and throat and into the stomach—for several weeks while the pancreas heals.

Before leaving the hospital, the person will be advised not to smoke, drink alcoholic beverages, or eat fatty meals. In some cases, the cause of the pancreatitis is clear, but in others, more tests are needed after the person is discharged and the pancreas is healed.

What is therapeutic endoscopic retrograde cholangiopancreatography (ERCP)?

ERCP is a specialized technique used to view the pancreas, gallbladder, and bile ducts and treat complications of acute and chronic pancreatitis—gallstones, narrowing or blockage of the pancreatic duct or bile ducts, leaks in the bile ducts, and pseudocysts—accumulations of fluid and tissue debris.

Soon after a person is admitted to the hospital with suspected narrowing of the pancreatic duct or bile ducts, a physician with specialized training performs ERCP.

After lightly sedating the patient and giving medication to numb the throat, the doctor inserts an endoscope—a long, flexible, lighted tube with a camera—through the mouth, throat, and stomach into the small intestine. The endoscope is connected to a computer and screen. The doctor guides the endoscope and injects a special dye into the pancreatic or bile ducts that helps the pancreas, gallbladder, and bile ducts appear on the screen while x rays are taken.

The following procedures can be performed using ERCP:

- **Sphincterotomy:** Using a small wire on the endoscope, the doctor finds the muscle that surrounds the pancreatic duct or bile ducts and makes a tiny cut to enlarge the duct opening. When a pseudocyst is present, the duct is drained.

- **Gallstone Removal:** The endoscope is used to remove pancreatic or bile duct stones with a tiny basket. Gallstone removal is sometimes performed along with a sphincterotomy.

- **Stent Placement:** Using the endoscope, the doctor places a tiny piece of plastic or metal that looks like a straw in a narrowed pancreatic or bile duct to keep it open.

- **Balloon Dilatation:** Some endoscopes have a small balloon that the doctor uses to dilate, or stretch, a narrowed pancreatic or bile duct. A temporary stent may be placed for a few months to keep the duct open.

People who undergo therapeutic ERCP are at slight risk for complications, including severe pancreatitis, infection, bowel perforation, or bleeding. Complications of ERCP are more common in people with acute or recurrent pancreatitis. A patient who experiences fever, trouble swallowing, or increased throat, chest, or abdominal pain after the procedure should notify a doctor immediately.

Gallstones that cause acute pancreatitis require surgical removal of the stones and the gall-bladder. If the pancreatitis is mild, gallbladder removal—called cholecystectomy—may proceed while the person is in the hospital. If the pancreatitis is severe, gallstones may be removed using therapeutic endoscopic retrograde cholangiopancreatography (ERCP)—a specialized technique used to view the pancreas, gallbladder, and bile ducts and treat complications of acute and chronic pancreatitis. Cholecystectomy is delayed for a month or more to allow for full recovery.

If an infection develops, ERCP or surgery may be needed to drain the infected area, also called an abscess. Exploratory surgery may also be necessary to find the source of any bleeding, to rule out conditions that resemble pancreatitis, or to remove severely damaged pancreatic tissue.

Pseudocysts—accumulations of fluid and tissue debris—that may develop in the pancreas can be drained using ERCP or EUS. If pseudocysts are left untreated, enzymes and toxins can enter the bloodstream and affect the heart, lungs, kidneys, or other organs.

Acute pancreatitis sometimes causes kidney failure. People with kidney failure need blood-cleansing treatments called dialysis or a kidney transplant.

In rare cases, acute pancreatitis can cause breathing problems. Hypoxia, a condition that occurs when body cells and tissues do not get enough oxygen, can develop. Doctors treat hypoxia by giving oxygen to the patient. Some people still experience lung failure—even with oxygen—and require a respirator for a while to help them breathe.

What is chronic pancreatitis?

Chronic pancreatitis is inflammation of the pancreas that does not heal or improve—it gets worse over time and leads to permanent damage. Chronic pancreatitis, like acute pancreatitis, occurs when digestive enzymes attack the pancreas and nearby tissues, causing episodes of pain. Chronic pancreatitis often develops in people who are between the ages of 30 and 40.

The most common cause of chronic pancreatitis is many years of heavy alcohol use. The chronic form of pancreatitis can be triggered by one acute attack that damages the pancreatic duct. The damaged duct causes the pancreas to become inflamed. Scar tissue develops and the pancreas is slowly destroyed.

Other causes of chronic pancreatitis are hereditary disorders of the pancreas; cystic fibrosis—the most common inherited disorder leading to chronic pancreatitis; hypercalcemia—high levels of calcium in the blood; hyperlipidemia or hypertriglyceridemia—high levels of blood fats; some medicines; and certain autoimmune conditions. Sometimes the cause is unknown.

Hereditary pancreatitis can present in a person younger than age 30, but it might not be diagnosed for several years. Episodes of abdominal pain and diarrhea lasting several days come and go over time and can progress to chronic pancreatitis. A diagnosis of hereditary pancreatitis is likely if the person has two or more family members with pancreatitis in more than one generation.

What are the symptoms of chronic pancreatitis?

Most people with chronic pancreatitis experience upper abdominal pain, although some people have no pain at all. The pain may spread to the back, feel worse when eating or drinking, and become constant and disabling. In some cases, abdominal pain goes away as the condition worsens, most likely because the pancreas is no longer making digestive enzymes. Other symptoms include nausea, vomiting, weight loss, diarrhea, and oily stools.

People with chronic pancreatitis often lose weight, even when their appetite and eating habits are normal. The weight loss occurs because the body does not secrete enough pancreatic enzymes to digest food, so nutrients are not absorbed normally. Poor digestion leads to malnutrition due to excretion of fat in the stool.

How is chronic pancreatitis diagnosed?

Chronic pancreatitis is often confused with acute pancreatitis because the symptoms are similar. As with acute pancreatitis, the doctor will conduct a thorough medical history and physical examination. Blood tests may help the doctor know if the pancreas is still making enough digestive enzymes, but sometimes these enzymes appear normal even though the person has chronic pancreatitis.

In more advanced stages of pancreatitis, when malabsorption and diabetes can occur, the doctor may order blood, urine, and stool tests to help diagnose chronic pancreatitis and monitor its progression.

After ordering x-rays of the abdomen, the doctor will conduct one or more of the tests used to diagnose acute pancreatitis—abdominal ultrasound, CT scan, EUS, and MRCP.

How is chronic pancreatitis treated?

Treatment for chronic pancreatitis may require hospitalization for pain management, IV hydration, and nutritional support. Nasogastric feedings may be necessary for several weeks if the person continues to lose weight.

When a normal diet is resumed, the doctor may prescribe synthetic pancreatic enzymes if the pancreas does not secrete enough of its own. The enzymes should be taken with every meal to help the person digest food and regain some weight. The next step is to plan a nutritious diet that is low in fat and includes small, frequent meals. A dietitian can assist in developing a meal plan. Drinking plenty of fluids and limiting caffeinated beverages is also important.

People with chronic pancreatitis are strongly advised not to smoke or consume alcoholic beverages, even if the pancreatitis is mild or in the early stages.

What complications may accompany chronic pancreatitis?

People with chronic pancreatitis who continue to consume large amounts of alcohol may develop sudden bouts of severe abdominal pain.

As with acute pancreatitis, ERCP is used to identify and treat complications associated with chronic pancreatitis such as gallstones, pseudocysts, and narrowing or obstruction of the ducts. Chronic pancreatitis also can lead to calcification of the pancreas, which means the pancreatic tissue hardens from deposits of insoluble calcium salts. Surgery may be necessary to remove part of the pancreas.

In cases involving persistent pain, surgery or other procedures are sometimes recommended to block the nerves in the abdominal area that cause pain.

Points To Remember

- Pancreatitis is inflammation of the pancreas, causing digestive enzymes to become active inside the pancreas and damage pancreatic tissue.
- Pancreatitis has two forms: acute and chronic.
- Common causes of pancreatitis are gallstones and heavy alcohol use.
- Sometimes the cause of pancreatitis cannot be found.
- Symptoms of acute pancreatitis include abdominal pain, nausea, vomiting, fever, and a rapid pulse.
- Treatment for acute pancreatitis includes intravenous (IV) fluids, antibiotics, and pain medications. Surgery is sometimes needed to treat complications.
- Acute pancreatitis can become chronic if pancreatic tissue is permanently destroyed and scarring develops.
- Symptoms of chronic pancreatitis include abdominal pain, nausea, vomiting, weight loss, diarrhea, and oily stools.
- Treatment for chronic pancreatitis may involve IV fluids; pain medication; a low-fat, nutritious diet; and enzyme supplements. Surgery may be necessary to remove part of the pancreas.

When pancreatic tissue is destroyed in chronic pancreatitis and the insulin-producing cells of the pancreas, called beta cells, have been damaged, diabetes may develop. People with a family history of diabetes are more likely to develop the disease. If diabetes occurs, insulin or other medicines are needed to keep blood glucose at normal levels. A health care provider works with the patient to develop a regimen of medication, diet, and frequent blood glucose monitoring.

How common is pancreatitis in children?

Chronic pancreatitis in children is rare. Trauma to the pancreas and hereditary pancreatitis are two known causes of childhood pancreatitis. Children with cystic fibrosis—a progressive and incurable lung disease—may be at risk of developing pancreatitis. But more often the cause of pancreatitis in children is unknown.

Chapter 22

Alcohol-Associated Brain Damage

There are few poisons that people take willingly, but alcohol has been popular for thousands of years. Some people report that mild alcohol poisoning (intoxication) can be enjoyable, but larger amounts permanently damage the brain and nervous system in a number of ways.

Fetal Alcohol Syndrome

Alcohol-related brain damage can start very early in life, even before birth. Fetal alcohol syndrome (FAS) is a collection of abnormalities seen in children born to women who drink alcohol during pregnancy. Signs of the condition are often apparent at birth, and may persist throughout life. FAS infants' faces are often abnormal, with oddly shaped eyes and lips, and relatively small heads. Heart defects and other physical abnormalities are also frequently present. Features vary from infant to infant, and not all may be present in all children with FAS.

Motor and intellectual development is usually delayed in children with FAS, and intelligence may be well below normal. There can be a wide range of severity, however, ranging from minimal to completely disabling. The degree of impairment tends to relate to the amount of alcohol consumed by the mother during pregnancy, but this isn't completely predictable.

It is not clear exactly how much alcohol is required to cause FAS, and this probably is not the same for all women. Timing is also probably important. Use during the first three months appears to be the most harmful.

Studies of women who have given birth to children with FAS provide some estimates, but a study to determine the minimum alcohol dose required to cause harm could never be

About This Chapter: The text in this chapter was written by David A. Cooke, MD, FACP. © 2013 Omnigraphics, Inc.

performed for ethical reasons. Because of this, most experts advise pregnant women to avoid alcohol completely.

Developmental Brain Damage

Alcohol use during childhood and adolescence also affects brain development. The brain grows rapidly during childhood and the teen years. It appears that the brain is particularly sensitive to damage from alcohol during these periods of life.

Heavy alcohol use at early ages reduces intelligence and IQ scores. Unfortunately, this is permanent, and does not improve even when alcohol is stopped.

Brain Atrophy

Prolonged alcohol use leads to shrinkage of the brain. Many studies comparing the brains of drinkers to nondrinkers by different methods have yielded the same results: drinkers' brains are smaller on CT and MRI imaging and weigh less at autopsy. Microscopic exams of brain samples show significant loss of nerve fibers, particularly in the brain regions involved in decision making. Heavier drinkers have more brain shrinkage and more severe nerve loss.

The long term effects of alcohol on brain size closely mirror impacts on brain function. Drinkers perform poorly on tests of intellectual performance compared to nondrinkers, and severity of impairment relates to the level of alcohol use. While it has not been proven that the brain shrinkage is the direct cause of poorer mental function, evidence strongly points to this relationship.

Newer imaging techniques such as functional MRI imaging show metabolic abnormalities in regions of drinkers' brains, which match the areas that atrophy over time. Interestingly, these abnormalities partially reverse in people who stop drinking. This suggests that some alcohol-related damage may be reversible, although other elements are clearly permanent.

In addition to effects on brain regions involved in memory, reasoning, and decision-making, alcohol damages the cerebellum, which has important functions in movement, balance, and coordination. These findings are not surprising to neurologists, who have long known that heavy drinkers may be unsteady and stagger, even when they haven't been drinking. Alcohol use can permanently impair balance.

Some researchers have commented that the brain changes seen in heavy drinkers look very much those that occur with aging. One theory of alcoholic brain damage is that it prematurely ages the brain, and this does fit with many scientific observations. If this is correct, heavy alcohol use can cause a 40 year old to have the brain of an 80 year old.

Wernicke-Korsakoff Syndrome

Wernicke encephalopathy and Korsakoff syndrome are two closely related brain conditions that are strongly associated with heavy alcohol use. They are often referred to as Wernicke-Korsakoff syndrome, because they have the same underlying cause, and features may overlap.

Wernicke-Korsakoff syndrome is mostly seen in alcoholics, but unlike other forms of alcoholic brain damage, alcohol is only an indirect cause. It develops when there is a critical deficiency in the brain of vitamin B1 (thiamine), which is common among alcoholics for multiple reasons. Some alcoholics substitute alcohol for food, particularly during binges, and may not get adequate thiamine in their diet. Alcohol directly reduces intestinal absorption of thiamine from food, and liver damage from alcohol reduces the body's ability to store the vitamin. Alcohol also interferes with nerve cells' ability to properly use thiamine. If brain thiamine levels drop low enough, Wernicke-Korsakoff syndrome develops.

It often presents initially with confusion, tremor, difficulty walking, and abnormal eye movements. This may lead to a wide, staggering gait and double vision. This phase is known as Wernicke encephalopathy. However, because many of the symptoms are similar to alcohol withdrawal, the diagnosis is often missed.

Without treatment, Wernicke encephalopathy usually leads to Korsakoff syndrome. Portions of the brain needed to create new memories collapse and die. People with Korsakoff syndrome develop severe, generalized amnesia, and cannot remember anything that happens after the disease's onset. Without memory of events more than a couple of minutes distant, they are often found out when they concoct elaborate and ridiculous stories from what they see around them.

If recognized and treated promptly, Wernicke-Korsakoff syndrome is treated with IV infusions of thiamine, and may be reversible. When heavy drinkers are admitted to the hospital, medical teams often administer IV thiamine as a precaution to prevent the condition. However, if not treated quickly enough, the brain impairments become permanent, and the affected person will never be able to live independently again.

Alcoholic Neuropathy

While many nerve cells are short, measured in micrometers, there are others that are extremely long. In a six foot tall person, single nerve cells may stretch over three feet from the spinal cord to the tips of the toes. Supporting cells this large is difficult, so the longest nerve cells in the body are most affected by toxins. Death of these cells is known as neuropathy.

The direct toxic effects of alcohol can kill long nerve fibers. Deficiencies in B vitamins that often accompany heavy alcohol use may add to the damage. The combination of alcoholic damage and vitamin deficiency may cause more severe neuropathy than either alone, especially if combined with other diseases that cause neuropathy such as diabetes.

Alcoholic neuropathy starts with loss of sensation in the toes. Initially, only the tips may be affected, but with continued use, the loss of feeling can extend upwards. In severe cases, someone with alcoholic peripheral neuropathy may be unable to feel anything below the knees. In advanced disease, neuropathy can also affect the fingers and hands, as they are also served by very long nerve fibers.

Alcoholic neuropathy can be more than just an inconvenience. Without pain sensation, a person can walk around with a shard of broken glass in their foot for days, without noticing until there is a severe infection. People with advanced neuropathy often end up needing toes amputated due to serious injuries, and sometimes they lose their feet.

Lack of sensation can also seriously interfere with walking. Without sensation in the feet, it is very difficult to maintain balance and avoid falling. People with bad alcoholic neuropathy may require walkers or wheelchairs to get about.

In some cases, alcohol neuropathy is quite painful. Some people simply notice numbness, but others feel constant burning or pains like electric shocks in the affected areas.

Other Toxic And Nutritional Neuropathies

While the conditions discussed above are the most commonly seen forms of alcohol-related brain and nerve injury, others are known to occur. Most are believed to be the result of the combined toxic effects of alcohol and nutritional deficiencies related to alcohol use. Sometimes, alcoholics will drink substances that have contaminants that greatly add to the damage.

Optic neuropathy is known to occur in some alcoholics. This involves damage to the nerve cells in the retinas, the light-sensing portions of the eye. Optic neuropathy can lead to varying degrees of visual impairment, and occasionally can cause complete blindness. This is most common with consumption of methanol (wood alcohol), but can occur with ordinary alcohol alone.

Summary

While the effects of alcohol intoxication resolve in a matter of hours, alcohol can have a variety of long-term effects on the brain and nervous system. Prolonged use can lead to a number of different kinds of brain and nerve damage. While risk of damage generally relates to level of alcohol use, it isn't completely predictable, and some people suffer serious harm from levels that don't cause problem for others. Stopping alcohol use can help reverse some kinds of alcoholic nerve damage, but many forms are permanent.

Chapter 23

Bone Health And Alcohol Use

Alcoholism And Recovery

According to the National Institute on Alcohol Abuse and Alcoholism (NIAAA), nearly 17.6 million Americans—or one in twelve adults—abuse alcohol or are alcoholic. Alcoholism is a disease characterized by a dependency on alcohol. Because alcohol affects almost every organ in the body, chronic heavy drinking is associated with many serious health problems, including pancreatitis, liver disease, heart disease, cancer, and osteoporosis.

Maintaining sobriety is undoubtedly the most important health goal for individuals recovering from alcoholism. However, attention to other aspects of health, including bone health, can help increase the likelihood of a healthy future, free from the devastating consequences of osteoporosis and fracture.

What Is Osteoporosis?

Osteoporosis is a condition in which bones become less dense and more likely to fracture. Fractures from osteoporosis can result in significant pain and disability. In the United States, more than 40 million people either already have osteoporosis or are at high risk due to low bone mass.

Risk factors for developing osteoporosis include thinness or small frame, being postmenopausal and particularly having had early menopause, abnormal absence of menstrual periods (amenorrhea), and prolonged use of certain medications, such as those used to treat lupus, asthma, thyroid deficiencies, and seizures. Other risk factors are low calcium intake, lack of physical activity, smoking, and excessive alcohol intake.

About This Chapter: "What People Recovering from Alcoholism Need to Know About Osteoporosis," National Institute of Arthritis and Musculoskeletal and Skin Diseases (www.niams.nih.gov), January 2012.

Osteoporosis often can be prevented. It is known as a silent disease because, if undetected, bone loss can progress for many years without symptoms until a fracture occurs. Osteoporosis has been called a childhood disease with old age consequences because building healthy bones in one's youth helps prevent osteoporosis and fractures later in life. However, it is never too late to adopt new habits for healthy bones.

The Link Between Alcohol And Osteoporosis

Alcohol negatively affects bone health for several reasons. To begin with, excessive alcohol interferes with the balance of calcium, an essential nutrient for healthy bones. It also increases parathyroid hormone levels, which in turn reduce the body's calcium reserves. Calcium balance is further disrupted by alcohol's ability to interfere with the production of vitamin D, a vitamin essential for calcium absorption.

In addition, chronic heavy drinking can cause hormone deficiencies in men and women. Men with alcoholism tend to produce less testosterone, a hormone linked to the production of osteoblasts (the cells that stimulate bone formation). In women, chronic alcohol exposure often produces irregular menstrual cycles, a factor that reduces estrogen levels, increasing the risk for osteoporosis. Also, cortisol levels tend to be elevated in people with alcoholism. Cortisol is known to decrease bone formation and increase bone breakdown.

Because of the effects of alcohol on balance and gait, people with alcoholism tend to fall more frequently than those without the disorder. Heavy alcohol consumption has been linked to an increase in the risk of fracture, including the most serious kind—hip fracture. Vertebral fractures are also more common in those who abuse alcohol.

Alcohol, Osteoporosis, And Men

There is a wealth of evidence that alcohol abuse may decrease bone density and lead to an increase in fractures. Low bone mass is common in men who seek medical help for alcohol abuse.

In cases where bone loss is linked to alcohol abuse, the first goal of treatment is to help the patient stop, or at least reduce, his consumption of alcohol. More research is needed to determine whether bone lost to alcohol abuse will rebuild once drinking stops, or even whether further damage will be prevented. It is clear, though, that alcohol abuse causes many other health and social problems, so quitting is ideal. A treatment plan may also include a balanced diet with lots of calcium- and vitamin D-rich foods, a program of physical exercise, and smoking cessation.

Source: Excerpted from "Osteoporosis in Men," National Institute of Arthritis and Musculoskeletal and Skin Diseases (www.niams.nih.gov), January 2012.

Osteoporosis Management Strategies

The most effective strategy for alcohol-induced bone loss is abstinence. People with alcoholism who abstain from drinking tend to have a rapid recovery of osteoblastic (bone-building) activity. Some studies have even found that lost bone can be partially restored when alcohol abuse ends.

Nutrition: Because of the negative nutritional effects of chronic alcohol use, people recovering from alcoholism should make healthy nutritional habits a top priority. As far as bone health is concerned, a well-balanced diet rich in calcium and vitamin D is critical. Good sources of calcium include low-fat dairy products; dark green, leafy vegetables; and calcium-fortified foods and beverages. Supplements can help ensure that you get adequate amounts of calcium each day, especially in people with a proven milk allergy. The Institute of Medicine recommends a daily calcium intake of 1,000 mg (milligrams) for men and women up to age 50. Women over age 50 and men over age 70 should increase their intake to 1,200 mg daily.

Vitamin D plays an important role in calcium absorption and bone health. Food sources of vitamin D include egg yolks, saltwater fish, and liver. Many people, especially those who are older or housebound, may need vitamin D supplements to achieve the recommended intake of 600 to 800 IU (International Units) each day.

Exercise: Like muscle, bone is living tissue that responds to exercise by becoming stronger. The best exercise for your bones is weight-bearing exercise that forces you to work against gravity. Some examples include walking, climbing stairs, weight training, and dancing. Regular exercise, such as walking, may help prevent bone loss and will provide many other health benefits.

Healthy Lifestyle: Smoking is bad for bones as well as the heart and lungs. Women who smoke tend to go through menopause earlier, resulting in earlier reduction in levels of the bone-preserving hormone estrogen and triggering earlier bone loss. In addition, smokers may absorb less calcium from their diets. Studies suggest that in people recovering from alcoholism, smoking cessation may actually enhance abstinence from drinking. Many suspect that smokers who abuse alcohol tend to be more dependent on nicotine than those who don't; therefore, a formal smoking cessation program may be a worthwhile investment for individuals in recovery. Alcohol also can have a negative effect on bone health. Those who drink heavily are more prone to bone loss and fracture, because of both poor nutrition and increased risk of falling.

Bone Density Test: A bone mineral density (BMD) test measures bone density in various parts of the body. This safe and painless test can detect osteoporosis before a fracture occurs and can predict one's chances of fracturing in the future. The BMD test can help determine whether medication should be considered. Individuals in recovery are encouraged to talk to their health care providers about whether they might be candidates for a BMD test.

Medication: Several medications are available for the prevention and/or treatment of osteoporosis, including: bisphosphonates; estrogen agonists/antagonists (also called selective estrogen receptor modulators or SERMS); calcitonin; parathyroid hormone; estrogen therapy; hormone therapy; and a recently approved RANK ligand (RANKL) inhibitor.

Chapter 24

Alcohol Use And Cancer Risk

Alcohol Consumption And Cancer

Drinking alcohol increases the risk of cancers of the mouth, esophagus, pharynx, larynx, and liver in men and women, and of breast cancer in women. In general, these risks increase after about one daily drink for women and two daily drinks for men. (A drink is defined as 12 ounces of regular beer, 5 ounces of wine, or 1.5 ounces of 80-proof liquor.)

The chances of getting liver cancer increase markedly with five or more drinks per day. Heavy alcohol use may also increase the risk of colorectal cancer and leads to greater increases in risk for most of the alcohol-related cancers. The earlier long-term, heavy alcohol use begins, the greater the cancer risk. Also, using alcohol with tobacco is riskier than using either one alone because it further increases the chances of getting cancers of the mouth, throat, and esophagus.

Some studies suggest that alcohol consumption is associated with a lower risk of some non-cancer health conditions. However, it is not recommended that anyone begin drinking or drink more frequently on the basis of health considerations.

About This Chapter: This chapter includes excerpts from the following documents produced by the National Cancer Institute (NCI; www.cancer.gov): "Cancer Trends Progress Report: Alcohol Consumption," June 20, 2012; "Fact Sheet: Head and Neck Cancers," April 17, 2012; "What You Need to Know about Breast Cancer," October 15, 2009; and "What You Need to Know about Liver Cancer," April 29, 2009. The chapter concludes with excerpts from "Other Ways to Reduce Cancer Risk," Centers for Disease Control and Prevention (www.cdc.gov), February 7, 2012.

Cancer Cells

Cancer begins in cells, the building blocks that make up tissues. Tissues make up the organs of the body, the breasts, and other parts of the body.

Normal cells grow and divide to form new cells as the body needs them. When normal cells grow old or get damaged, they die, and new cells take their place.

Sometimes, this process goes wrong. New cells form when the body doesn't need them, and old or damaged cells don't die as they should. The buildup of extra cells often forms a mass of tissue called a lump, nodule, growth, or tumor.

Source: NCI, April 29, 2009 and October 15, 2009.

Head And Neck Cancers

Cancers that are known collectively as head and neck cancers usually begin in the squamous cells that line the moist, mucosal surfaces inside the head and neck (for example, inside the mouth, the nose, and the throat). These squamous cell cancers are often referred to as squamous cell carcinomas of the head and neck. Head and neck cancers can also begin in the salivary glands, but salivary gland cancers are relatively uncommon. Salivary glands contain many different types of cells that can become cancerous, so there are many different types of salivary gland cancer.

Cancers of the head and neck are further categorized by the area of the head or neck in which they begin. Cancers of the brain, the eye, the esophagus, and the thyroid gland, as well as those of the scalp, skin, muscles, and bones of the head and neck, are not usually classified as head and neck cancers.

Oral Cavity Cancer

The oral cavity includes the lips, the front two-thirds of the tongue, the gums, the lining inside the cheeks and lips, the floor (bottom) of the mouth under the tongue, the hard palate (bony top of the mouth), and the small area of the gum behind the wisdom teeth. Symptoms of oral cavity cancer include a white or red patch on the gums, the tongue, or the lining of the mouth; a swelling of the jaw that causes dentures to fit poorly or become uncomfortable; and unusual bleeding or pain in the mouth.

The following risk factors have been identified for oral cavity cancer:

- The use of alcohol or tobacco is an important risk factor.

- Poor oral hygiene and missing teeth may be weak risk factors for cancers of the oral cavity.

- Use of mouthwash that has a high alcohol content is a possible, but not proven, risk factor.

- Immigrants from Southeast Asia who use paan (betel quid) in the mouth should be aware that this habit has been strongly associated with an increased risk of oral cancer.

- Consumption of mate, a tea-like beverage habitually consumed by South Americans, has been associated with an increased risk of cancers of the mouth, the throat, the esophagus, and the larynx.

Pharyngeal Cancer

The pharynx is a hollow tube about five inches long that starts behind the nose and leads to the esophagus. It has three parts:

- **Nasopharynx:** The upper part of the pharynx, behind the nose.

- **Oropharynx:** The middle part of the pharynx, including the soft palate (the back of the mouth), the base of the tongue, and the tonsils.

- **Hypopharynx:** The lower part of the pharynx.

Symptoms of pharyngeal cancer include trouble breathing or speaking; pain when swallowing; pain in the neck or the throat that does not go away; frequent headaches, pain, or ringing in the ears; or trouble hearing.

The use of alcohol or tobacco is a risk factor for pharyngeal cancer. Asian ancestry, particularly Chinese, is a risk factor for nasopharyngeal cancer, along with Epstein-Barr virus infection, occupational exposure to wood dust, and consumption of certain preserved or salted foods during childhood. Human papillomavirus (HPV) infection is also known to cause oropharyngeal cancer.

Laryngeal Cancer

The larynx, also called the *voice box*, is a short passageway formed by cartilage just below the pharynx in the neck. The larynx contains the vocal cords. It also has a small piece of tissue, called the epiglottis, which moves to cover the larynx to prevent food from entering the air passages. The symptoms of laryngeal cancer include pain when swallowing or ear pain.

The use of alcohol or tobacco is a risk factor for laryngeal cancer. Certain industrial exposures, including exposures to asbestos and synthetic fibers, have been associated with cancer of the larynx, but the increase in risk remains controversial. People working in certain jobs in the construction, metal, textile, ceramic, logging, and food industries may have an increased risk of cancer of the larynx. The consumption of mate, has also been associated with an increased risk of cancer of the larynx.

Causes Of Head And Neck Cancers

The most important risk factors for head and neck cancers are alcohol and tobacco use (including use of smokeless tobacco, sometimes called *chewing tobacco* or *snuff*). These risk factors are particularly important for cancers of the oral cavity, oropharynx, hypopharynx, and larynx. At least 75 percent of head and neck cancers are caused by tobacco and alcohol use. People who use both tobacco and alcohol are at greater risk of developing these cancers than

---

Alcohol-Induced Flush Warns Of Esophageal Cancer Risk

Asian flush, a response to alcoholic beverages caused by a buildup of acetaldehyde, is most often seen in Japanese, Chinese, and Koreans who are unable to metabolize alcohol effectively. It is also strongly associated with risk for esophageal cancer: People who turn red after drinking have a dramatically higher risk of developing the disease than those who don't flush.

In the March 2009 issue of *PLoS Medicine*, study authors Dr. Philip Brooks of the National Institute on Alcohol Abuse and Alcoholism, and his collaborators at Duke University and the National Hospital Organization Kurihama Alcoholism Center in Japan wrote that because flushing is easily apparent and also strongly linked with cancer risk, it should be a routine cancer screening factor in primary care settings.

They noted that 36 percent of East Asians, or approximately 540 million people worldwide, carry a defective copy of the gene for aldehyde dehydrogenase 2 (ALDH2), the enzyme that helps break down acetaldehyde, a product of ethanol metabolism, into acetate. Acetaldehyde is strongly carcinogenic, the authors explained.

People who carry two defective copies of the ALDH2 gene are usually unable to drink significant amounts of alcohol due to the severity of their reaction. However, those who have only one defective copy of the gene can develop tolerance, and prospective studies have shown that the risk for developing cancers in the upper aerodigestive tract is approximately 12 times higher in these individuals. Furthermore, because acetaldehyde lingers in saliva, particularly in those who smoke, they are at an even greater risk for cancer.

Pointing out other social trends that pose increased risk among this population, the authors wrote, "Clinicians need to be aware of the risk of esophageal cancer from alcohol consumption in their ALDH2-deficient patients…[and should] determine whether an individual of East Asian descent is ALDH2 deficient simply by asking whether they have experienced the alcohol flushing response."

Source: "Alcohol-induced Flush Warns of Esophageal Cancer, Risk," *NCI Cancer Bulletin*, Vol. 6, No. 7, April 7, 2009.

people who use either tobacco or alcohol alone. Tobacco and alcohol use are not risk factors for salivary gland cancers.

Infection with human papillomavirus (HPV) is a risk factor for some types of head and neck cancers, particularly oropharyngeal cancer that involves the tonsils or the base of the tongue. In the United States, the incidence of oropharyngeal cancers caused by HPV infection is increasing, while the incidence of oropharyngeal cancers related to other causes is falling.

Signs And Symptoms Of Head And Neck Cancers

The signs and symptoms of head and neck cancers may include a lump or a sore that does not heal, a sore throat that does not go away, difficulty in swallowing, and a change or hoarseness in the voice. These symptoms may also be caused by other, less serious conditions. It is important to check with a doctor or dentist about any of these symptoms.

Breast Cancer

Inside a woman's breast are 15 to 20 sections called lobes. Each lobe is made of many smaller sections called lobules. Lobules have groups of tiny glands that can make milk. After a baby is born, a woman's breast milk flows from the lobules through thin tubes called ducts to the nipple. Fat and fibrous tissue fill the spaces between the lobules and ducts.

The breasts also contain lymph vessels. These vessels are connected to small, round masses of tissue called lymph nodes. Groups of lymph nodes are near the breast in the underarm (axilla), above the collarbone, and in the chest behind the breastbone.

Benign And Malignant Breast Tumors

Tumors in the breast can be benign (not cancer) or malignant (cancer). Benign tumors are not as harmful as malignant tumors. Benign tumors are rarely a threat to life. They can be removed and usually don't grow back. They don't invade the tissues around them and don't spread to other parts of the body.

Malignant tumors, on the other hand, may be a threat to life. They often can be removed, but sometimes they grow back. They can invade and damage nearby organs and tissues (such as the chest wall) and can spread to other parts of the body.

Breast cancer cells can spread by breaking away from the original tumor. They enter blood vessels or lymph vessels, which branch into all the tissues of the body. The cancer cells may be found in lymph nodes near the breast. The cancer cells may attach to other tissues and grow to form new tumors that may damage those tissues. The spread of cancer is called metastasis.

Alcohol Consumption And Breast Disease

A team from Brigham and Women's Hospital and Harvard Medical School in Boston, and Washington University School of Medicine in St. Louis investigated childhood and adolescent risk factors for benign breast disease among girls with a family history of breast cancer. Benign breast disease, a large class of breast ailments that can cause breast lumps or breast pain, is a known risk factor for breast cancer. The authors found that among adolescent girls with a family history of breast cancer (or maternal benign breast disease), there was a significant association between amount of alcohol consumed and further increased risk of getting benign breast disease as young women.

Source: "Team from Harvard and Wash U. Studies Adolescent Alcohol Consumption and Breast Cancer," National Cancer Institute (www.cancer.gov), November 14, 2011.

Breast Cancer Risk Factors

No one knows the exact causes of breast cancer. Doctors seldom know why one woman develops breast cancer and another doesn't. Doctors do know that bumping, bruising, or touching the breast does not cause cancer. And breast cancer is not contagious. You can't catch it from another person.

Doctors also know that women with certain risk factors are more likely than others to develop breast cancer. A risk factor is something that may increase the chance of getting a disease.

Some risk factors (such as drinking alcohol) can be avoided. But most risk factors (such as having a family history of breast cancer) can't be avoided. Studies have found the following risk factors for breast cancer:

- **Age:** The chance of getting breast cancer increases as you get older. Most women are over 60 years old when they are diagnosed.

- **Personal Health History:** Having breast cancer in one breast increases your risk of getting cancer in your other breast. Also, having certain types of abnormal breast cells (atypical hyperplasia, lobular carcinoma in situ [LCIS], or ductal carcinoma in situ [DCIS]) increases the risk of invasive breast cancer. These conditions are found with a breast biopsy.

- **Family Health History:** Your risk of breast cancer is higher if your mother, father, sister, or daughter had breast cancer. The risk is even higher if your family member had breast cancer before age 50. Having other relatives (in either your mother's or father's family) with breast cancer or ovarian cancer may also increase your risk.

- **Certain Genome Changes:** Changes in certain genes, such as BRCA1 or BRCA2, substantially increase the risk of breast cancer. Tests can sometimes show the presence of these rare, specific gene changes in families with many women who have had breast cancer, and health care providers may suggest ways to try to reduce the risk of breast cancer or to improve the detection of this disease in women who have these genetic changes. Also, researchers have found specific regions on certain chromosomes that are linked to the risk of breast cancer. If a woman has a genetic change in one or more of these regions, the risk of breast cancer may be slightly increased. The risk increases with the number of genetic changes that are found. Although these genetic changes are more common among women than BRCA1 or BRCA2, the risk of breast cancer is far lower.

- **Radiation Therapy To The Chest:** Women who had radiation therapy to the chest (including the breasts) before age 30 are at an increased risk of breast cancer. This includes women treated with radiation for Hodgkin lymphoma. Studies show that the younger a woman was when she received radiation treatment, the higher her risk of breast cancer later in life.

- **Reproductive And Menstrual History:** The older a woman is when she has her first child, the greater her chance of breast cancer. Women who never had children are at an increased risk of breast cancer. Women who had their first menstrual period before age 12 are at an increased risk of breast cancer. Women who went through menopause after age 55 are at an increased risk of breast cancer. Women who take menopausal hormone therapy for many years have an increased risk of breast cancer.

- **Race:** In the United States, breast cancer is diagnosed more often in white women than in African American/black, Hispanic/Latina, Asian/Pacific Islander, or American Indian/Alaska Native women.

- **Breast Density:** Breasts appear on a mammogram (breast x-ray) as having areas of dense and fatty (not dense) tissue. Women whose mammograms show a larger area of dense tissue than the mammograms of women of the same age are at increased risk of breast cancer.

- **History Of Taking DES:** DES was given to some pregnant women in the United States between about 1940 and 1971. (It is no longer given to pregnant women.) Women who took DES during pregnancy may have a slightly increased risk of breast cancer. The possible effects on their daughters are under study.

- **Being Overweight Or Obese After Menopause:** The chance of getting breast cancer after menopause is higher in women who are overweight or obese.

- **Lack Of Physical Activity:** Women who are physically inactive throughout life may have an increased risk of breast cancer.

- **Drinking Alcohol:** Studies suggest that the more alcohol a woman drinks, the greater her risk of breast cancer.

Having a risk factor does not mean that a woman will get breast cancer. Most women who have risk factors never develop breast cancer.

Many other possible risk factors have been studied. For example, researchers are studying whether women who have a diet high in fat or who are exposed to certain substances in the environment have an increased risk of breast cancer. Researchers continue to study these and other possible risk factors.

Liver Cancer

The liver is the largest organ inside your abdomen. It's found behind your ribs on the right side of your body.

The liver does important work to keep you healthy. It removes harmful substances from the blood. It makes enzymes and bile that help digest food. It also converts food into substances needed for life and growth.

The liver gets its supply of blood from two vessels. Most of its blood comes from the hepatic portal vein. The rest comes from the hepatic artery.

Benign And Malignant Liver Tumors

Growths in the liver can be benign (not cancer) or malignant (cancer). Benign tumors are not as harmful as malignant tumors. Benign tumors are rarely a threat to life. They can be removed and usually don't grow back. Benign tumors don't invade the tissues around them and don't spread to other parts of the body.

Malignant growths may be a threat to life. They sometimes can be removed but can grow back. Malignant tumors can invade and damage nearby tissues and organs (such as the stomach or intestine). They can also spread to other parts of the body.

Most primary liver cancers begin in hepatocytes (liver cells). This type of cancer is called hepatocellular carcinoma or malignant hepatoma.

Liver cancer cells can spread by breaking away from the original tumor. They mainly spread by entering blood vessels, but liver cancer cells can also be found in lymph nodes. The cancer cells may attach to other tissues and grow to form new tumors that may damage those tissues.

Risk Factors For Liver Cancer

Doctors can't always explain why one person gets liver cancer and another doesn't. However, we do know that people with certain risk factors may be more likely than others to develop liver cancer. A risk factor is something that may increase the chance of getting a disease. Studies have found the following risk factors for liver cancer:

- **Hepatitis**: Infection with hepatitis B virus (HBV) or hepatitis C virus (HCV) can increase the risk of liver cancer. Liver cancer can develop after many years of infection with either of these viruses. Around the world, infection with HBV or HCV is the main cause of liver cancer. HBV and HCV can be passed from person to person through blood (such as by sharing needles) or sexual contact. An infant may catch these viruses from an infected mother. Although HBV and HCV infections are contagious diseases, liver cancer is not. You can't catch liver cancer from another person. HBV and HCV infections may not cause symptoms, but blood tests can show whether either virus is present. If so, the doctor may suggest treatment. Also, the doctor may discuss ways to avoid infecting other people. In people who are not already infected with HBV, hepatitis B vaccine can prevent HBV infection. Researchers are working to develop a vaccine to prevent HCV infection.

- **Heavy Alcohol Use:** Having more than two drinks of alcohol each day for many years increases the risk of liver cancer and certain other cancers. The risk increases with the amount of alcohol that a person drinks.

- **Aflatoxin:** Liver cancer can be caused by aflatoxin, a harmful substance made by certain types of mold. Aflatoxin can form on peanuts, corn, and other nuts and grains. In parts of Asia and Africa, levels of aflatoxin are high. However, the United States has safety measures limiting aflatoxin in the food supply.

- **Iron Storage Disease:** Liver cancer may develop among people with a disease that causes the body to store too much iron in the liver and other organs.

- **Cirrhosis:** Cirrhosis is a serious disease that develops when liver cells are damaged and replaced with scar tissue. Many exposures cause cirrhosis, including HBV or HCV infection, heavy alcohol use, too much iron stored in the liver, certain drugs, and certain parasites. Almost all cases of liver cancer in the United States occur in people who first had cirrhosis, usually resulting from hepatitis B or C infection, or from heavy alcohol use.

- **Obesity And Diabetes:** Studies have shown that obesity and diabetes may be important risk factors for liver cancer.

The more risk factors a person has, the greater the chance that liver cancer will develop. However, many people with known risk factors for liver cancer don't develop the disease.

Ways To Reduce Cancer Risk

You can reduce your risk of getting cancer in a variety of ways, including keeping a healthy weight, avoiding tobacco, limiting the amount of alcohol you drink, and protecting your skin from the sun.

Keeping A Healthy Weight

Research has shown that being overweight or obese substantially raises a person's risk of getting endometrial (uterine), breast, prostate, and colorectal cancers. Overweight is defined as a body mass index (BMI) of 25 to 29, and obesity is defined as a BMI of 30 or higher.

Avoiding Tobacco

Lung cancer is the leading cause of cancer death, and cigarette smoking causes almost all cases. Compared to nonsmokers, men who smoke are about 23 times more likely to develop lung cancer and women who smoke are about 13 times more likely. Smoking causes about 90% of lung cancer deaths in men and almost 80% in women. Smoking also causes cancer of the voice box (larynx), mouth and throat, esophagus, bladder, kidney, pancreas, cervix, and stomach, and causes acute myeloid leukemia.

People who are exposed to secondhand smoke at home or at work increase their risk of developing lung cancer by 20% to 30%. Concentrations of many cancer-causing and toxic chemicals are higher in secondhand smoke than in the smoke inhaled by smokers.

Limiting Alcohol Intake

Studies around the world have shown that drinking alcohol regularly increases the risk of getting mouth, voice box, and throat cancers. Daily consumption of around 50g of alcohol doubles or triples the risk for these cancers, compared with the risk in nondrinkers.

A large number of studies provide strong evidence that drinking alcohol is a risk factor for primary liver cancer, and more than 100 studies have found an increased risk of breast cancer with increasing alcohol intake. The link between alcohol consumption and colorectal (colon) cancer has been reported in more than 50 studies.

Protecting Your Skin From The Sun

Skin cancer is the most common form of cancer in the United States. Exposure to the sun's ultraviolet (UV) rays appears to be the most important environmental factor involved with developing skin cancer. To help prevent skin cancer while still having fun outdoors, protect yourself by seeking shade, applying sunscreen, and wearing sun-protective clothing, a hat, and sunglasses.

Chapter 25

Fetal Alcohol Spectrum Disorders

Facts About FASDs

Fetal alcohol spectrum disorders (FASDs) are a group of conditions that can occur in a person whose mother drank alcohol during pregnancy. These effects can include physical problems and problems with behavior and learning. Often, a person with an FASD has a mix of these problems.

Signs And Symptoms

FASDs refer to the whole range of effects that can happen to a person whose mother drank alcohol during pregnancy. These conditions can affect each person in different ways, and can range from mild to severe.

A person with an FASD might have these characteristics and concerns:

Abnormal facial features, such as a smooth ridge between the nose and upper lip (this ridge is called the philtrum)

- Small head size
- Shorter-than-average height
- Low body weight
- Poor coordination

About This Chapter: This chapter includes excerpts from the following documents produced by the Centers for Disease Control and Prevention (www.cdc.gov): "Facts about FASDs," September 11, 2011; "Alcohol Use in Pregnancy," October 6, 2010; "Diagnosis," October 6, 2010; "Treatments," August 19, 2011; and "Secondary Conditions," October 6, 2010.

- Hyperactive behavior

- Difficulty paying attention

- Poor memory

- Difficulty in school (especially with math)

- Learning disabilities

- Speech and language delays

- Intellectual disability or low IQ

- Poor reasoning and judgment skills

- Sleep and sucking problems as a baby

- Vision or hearing problems

- Problems with the heart, kidneys, or bones

Types Of FASDs

Different terms are used to describe FASDs, depending on the type of symptoms.

- **Fetal Alcohol Syndrome (FAS):** FAS represents the severe end of the FASD spectrum. Fetal death is the most extreme outcome from drinking alcohol during pregnancy. People with FAS might have abnormal facial features, growth problems, and central nervous system (CNS) problems. People with FAS can have problems with learning, memory, attention span, communication, vision, or hearing. They might have a mix of these problems. People with FAS often have a hard time in school and trouble getting along with others.

- **Alcohol-Related Neurodevelopmental Disorder (ARND):** People with ARND might have intellectual disabilities and problems with behavior and learning. They might do poorly in school and have difficulties with math, memory, attention, judgment, and poor impulse control.

- **Alcohol-Related Birth Defects (ARBD):** People with ARBD might have problems with the heart, kidneys, or bones or with hearing. They might have a mix of these.

The term fetal alcohol effects (FAE) was previously used to describe intellectual disabilities and problems with behavior and learning in a person whose mother drank alcohol during pregnancy. In 1996, the Institute of Medicine (IOM) replaced FAE with the terms alcohol-related neurodevelopmental disorder (ARND) and alcohol-related birth defects (ARBD).

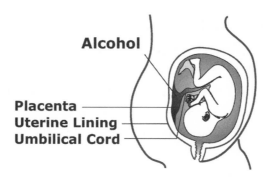

Figure 25.1. Transmission of alcohol to the fetus (Source: "Effects of Alcohol on a Fetus," Substance Abuse and Mental Health Services Administration, 2007).

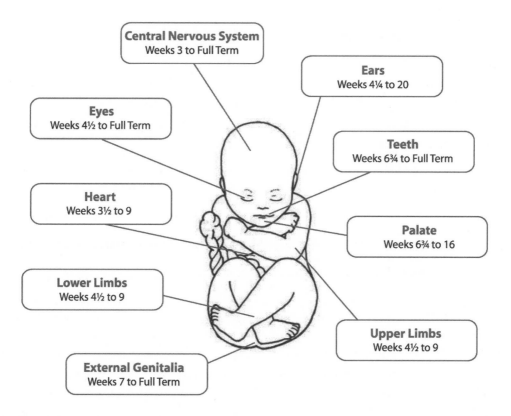

Figure 25.2. Periods of fetal development (Source: "Effects of Alcohol on a Fetus," Substance Abuse and Mental Health Services Administration, 2007).

Alcohol Use In Pregnancy

There is no known safe amount of alcohol to drink while pregnant. There is also no safe time during pregnancy to drink and no safe kind of alcohol. The CDC urges pregnant women not to drink alcohol any time during pregnancy. Women also should not drink alcohol if they are planning to become pregnant or are sexually active and do not use effective birth control. FASDs are 100% preventable. If a woman doesn't drink alcohol while she is pregnant, her child cannot have an FASD.

Why Alcohol Is Dangerous

When a pregnant woman drinks alcohol, so does her unborn baby. Alcohol in the mother's blood passes through the placenta to the baby through the umbilical cord. Drinking alcohol during pregnancy can cause miscarriage, stillbirth, and a range of lifelong disorders, known as fetal alcohol spectrum disorders (FASDs).

When Alcohol Is Dangerous

There is no known safe time to drink alcohol during pregnancy. Drinking alcohol in the first three months of pregnancy can cause the baby to have abnormal facial features. Growth and central nervous system problems (for example, low birthweight, behavioral problems) can occur from drinking alcohol anytime during pregnancy. The baby's brain is developing throughout pregnancy and can be damaged at any time.

If a woman is drinking alcohol during pregnancy, it is never too late to stop. The sooner a woman stops drinking, the better it will be for both her baby and herself.

The Difficulty Diagnosing Fetal Alcohol Spectrum Disorders

The term fetal alcohol spectrum disorders (FASDs) is not meant for use as a clinical diagnosis. The Centers for Disease Control and Prevention (CDC) worked with a group of experts and organizations to review the research and develop guidelines for diagnosing fetal alcohol syndrome (FAS). The guidelines were developed for FAS only. CDC and its partners are working to put together diagnostic criteria for other FASDs, such as ARND. Clinical and scientific research on these conditions is going on now.

Diagnosing FAS can be hard because there is no medical test, like a blood test, for it. And other disorders, such as ADHD (attention-deficit/hyperactivity disorder) and Williams syndrome, have some symptoms like FAS.

Source: CDC, September 11, 2011.

Diagnosis Of Fetal Alcohol Syndrome

Deciding if a child has fetal alcohol syndrome (FAS) takes several steps. There is no one test to diagnose FAS, and many other disorders can have similar symptoms. Following is an overview of the diagnostic guidelines for FAS. These criteria have been simplified for a general audience. They are listed here for information purposes and should be used only by trained health care professionals to diagnose or treat FAS.

Healthcare professionals look for the following signs and symptoms when diagnosing FAS:

Abnormal Facial Features

A person with FAS has three distinct facial features:

- Smooth ridge between the nose and upper lip (smooth philtrum)

- Thin upper lip

- Short distance between the inner and outer corners of the eyes, giving the eyes a wide-spaced appearance.

Growth Problems

Children with FAS have height, weight, or both that are lower than normal (at or below the 10th percentile). These growth issues might occur even before birth. For some children with FAS, growth problems resolve themselves early in life.

Central Nervous System Problems

The central nervous system is made up of the brain and spinal cord. It controls all the workings of the body. When something goes wrong with a part of the nervous system, a person can have trouble moving, speaking, or learning. He or she can also have problems with memory, senses, or social skills. There are three categories of central nervous system problems:

Structural: FAS can cause differences in the structure of the brain. There are two general signs of structural differences: smaller-than-normal head size for the person's overall height and weight (at or below the 10th percentile) and significant changes in the structure of the brain as seen on brain scans such as MRIs or CT scans.

Neurologic: There are problems with the nervous system that cannot be linked to another cause. Examples include poor coordination, poor muscle control, and problems with sucking as a baby.

Functional: The person's ability to function is well below what's expected for his or her age, schooling, or circumstances. To be diagnosed with FAS, a person must have cognitive deficits (for example, low IQ or significant developmental delay in children who are too young for an IQ assessment) or problems in at least three of the following areas:

- **Cognitive Deficits Or Developmental Delays:** Examples include specific learning disabilities (especially math), poor grades in school, performance differences between verbal and nonverbal skills, and slowed movements or reactions.

- **Executive Functioning Deficits:** These deficits involve the thinking processes that help a person manage life tasks. Such deficits include poor organization and planning, lack of inhibition, difficulty grasping cause and effect, difficulty following multistep directions, difficulty doing things in a new way or thinking of things in a new way, poor judgment, and inability to apply knowledge to new situations.

- **Motor Functioning Delays:** These delays affect how a person controls his or her muscles. Examples include delay in walking (gross motor skills), difficulty writing or drawing (fine motor skills), clumsiness, balance problems, tremors, difficulty coordinating hands and fingers (dexterity), and poor sucking in babies.

- **Attention Problems Or Hyperactivity:** A child with these problems might be described as "busy," overly active, inattentive, easily distracted, or having difficulty calming down, completing tasks, or moving from one activity to the next. Parents might report that their child's attention changes from day to day (for example, "on" and "off" days).

- **Problems With Social Skills:** A child with social skills problems might lack a fear of strangers, be easily taken advantage of, prefer younger friends, be immature, show inappropriate sexual behaviors, and have trouble understanding how others feel.

- **Other Problems:** Other problems can include sensitivity to taste or touch, difficulty reading facial expression, and difficulty responding appropriately to common parenting practices (for example, not understanding cause-and-effect discipline)

Mother's Alcohol Use During Pregnancy

Confirmed alcohol use during pregnancy can strengthen the case for FAS diagnosis. Confirmed absence of alcohol exposure would rule out the FAS diagnosis. It's helpful to know whether or not the person's mother drank alcohol during pregnancy. But confirmed alcohol use during pregnancy is not needed if the child meets the other criteria.

Summary: Criteria For FAS Diagnosis

A diagnosis of FAS requires the presence of all three of the following findings:

- All three facial features

- Growth deficits

- Central nervous system problems. A person could meet the central nervous system criteria for FAS diagnosis if there is a problem with the brain structure, even if there are no signs of functional problems.

Treatments For Fetal Alcohol Spectrum Disorders

No two people with an FASD are exactly alike. FASDs can include physical or intellectual disabilities, as well as problems with behavior and learning. These symptoms can range from mild to severe. Treatment services for people with FASDs should be different for each person depending on the symptoms.

Early Intervention Services

There is no cure for FASDs, but research shows that early intervention treatment services can improve a child's development. Early intervention services help children from birth to three years of age (36 months) learn important skills. Services include therapy to help the child talk, walk, and interact with others.

FASD Treatment Overview

FASDs last a lifetime. There is no cure for FASDs, but early intervention treatment services can improve a child's development.

There are many types of treatment options, including medication to help with some symptoms, behavior and education therapy, parent training, and other alternative approaches. No one treatment is right for every child. Good treatment plans will include close monitoring, follow-ups, and changes as needed along the way.

Also, "protective factors" can help reduce the effects of FASDs and help people with these conditions reach their full potential. Protective factors include diagnosis before six years of age; loving, nurturing, and stable home environment during the school years; absence of violence; and involvement in special education and social services.

Source: CDC, September 11, 2011.

Even if a child has not received a diagnosis, he or she might qualify for early intervention treatment services. The Individuals with Disabilities Education Act (IDEA) says that children younger than three years of age who are at risk of having developmental delays may be eligible for services. The early intervention system in the child's state will help have the child evaluated and provide services if the child qualifies.

In addition, treatment for particular symptoms, such as speech therapy for language delays, often does not need to wait for a formal diagnosis.

Protective Factors

Studies have shown that some protective factors can help reduce the effects of FASDs and help people with these conditions reach their full potential. Protective factors include the following:

Early Diagnosis: A child who is diagnosed at a young age can be placed in appropriate educational classes and get the social services needed to help the child and his or her family. Early diagnosis also helps families and school staff to understand why the child might act or react differently from other children sometimes.

Special Education And Social Services: Children who receive special education geared towards their specific needs and learning style are more likely to reach their full potential. Children with FASDs have a wide range of behaviors and challenges that might need to be addressed. Special education programs can better meet each child's needs. In addition, families of children with FASDs who receive social services, such as counseling or respite care have more positive experiences than families who do not receive such services.

Loving, Nurturing, And Stable Home Environment: Children with FASDs can be more sensitive than other children to disruptions, changes in lifestyle or routines, and harmful relationships. Therefore, having a loving, stable home life is very important for a child with an FASD. In addition, community and family support can help prevent secondary conditions, such as criminal behavior, unemployment, and incomplete education.

Absence Of Violence: People with FASDs who live in stable, non-abusive households or who do not become involved in youth violence are much less likely to develop secondary conditions than children who have been exposed to violence in their lives. Children with FASDs need to be taught other ways of showing their anger or frustration.

Types Of Treatments

Many types of treatments are available for people with FASDs. They can generally be broken down into five categories: medical care; medication; behavior and education therapy; parent training; and alternative approaches.

Medical Care: People with FASDs have the same health and medical needs as people without FASDs. Like everyone else, they need well-baby care, vaccinations, good nutrition, exercise, hygiene, and basic medical care. But, for people with FASDs, concerns specific to the disorder must also be monitored and addressed either by a current doctor or through referral to a specialist. The types of treatments needed will be different for each person and depend upon the person's symptoms.

Types of medical specialists might include the following:

- Pediatrician
- Primary care provider
- Dysmorphologist
- Otolaryngologist
- Audiologist
- Immunologist
- Neurologist
- Mental health professionals (child psychiatrist and psychologist, school psychologist, behavior management specialist)
- Ophthalmologist
- Plastic surgeon
- Endocrinologist
- Gastroenterologist
- Nutritionist
- Geneticist
- Speech-language pathologist
- Occupational therapist
- Physical therapist

Medication: No medications have been approved specifically to treat FASDs. But, several medications can help improve some of the symptoms of FASDs. For example, medication might help manage high energy levels, inability to focus, or depression. Following are some examples of medications used to treat FASD symptoms:

- **Stimulants:** This type of medication is used to treat symptoms such as hyperactivity, problems paying attention, and poor impulse control, as well as other behavior issues.

- **Antidepressants:** This type of medication is used to treat symptoms such as sad mood, loss of interest, sleep problems, school disruption, negativity, irritability, aggression, and anti-social behaviors.

- **Neuroleptics:** This type of medication is used to treat symptoms such as aggression, anxiety, and certain other behavior problems.

- **Anti-Anxiety Drugs:** This type of medication is used to treat symptoms of anxiety.

Medications can affect each child differently. One medication might work well for one child, but not for another. To find the right treatment, the doctor might try different medications and doses.

Behavior And Education Therapy: Behavior and education therapy can be an important part of treatment for children with FASDs. Although there are many different types of therapy for children with developmental disabilities, only a few have been scientifically tested specifically for children with FASDs.

Following are behavior and education therapies that have been shown to be effective for some children with FASDs:

- **Friendship Training:** Many children with FASDs have a hard time making friends, keeping friends, and socializing with others. Friendship training teaches children with FASDs how to interact with friends, how to enter a group of children already playing, how to arrange and handle in-home play dates, and how to avoid and work out conflicts. A research study found that this type of training could significantly improve children's social skills and reduce problem behaviors.

- **Specialized Math Tutoring:** A research study found that special teaching methods and tools can help improve math knowledge and skills in children with FASDs.

- **Executive Functioning Training:** This type of training teaches behavioral awareness and self-control and improves executive functioning skills, such as memory, cause and effect, reasoning, planning, and problem solving.

- **Parent-Child Interaction Therapy:** This type of therapy aims to improve parent-child relationships, create a positive discipline program, and reduce behavior problems in children with FASDs. Parents learn new skills from a coach. A research study found significant decrease in parent distress and child behavior problems.

- **Parenting And Behavior Management Training:** The behavior and learning problems that affect children with FASDs can lead to high levels of stress for the children's parents. This training can improve caregiver comfort, meet family needs, and reduce child problem behaviors.

Parent Training: Children with FASDs might not respond to the usual parenting practices. Parent training has been successful in educating parents about their child's disability and about ways to teach their child many skills and help them cope with their FASD-related symptoms. Parent training can be done in groups or with individual families. Such programs are offered by therapists or in special classes.

Families might need support from a family counselor or therapist. Parents might also benefit from local support groups, in which parents of children with FASDs can discuss concerns, ask questions, and find encouragement.

Alternative Approaches: With any disability, injury, or medical condition, many untested therapies become known and are promoted by informal networks. These therapies are referred to as alternative treatments.

Some of the alternative treatments used for people with FASDs include biofeedback; auditory training; relaxation therapy, visual imagery, and meditation (especially for sleep problems and anxiety); creative art therapy; yoga and exercise; acupuncture and acupressure; massage, Reiki, and energy healing; vitamins, herbal supplements, and homeopathy; and animal-assisted therapy.

Secondary Conditions

Fetal alcohol spectrum disorders (FASDs) often lead to other disorders, called *secondary conditions*. Secondary conditions are problems that a person is not born with, but might get as a result of having an FASD. These conditions can be improved or prevented with appropriate treatments for children and adults with FASDs and their families. Following are some of the secondary conditions that have been found to be associated with FASDs.

Mental Health Problems

Several studies have shown an increased risk for cognitive disorders (for example, problems with memory), mental illness, or psychological problems among people with FASDs. These are the most frequently diagnosed disorders:

- Attention problems, including attention-deficit/hyperactivity disorder (ADHD)
- Conduct disorder (aggression toward others and serious violations of rules, laws, and social norms)

- Alcohol or drug dependence
- Depression

Other psychiatric problems, such as anxiety disorders, eating disorders, and posttraumatic stress disorder, have also been reported for some patients.

Disrupted School Experience

Children with FASDs are at a higher risk for being suspended, expelled, or dropping out of school. Difficulty getting along with other children, poor relationships with teachers, and truancy are some of the reasons that lead to their removal from the school setting. Many children with FASDs remain in school but have negative experiences because of their behavioral challenges.

In a 2004 study, disrupted school experience was reported for 14% of school children and 61% of adolescents and adults with FASDs. About 53% of the adolescents with FASDs had been suspended from school, 29% had been expelled, and 25% had dropped out.

Trouble With The Law

Teenagers and adults with FASDs are at a higher risk for having interactions with police, authorities, or the judicial system. Difficulty controlling anger and frustration, combined with problems understanding the motives of others, result in many people with FASDs being involved in violent or explosive situations. People with FASDs can be very easy to persuade and manipulate, which can lead to their taking part in illegal acts without being aware of it. Trouble with the law is reported overall for 14% of children and 60% of adolescents and adults with FASDs.

Inappropriate Sexual Behavior

People with FASDs are at higher risk for showing inappropriate sexual behavior, such as inappropriate advances and inappropriate touching. If the person with an FASD is also a victim of violence, the risk of participating in sexually inappropriate behavior increases. Inappropriate sexual behaviors increase slightly with age from 39% in children to 48% in adolescents and 52% in adults with FASDs.

Alcohol And Drug Problems

Studies suggest that more than a third of people with FASDs have had problems with alcohol or drugs, with more than half of that requiring inpatient treatment.

Dependent Living And Problems With Employment Over 21 Years

Adults with FASDs generally have difficulty sustaining employment or living independently in their communities.

Part Four
Mental Health And Behavioral Risks Associated With Alcohol

Chapter 26

Alcohol And Mental Health

Some teens struggle with alcohol abuse and others suffer from mental health disorders. Some teens have both.

A teen with a drinking problem is more likely than other teens to also have a mental disorder. The opposite is true as well. A teen with a mental health condition is more likely to abuse alcohol.

Mental Health Issues That Affect Teens

Mental health is not just about whether someone does or does not have a mental illness. Emotions—like being worried or stressed or just being in a down mood—affect everyone. Social concerns—like fitting in and having relationships—are often hard to deal with. That's normal. Being a teen can be stressful.

But some teens have mental health problems that go beyond what's typical. They are troubled by intense feelings that are too much to handle. Or they experience a severe lack of feelings and expression. Teens with certain conditions behave in a way that disrupts their own lives and others' lives. They can have uncontrollable thoughts that are disturbing and even frightening.

Mental health disorders can be continual—teens are never free of symptoms. But some disorders are intermittent or cyclical. Symptoms go away or come in waves and are stronger at some periods than others. Episodes can last days, weeks, or months at a time.

Teens with mental disorders can't control these feelings, behaviors, or thoughts on their own, try as they might. It isn't a question of having enough willpower or self-discipline. They need professional help to find out what condition they have. Then they need treatment.

About This Chapter: "Alcohol and Mental Health," by Lisa Esposito, reviewed by David A. Cooke, MD, FACP. December 2012. © 2013 Omnigraphics, Inc.

Some of the mental health conditions that can affect teens are described below.

Anxiety Disorder

Anxiety disorder is a condition of overwhelming anxiety. Fears and worries fill a person's thoughts. Teens with anxiety disorder may suffer from headaches, stomachaches, and muscle cramps. Some experience episodes of blushing, trembling, sweating, and rapid, shallow breathing (hyperventilating). Anxiety disorders can interfere with a person's ability to attend school and take part in activities.

Attention-Deficit/Hyperactivity Disorder (ADHD)

ADHD starts in early childhood and may continue into the teen years. Besides having trouble paying attention and being restlessness, signs include being easily distracted and forgetting things, having trouble following directions or finishing tasks (like homework), often losing possessions, and blurting out comments. Teens with ADHD are more likely to take dangerous risks, and they have more car accidents than other teens.[1] Teens with ADHD are also at significantly increased risk for developing addiction to alcohol and other drugs.

Bipolar Disorder (Manic-Depressive Illness)

Bipolar disorder is a major psychiatric illness involving sharp mood swings. During a manic phase, people are extremely upbeat, happy and, active. They may talk quickly on a variety of subjects at once. In a depressive phase, they are really sad and much less active. These phases are much more intense than normal moodiness. Bipolar disorder can disrupt how teens function at school, at home, and with friends. If not treated, it can lead to self-harm and suicide attempts. About 2.5 percent of U.S. teens have bipolar disorder.[2]

Conduct Disorder

Conduct disorder involves behaviors that are antisocial and violate other people's rights. Teens who have it can be aggressive, violent, destructive, or deceitful. They break rules and sometimes laws.[3] Behaviors range from lying, running away, and truancy to bullying, cruelty to people or animals, vandalism, stealing, intimidation, and rape. Growing up in poverty or in a troubled family raises a teen's risk for developing conduct disorder.

Depression

People with depression feel sad almost all the time. Depression saps their energy. It affects their sleep and makes it hard to pay attention in school. Activities they used to enjoy no longer seem interesting. Depressed teens are more likely to think about death and they're at higher risk for suicide. When teens say they want to die or kill themselves, it is an emergency. They need immediate professional help.

Self-Injury

Self-injury includes cutting, carving, burning, branding, skin picking, hair pulling, biting, and head banging. Some teens who do this say it helps relieve the pressure they feel inside from stress, pain, fear, or anger. Most teens grow out of self-injury although the physical scars can be permanent. Self-injury can be a symptom of other mental health conditions including depression and bipolar disorder.

Social Phobia

Social phobia is a type of anxiety disorder. It's an excessive and constant fear of meeting new people or embarrassing yourself in a social situation. Teens with social phobia tend to steer clear of groups and avoid making efforts to have friends. Fear of situations like attending a party, having to speak up in class, or work on a group project can spur anxiety attacks. These include heart racing and pounding, shortness of breath, dizziness, and nausea.

Schizophrenia

Schizophrenia is a severe mental illness which causes difficulties with coherent thought and maintaining connections to reality. People with schizophrenia can experience hallucinations (such as hearing voices) or delusions (strong beliefs that go against reality). They act or speak in strange or unpredictable ways. They may become violent or catatonic (such as not moving for days). They may lose motivation, energy, or interest in activities or people. They may develop flat facial expressions and speech patterns that make them appear emotionless. They may no longer dress or groom themselves properly and have trouble going about the normal routines of their day. School changes—like smaller, special classes— often become necessary.[4]

Suicide

Suicide is the third-leading cause of death in people ages 10 to 24.[5] Depression and other disorders—including alcohol and drug abuse—put teens at higher risk for suicide. Warning signs include talking about dying and marked changes in personality, behavior, sleep, or eating habits. Teens who are suicidal express low self-esteem and hopelessness. When teens who are already vulnerable go through a loss—like parents divorcing or breaking up with a boyfriend or girlfriend—suicide risk is higher.

Dual Diagnosis

Dual diagnosis is the official term for having a psychiatric illness and an alcohol or other substance abuse disorder. Comorbidity and co-occurring disorders also mean having two such illnesses at the same time. One example would be a teen with bipolar disorder who is also dependent on alcohol. As hard as it is to deal with a single disorder, having two complicates life even more. Drinking makes the mental health problem worse. Mental illness makes the drinking problem worse. It takes effort to sort out which conditions a teen has and figure out the right treatment for both.

How Mental Illness Affects Alcohol Use

It's true that many adolescents experiment with alcohol. But teens struggling with mental health issues are more likely to drink alcohol. They have different patterns to their drinking. They tend to start drinking at a younger age and are more likely to drink heavily. Binge drinking is more common. Bingeing can lead to alcohol poisoning. This is a medical emergency that can result in coma and even death.

Self-Medication

Teens with mental health issues may drink to self-medicate. They may not realize that they have a specific mental disorder. But they drink to try and change the unbearable way they feel.

This doesn't apply to all disorders. A 2011 study found that teens with general anxiety were almost three times as likely as others to become frequent drinkers. But the opposite was true for teens with social phobia. They were less likely to become heavy drinkers than other teens.[6]

A few studies suggest that girls who are physically or sexually abused are more likely to later develop drinking problems. However, this has not been shown in boys.

Genetics

Parents pass on their genes to their children. Genes affect the color of a person's eyes, how tall they grow, and whether they have certain medical conditions. The genes a child inherits can affect lifelong mental health. Bipolar disorder and schizophrenia run in families. Teens who have a parent, brother, or sister with these conditions are at higher risk for developing them.

Research suggests that some of the same genes that affect mental illnesses also are related to alcohol use and disorders. Genes are thought to influence how early drinking starts and how likely a drinker is to become addicted to alcohol.

Stress Drinking Linked To Early Alcohol Use

People who begin drinking at a young age also may drink heavily during stressful events later in life. Results from a recent study published in the June 2011 issue of *Alcoholism: Clinical & Experimental Research* found an interaction between an early age of first drink and drinking patterns later in adulthood.

The research team examined data from the Mannheim Study of Children at Risk, a German-based longitudinal study that tracked the outcome of early risk factors from infancy through young adulthood. Participants surveyed at ages 15 and 19 reported the age when they first had more than just a few sips of alcohol. The earliest age of first drink in the study was 8 years old, and about half of the participants began drinking before age 14.

At age 22, participants answered questions about their drinking behavior, including how many days in the past month they drank alcohol and how much they drank on those occasions. The researchers also asked questions about whether participants experienced major stressful life events, including family, health, job, and legal troubles, and daily hassles, such as bad weather or sleep problems.

Results showed stress doesn't necessarily cause people to drink more often but it does cause them to drink larger quantities when they do drink. Daily hassles proved to be unrelated to drinking behavior.

In addition, the age of first drink had a significant influence on both the number of drinking days and the total amount of alcohol consumed in the last month. People with an earlier age of first drink had more frequent and higher consumption levels than people who began drinking at an older age.

Dorothea Blomeyer, a first author on the study, hypothesizes that adolescents who drink may learn to use alcohol as a way of dealing with stress. As a result, Blomeyer explains, "This study extends our knowledge on how the connection between early age of first drink and later drinking problems might develop."

Source: From "Stress Drinking Linked to Early Alcohol Use," *Spectrum*, National Institute on Alcohol Abuse and Alcoholism (www.niaaa.nih.gov), Vol. 3, Issue 2, June 2011.

However, teens' drinking choices also are deeply affected by what they see and experience as they grow up. Parents' own drinking and attitudes toward alcohol make a big impression. The society in which teens live—how drinking is viewed—and the friends they have affect teen drinking than genes, research suggests.

On the other hand, living in a healthy environment can help teens compensate for a higher genetic risk of alcohol problems.

Drinking And Mental Health Conditions: The Connection

- People with anxiety are 1.5 times more likely to be addicted to alcohol.[7]

- People with depression have a 1.9 time higher risk of being addicted to alcohol.[7]

- Depression and alcohol abuse both raise the risk for suicide.[7]

- Of high school students who consider suicide, nearly twice as many have used alcohol.[8]

- Of high school students ever treated for a mental health problem, 11 percent also have an alcohol use disorder, compared with 5 percent without a mental health problem.[8]

Source: Lisa Esposito.

Family And Childhood Circumstances

If one or both of a teen's biological parents is alcoholic, that teen is at a higher risk for having a drinking problem. Bad relationships with parents also place children at risk for alcohol issues. This includes parents who don't support or communicate calmly with their children. Extremes of discipline—too much or too little—are harmful. Parents who show no concern about what children do or where they go can make underage drinking more likely. So can parental disciplinary styles that are inconsistent or involve hostile, rejecting, or harsh tactics. Child abuse and child neglect raise the risk for alcohol dependence. So does bullying by peers.

Personality Traits

How children act at a young age may predict their alcohol use as teens. Certain personality traits seem to put kids at higher risk. These include being disruptive, fearless, aggressive, impulsive, quick-tempered, very irritable, or hard to control.[9]

Having low self-esteem is also tied to a higher risk of drinking problems.

These traits don't guarantee that a child will someday have drinking problems. But they could mean a child is more vulnerable.

Vicious Cycle

A study of college students uncovered two types of heavy drinkers.[10] One group drinks for stimulation—for the high. Drinking is a big part of their social interaction. This group is more likely to participate in drinking games or contests that can result in alcohol poisoning.

The other group drinks to reduce tension and stress: to feel better. Depressed or anxious teens who drink might feel less sad, stressed, or isolated at first. But as they drink more to recapture that state of mind, the short-term benefits go away. Heavy drinking leaves them feeling even more depressed, hopeless, and alone.

As drinkers need increasingly more alcohol to feel the same effects, dependence becomes a risk.

How Alcohol Affects Mental Health

About 20 percent of people in the general population have a mental illness. But up to 37 percent of alcohol abusers have a mental illness.[11] It's not always clear which problem comes first.

Heavy drinkers sometimes abuse illegal drugs and prescription drugs. Narcotic painkillers are a type of prescription drug that can cause addiction. They can also lead to overdose.

Alcohol abuse can cause sleep disturbance and may affect learning and memory. Starting to drink before age 15 raises the odds for later alcohol dependence.

Brain Connection

The teen brain is still developing. In some areas—like learning ability—it's as mature as the adult brain. But in other areas—like controlling impulses and making decisions—the teen brain isn't fully mature. That can affect the decision teens make about drinking.[12] Drinking can harm teens' growing brains, including areas involved in mental health disorders. (See Chapter 12 to learn more about how the brain develops.)

Some chemicals in the brain affect people's moods and their mental health. Studies have found that people who abuse alcohol and drugs may have different amount of these brain chemicals than other people.

Dopamine is a chemical that acts in the brain's reward and pleasure areas.[13] One study found changes in dopamine levels in patients who had both schizophrenia and addiction. Serotonin is a chemical that affects how happy people feel. Some studies have found smaller amounts of serotonin in people with depression. Serotonin may affect the brain's response to alcohol and alcohol abuse may reduce serotonin levels in the brain.

Suicide And Alcohol

Many people who are suicidal have experienced problems with alcohol. Alcohol abuse can also come before depression. And depressed people are more likely to commit suicide. So all three conditions overlap.

A 2010 survey of U.S. high school students looked at the connection between alcohol use and mental health.[14] It compared responses from teens who had ever used alcohol with those who had not. These were the results:

- Feeling alone or isolated: 24 percent of drinkers but only 19 percent of non-drinkers

- Feeling very sad or depressed: 23 percent of drinkers but only 13 percent of non-drinkers

- Thinking they will develop depression someday: 37 percent of drinkers and 23 percent of non-drinkers

- Having thoughts or plans of suicide: 16 percent of drinkers and 8.5 percent of non-drinkers

Teens who were currently drinking were twice as likely to have suicide thoughts or plans than non-drinkers. The worst risk was for teens with a disorder like alcohol dependence. They were nearly three times as like to think about or plan suicide.

Many studies show connections among depression and other mental illnesses, alcohol and drug abuse, and suicide. According to the American Psychological Association, more than 90 percent of people who die from suicide have such risk factors.[15]

Signs Of Disorders

The way people behave is a sign of their mental health. Teens with mental disorders or alcohol problems—or both—may show these some of these signs:

- School absences and bad or failing grades

- Fighting and assault

- Not participating in activities such as sports or clubs

- Legal issues, including drunk driving or hurting others

- Sexual activity at younger ages

- Sex without protection against pregnancy or diseases

- Unwanted sexual activity—sex that the teen didn't agree to

- Problems with memory

- Illegal or prescription drug abuse

Source: Lisa Esposito.

Alcohol In Co-Occurring Disorders

About one-fourth to one-third of people being treated in mental health facilities also have alcohol or drug disorders. And of people being treated for alcohol or drug addiction, one-half to three-fourths also have a mental health disorder.[16]

Some people with mental health disorders are more sensitive to alcohol's effects. People with dual diagnosis who stop drinking may be discouraged when other symptoms of the other disorder continue.

Treating Mental Illness And Alcoholism Dependence

Professional help is available for teens who show signs of a mental health or drinking disorder. Family physicians, pediatricians, and school guidance counselors are good starting points. They can refer teens to psychiatrist, psychologists, and recovery programs. Most insurance covers mental health treatment.

Teens receiving treatment for drug and alcohol abuse should also be checked for co-occurring mental health disorders.

The therapies listed below are used for teens with mental disorders, substance disorders, or both. Not all treatments are recommended for teens with dual diagnosis.

Counseling/Psychotherapy (Talk Therapy)

Talk therapy uses a special kind of conversation to help teens understand and deal with their mental health problems. This conversation takes place between teens and a therapist. Therapists can be psychiatrists, psychologists, or counselors. Psychiatrists are also licensed to prescribe medications when needed.

Choosing the best type of talk therapy depends on the mental health condition involved. Some methods help with a variety of conditions. The following methods are often used to help teens.

Cognitive behavior therapy (CBT) can help in anxiety, depression, alcohol, and drug disorders. It's used to change confused or distorted thinking that can cause troubling feelings and behaviors. First, teens learn to recognize their harmful thinking patterns. Then they identify more helpful ways of thinking. They use these new ways of thinking in their day-to-day lives and discuss the results with their therapist.

Crisis prevention includes crisis centers and hotlines for teens who need help right away. The National Suicide Prevention Lifeline takes calls 24 hours a day at 800-273-TALK (800-273-8255).

Dialectical behavior therapy (DBT) can work for older teens who self-injure or have suicidal thoughts. It helps them control the negative emotions that lead to harmful behaviors. Teens learn to use better coping strategies.

Individual counseling helps with depression and other mood disorders. This type of therapy treats symptoms like continual sadness. It can help teens in especially stressful times. The therapist and teen work to get rid of feelings of failure and self-blame that can come with depression.

Family therapy includes teens and parents, and sometimes brothers, sisters, and grandparents. Its goal is to help families communicate and support one another. It also helps parents and siblings understand what the teen is going through and how that affects the entire family.

Group therapy often involves several people with the same mental disorder meeting together with a therapist. It helps teens understand what they're going through and can improve their social skills. Group therapy is often used for teens with alcohol disorders.

Parent management training is a type of family therapy. It's useful when teens have conduct disorder. It can help when parents are unstable or not functioning well. Parents learn how to support healthy behavior in their children. They also learn more positive types of discipline.

School-based mental health services include screening programs to uncover mental health, alcohol, and drug issues. Easy access for students is one advantage. Some programs offer individual and group counseling for a variety of conditions. Staff can refer students to mental health care providers in the community.

Twelve-step programs like Alcoholics Anonymous (AA) help teens stop drinking. However, they may not be the best fit for a teen with dual diagnosis, but some 12-step programs have been created specifically for people with dual diagnosis.

Medication

Medications can help in many conditions. They're often used for ADHD, anxiety disorders, depression, schizophrenia, and bipolar disorder. Medication is usually not the only treatment. It is often combined with some kind of counseling.

Different kinds or classes of medications are used depending on the condition. Teens, families, and doctors need to watch for drug side effects. It may take several attempts to find the right medication or combination for the individual teen. Dosages may need to be adjusted.

Teens on antidepressant drugs need to be carefully monitored. In 2007, the Food and Drug Administration added a label warning on all medicines used to treat depression. A study had found that children and teens who take certain types of these drugs might be more likely to think about or attempt suicide, especially in the first few weeks of treatment.[17]

Treating Dual Diagnosis

Finding the right therapist and treatment for any mental health condition can be a challenge. When teens have dual diagnosis, families have even more factors to consider.

Treatment programs focused on alcohol abuse can conflict with mental disorder treatment. These programs sometimes discourage use of certain prescription medicines. Teens with dual diagnosis often have a condition, like bipolar disorder, that requires these medicines.

Some alcohol or drug abuse programs can involve group members confronting one another about their behavior. This may not be helpful for dual diagnosis. Confrontations can increase stress for teens with anxiety disorder or depression.

Some programs that treat mental disorders will not accept patients who are currently abusing alcohol or drugs. Before starting any kind of talk therapy, intoxicated teens need to get sober.

Detoxification means getting rid of alcohol (or drugs) in the body. It may take several days or a more than a week. Medications can help people get through detoxification.

Sequential therapy involves treating one condition at a time. After one condition is under control, treatment then focuses on the other. However, experts say it's better to start treating both conditions as soon as possible.

When a teen has dual diagnosis, more than one mental health care provider may be involved. All providers need to communicate with one another about the teen's progress and treatment plans. Professionals called case managers can help coordinate all this care.

Integrated therapy focuses on co-occurring conditions to make sure they are treated correctly and neither is ignored. The same therapist works on all conditions.

When possible, a combination of talk therapy and medication, along with support and self-help groups, is best for treating dual diagnosis. Even then, relapse—the return of symptoms—can occur. Mental health providers are trained to help teens get through relapse.

Programs focused on teens with dual diagnosis are increasing. Some take place in hospitals or in residential treatment centers where teens stay for a number of weeks. In addition to other treatments, teens are educated about their conditions and how to manage their medications.

Teens with dual diagnosis are also encouraged to exercise, take part in recreation and hobbies, and follow a healthy diet. Exercise eases stress, depression, and anxiety. Participating in activities helps teen make friends and improve their social skills. All this will support their efforts to restore their mental health.

Notes

1. Russell A. Barkley and D.J. Cox. A Review of Driving Risks and Impairments Associated With Attention-Deficit/Hyperactivity Disorder and the Effects of Stimulant Medication on Driving Performance, *Journal of Safety Research* 38 (2007).

2. Kathleen Merikangas and others. "Prevalence, Persistence, and Sociodemographic Correlates of DSM-IV Disorders in The National Comorbidity Survey Replication Adolescent Supplement." *Archives of General Psychiatry* 69(4) (April 2012).

3. American Academy of Child and Adolescent Psychiatry. "Your Adolescent: Conduct Disorders." 2010 brochure. Accessed Oct. 16, 2012. http://www.aacap.org/cs/root/ publication_store/your_adolescent_conduct_disorders

4. National Alliance on Mental Illness. "Early Onset Schizophrenia." (Arlington, VA: NAMI, July 2010). http://www.nami.org/Content/ContentGroups/Helpline1/Early_ Onset_Schizophrenia.htm

5. Centers for Disease Control and Prevention. "Suicide Prevention: Youth Suicide." (Atlanta: CDC, August 15, 2012). http://www.cdc.gov/violenceprevention/pub/youth_ suicide.htm

6. Sari Frojd and others. "Associations of Social Phobia and General Anxiety with Alcohol and Drug Use in a Community Sample of Adolescents." *Alcohol and Alcoholism* 46(2), 2011.

7. Institute of Alcohol Studies. "Alcohol And Mental Health: IAS Factsheet" (London: IAS, 2007). http://www.ias.org.uk/resources/factsheets/mentalhealth.pdf

8. National Center on Addiction and Substance Abuse at Columbia University (CASA). "Adolescent Substance Use: America's #1 Public Health Problem." Report (New York: CASA, June 2011). http://www.casacolumbia.org/templates/publications _reports.aspx

9. Newbury-Birch, Dorothy, et al. "Impact Of Alcohol Consumption on Young People: A Systematic Review Of Published Reviews." Department for Children, Schools, and Families (Nottingham, UK: Newcastle University, 2009). http://dera.ioe.ac.uk/ 11355/1/DCSF-RR067.pdf

10. Ibid.

11. See note 7 above.

12. National Institute of Mental Health. "The Teen Brain: Still Under Construction." (Bethesda, MD: NIMH, 2011). http://www.nimh.nih.gov/health/publications/the-teen-brain-still-under-construction/complete-index.shtml

13. National Institute on Drug Abuse. "Study Finds Combined Dopamine Dysfunction in Drug Addicted, Schizophrenic Patients" *Science Spotlight*, October 4, 2012. http://www.drugabuse.gov/news-events/news-releases/study-finds-combined-dopamine-dysfunction-in-drug-addicted-schizophrenic-patients

14. See note 8 above.

15. American Psychological Association. "Teen Suicide Is Preventable" (Washington: APA, 2012). Accessed October 10, 2012. http://www.apa.org/research/action/suicide.aspx

16. Hazelden. "Behavioral Health Evolution: Co-Occurring Disorders" (Center City, MN: Hazelden, 2011.) http://www.bhevolution.org/public/co-occurring_disorders.page

17. National Institute of Mental Health. "Antidepressant Medications for Children and Adolescents: Information for Parents and Caregivers" (Bethesda, MD: NIMH, nd). Accessed November 1, 2012. http://www.nimh.nih.gov/health/topics/child-and-adolescent-mental-health/antidepressant-medications-for-children-and-adolescents-information-for-parents-and-caregivers.shtml

Chapter 27

Alcohol And Suicide Risk

Being a teenager can be stressful. Pressure from school, work, family, and friends can build up to a point where the obstacles in life seem almost impossible to overcome. Teens sometimes turn to alcohol or thoughts of suicide as a way out. Suicide is the third most common cause of death for teens and young adults in the United States, and studies suggest that approximately one out of every ten teenagers attempts suicide.[1] It is an especially alarming major public health concern. Suicidal thoughts are dangerous enough, but mixed with alcohol abuse those thoughts may become even more lethal, and the use of alcohol can further contribute to negative emotions and suicidal behaviors.

Alcohol Use And Suicide Risk Factors

Alcohol abuse has been shown to be a major risk factor for suicide. About one-fourth of all suicides are attempted while a person is intoxicated by alcohol. Additionally, alcohol—sometimes in combination with other drugs—is involved in about one out of ten suicide-related visits to the emergency department.[2]

Alcohol can make someone feel uninhibited, which means he or she is more likely to do something that normally would not be done. Feeling uninhibited can make someone more likely to do something drastic or extreme, like attempt suicide.[3] Furthermore, alcohol can encourage feelings of depression and hopelessness in suicidal people. Alcohol may also reduce a person's ability to make reasonable judgments or smart choices and can make a person more aggressive.

About This Chapter: "Alcohol and Suicide Risk," by Zachary Klimecki, reviewed by David A. Cooke, MD, FACP. December 2012. © 2013 Omnigraphics, Inc.

Alcohol use has been shown to be a significant contributing factor for many unplanned suicides by teenagers. Unplanned suicide attempts occur when an individual dies by suicide without a specific, preconsidered plan and had only passing thoughts of suicide or none at all before attempting suicide. Planned suicides happen with far less frequency. Alcohol can put people who are at risk for suicidal behaviors in a state-of-mind that enables them to attempt an unplanned suicide. Teenagers who are prone to aggressive or impulsive behavior—such as those with behavioral disorders—and who drink may have an increased suicide risk.[4]

Help For People In Crisis

If you or someone you know is considering suicide, get help immediately. Call the National Suicide Prevention Hotline: 800-273-TALK (8255).

Stress At Home

Stresses in the home environment can place some teens at risk for alcohol abuse and suicidal thoughts. When teens endure abuse at the hands of family members, this can cause mental distress that potentially leads to dangerous behaviors. Some teens turn to alcohol to escape these and other problems. If someone in the house already abuses alcohol, this type of attempted escaping is more likely for two reasons: Alcohol may be more readily available, and teens with a family history of alcohol dependency may have an increased genetic risk for being susceptible to alcohol abuse themselves.

Likewise, a family history of suicide or mental illness can be a significant risk factor for mental illness and suicidal behavior in teens. Many psychiatric disorders, such as bipolar disorder, carry with them an increased risk of suicide. Teens who have undiagnosed psychiatric disorders may experience damaging periods of time in which their illnesses go untreated. As a result, negative behaviors like drinking and suicidal thinking can develop. Recognizing a family history of mental issues and problems with alcohol can help a teen in distress understand the related health concerns and receive the support needed before dangerous habits develop.

Because the first phase of alcohol intoxication gives a person a short-lasting sensation of wellbeing, teens with mental illnesses sometimes turn to alcohol as a way to self-medicate. In the long-term, drinking alcohol will not help the symptoms of mental illness and can complicate psychological treatments. Furthermore, alcohol can interact with some prescription medications in a life-threatening way.

Stress At School

Going to school can be a particularly stressful event for some teenagers. Teens often juggle a heavy class load and the demands of homework and extracurricular activities while trying to maintain a social life. These tasks can lead to increased pressures, especially for adolescents who do not know how to successfully manage the stress that surrounds them.

Some students may seek out alcohol as a way to distance themselves from their troubles. If alcohol is inappropriately used as a coping mechanism and teens find themselves too over-whelmed, their thoughts have the potential to drift towards suicide.

Along with the weight of academic life, students who are considered "different" may face additional adversity. Those who do no fit the mold may be made fun of, bullied, or harassed. These actions may have long-term damaging effects on teens' self-esteem and they can lead to negative behaviors among their victims. Teens may try drinking alcohol as a way to fit in, and friends may coerce them into drinking when they otherwise would have not bowed to the pressure. This combination of social pressures and low self-esteem in the face of negative behaviors can intensify suicidal thoughts.

Binge Drinking

Binge drinking has been associated with suicide attempts in teens. Binge drinking is the act of consuming a large amount of alcohol in a relatively short period of time. Drinking four (for females) or five (for males) or more alcoholic drinks within the timespan of a couple of hours is usually considered binge drinking. It is the most common form of excessive alcohol use in the United States. People younger than 21 consume alcohol by binge drinking 90% of the time. Teens who drink to cope with negative feelings are also more likely to binge drink.[5,6]

Although binge drinkers are commonly not alcoholics,[7] binge drinking is closely connected to the negative effects associated with alcohol, such as acting impulsively and losing inhibition. According to the 2011 National Youth Risk Behavior Survey, 21.9% of students across the United States had participated in binge drinking at least one day in the month before the survey.[8]

Alcoholism

According to the American Foundation for Suicide Prevention, alcohol dependence plays a role in almost 30% of all suicide deaths and 7% of alcoholics will die by suicide.[9] Men who attempt suicide are more likely than women to have a history of abusing alcohol. Alcoholics most often attempt suicide when problems occur in their personal relationships, like a break-up. Alcoholics who attempt suicide are more likely to also have underlying emotional problems or mental illness. A person with depression who develops a problem with alcohol has a higher chance of considering suicide and going through with it. Alcohol abuse can lead to changes in the brain that cause depression over time. Beyond emotional and environmental factors, suicidal behavior and alcoholism may also share common genetic trait.[10]

Other Risk Factors

Females are more likely to attempt suicide than males, but men are more likely to actually die by suicide. Males 15 to 19 years old die by suicide almost five times more often than females.[11] The 2011 National Youth Risk Behavior Survey reported that 15.8% of students seriously considered suicide at one point during the year before the survey.[12]

Alcohol can worsen certain factors that already put teens at risk for suicide. The following factors can generally increase suicide risk, whether or not alcohol or other substance abuse occurs:

- Physical abuse

- Emotional abuse

- Sexual abuse

- Depression

- Previous suicide attempts

- Violence in the home

- Guns in the home

- Family history of mental illness

- Family history of suicide[13]

Teens who have these risk factors are not necessarily suicidal, but still may be at risk. Recognizing problems that exist before they get out of control is an important step toward avoiding an alcohol-related suicide.

Prevention

If a friend or loved one has a problem with alcohol or suicidal thoughts, it is important that he or she gets help. People who are acting suicidal, should not be left alone. They need professional help.[14]

Sometimes it can be hard to recognize when someone has a problem, but there are several ways to spot someone who potentially needs help. A person who might be considering suicide may talk about the following:

- Wanting to die

- Having no reason to live

- Feeling trapped

- Being in a lot of pain

- Being a burden

People with suicidal thoughts may be looking for ways to kill themselves, sometimes by searching online. They may act recklessly, have extreme mood swings, and sleep constantly or very little. They may stop communication with friends and family and isolate themselves. They may start using drugs or drinking alcohol excessively.

By limiting the availability of substances that can be abused in the home, adults can help prevent teens from using alcohol and other drugs in lethal ways. Building social support networks for suicidal individuals can give them an outlet to openly express negative emotions that otherwise could lead to despair and suicidal thoughts. Family, friends, teachers, school administrators, counselors, and faith leaders can all play an active role in a support network that could save a person's life.[15] Interventions to assist people who abuse alcohol can also help prevent further alcohol-related injuries or suicide attempts.[16]

A variety of different therapies exist that can help suicidal people or those who have an alcohol problem. A type of psychotherapy called cognitive therapy assists people who are considering suicide by helping them acknowledge other options. Cognitive therapy has been shown to reduce rates of repeated suicide attempts by 50%. Some other types of therapy work better for specific groups of individuals, and for some people medications are used to help alleviate suicidal tendencies[17] (although some antidepressants must be used with caution, especially in teens, because they are associated with increasing suicide risks).

Helping an individual get needed care is extremely important. If you know someone who needs help make sure to speak up. Contact the National Suicide Prevention Hotline for help:

- National Suicide Prevention Hotline: 800-273-TALK (8255)

For more options, see the resources at the end of the book. If someone threatening to hurt him- or herself, is in immediate danger, or is injured by a suicide attempt, call 911.

Notes

1. Schilling, Elizabeth A., et al. Adolescent Alcohol Use, Suicidal Ideation, and Suicide Attempts. *Society for Adolescent Medicine*. 2009. http://www.jahonline.org/article/S1054-139X(08)00337-6/fulltext

2. Substance Abuse and Mental Health Services Administration, Office of Applied Studies. *The DAWN Report: Emergency Department Visits for Drug-Related Suicide Attempts by Adolescents: 2008* (Rockville, MD: SAMHSA, May 13, 2010). http://oas.samhsa.gov/2k10/DAWN001/SuicideAttemptsHTML.pdf

3. Center for Substance Abuse Treatment. Substance Abuse and Suicide Prevention: Evidence and Implications—A White Paper. DHHS Pub. No. SMA-08-4352 (Rockville, MD: Substance Abuse and Mental Health Services Administration, 2008). http://www.samhsa.gov/matrix2/508SuicidePreventionPaperFinal.pdf

4. American Foundation for Suicide Prevention. Facts and Figures (New York: AFPS, 2010). http://www.afsp.org/index.cfm?fuseaction=home.viewpage&page_id=050fea9f-b064-4092-b1135c3a70de1fda

5. See note 1 above.

6. Centers for Disease Control and Prevention. Binge Drinking (Atlanta: CDC, November 2012). http://www.cdc.gov/alcohol/fact-sheets/binge-drinking.htm

7. Ibid.

8. Centers for Disease Control and Prevention. Youth Risk Behavior Surveillance — United States, 2011. *MMWR*. 2012. http://www.cdc.gov/mmwr/pdf/ss/ss6104.pdf

9. See note 4 above.

10. Brady, John. The Association Between Alcohol Misuse And Suicidal Behaviour. *Alcohol & Alcoholism* Vol. 41, No. 5, pp. 473–478. August 2006. http://alcalc.oxfordjournals.org/content/41/5/473.full.pdf

11. National Institute of Mental Health. Suicide in the U.S.: Statistics and Prevention (Bethesda, MD: NIMH, September 27, 2010). http://www.nimh.nih.gov/health/publications/suicide-in-the-us-statistics-and-prevention/index.shtml

12. See note 8 above.

13. See note 11 above.

14. National Institute of Mental Health. Suicide: A Major, Preventable Mental Health Problem (Bethesda, MD: NIMH, 2012). http://www.nimh.nih.gov/health/publications/suicide-a-major-preventable-mental-health-problem-fact-sheet/suicide-a-major-preventable-mental-health-problem.shtml

15. National Center for Injury Prevention and Control, Division of Violence Prevention. Suicides Due to Alcohol and/or Drug Overdose: A Data Brief from the National Violent Death Reporting System (Atlanta: Centers for Disease Control and Prevention, National Center for Injury Prevention and Control, nd). Accessed November 14, 2012. http://www.cdc.gov/violenceprevention/pdf/NVDRS_Data_Brief-a.pdf

16. See note 10 above.

17. See note 11 above.

Chapter 28

How Addiction Develops

Not so long ago, people debated whether alcoholism, like other addictions, was a behavioral problem or a mental health disorder or disease. In other words, do some people simply choose to drink too much every day? Or does a person who is addicted to alcohol have no choice in the matter? Today scientists agree with the second point of view. Addiction is a progressive disease (meaning that it gets worse over time), and the addict has little control without ongoing support to break the habit and stay sober.

Nobody gets addicted to alcohol with occasional drinking or a single nightly cocktail, glass of wine, or bottle of beer. Alcohol addiction develops with repeated, heavy drinking. The problem keeps getting worse, because changes that occur in the brain make it difficult for the alcoholic to stop drinking.

Alcohol And The Brain

Because alcohol addiction is a disease of the brain, it's important to know how a healthy brain works. Inside the brain are billions of nerve cells, or neurons. The neurons send messages to each other by releasing chemicals called neurotransmitters. The neurotransmitters carry information to parts of nearby cells called receptors.

The chemicals in the brain must be in balance for everything to function normally. Alcohol upsets the balance of neurotransmitters. Alcohol has complex chemical effects on the brain, reducing the release of some neurotransmitters and leading to increased release of other neurotransmitters. These changes in brain chemistry lead to the pleasurable and undesired effects of alcohol intoxication.

About This Chapter: "How Addiction Develops," by Laurie Lewis, reviewed by David A. Cooke, MD, FACP, December 2012. © 2013 Omnigraphics, Inc.

The brain attempts to maintain chemical stability, so with repeated and prolonged exposure to alcohol, it will begin to alter its neurotransmitter production to compensate. Drinking a given amount of alcohol will no longer produce the same effects it once did, and a drinker may need to drink more to develop the same pleasurable effect. The drinker has developed tolerance, or lack of sensitivity to alcohol's effects. If a drinker is accustomed to daily alcohol use, withdrawal may also occur if alcohol is suddenly stopped. This is due to unopposed effects of the brain's compensatory mechanisms.

Factors That May Contribute To Addiction

- **Brain Chemicals:** Addiction is a disease occurring when chemicals that are naturally produced in the brain become off balance. These chemicals act as neurotransmitters, enabling brain cells to communicate with each other. The main chemical involved in addiction is dopamine, which plays a major role in the pleasure and reward circuits of the brain. Other naturally occurring chemical systems involved in addiction include opioids such as endorphins, which also are involved in reward and pleasure; glutamate, which influences the reward circuit and the ability to learn; gamma-aminobutyric acid (GABA), which helps regulate emotional states, anxiety, and response to stress; and corticotropin-releasing factor (CPF) and perhaps other chemicals involved in the response to stress. Eventually, medications that target these naturally occurring brain chemicals may be developed to help in the treatment of addiction.

Addiction Is A Disease

"Addiction fits all the criteria for a disease," says Harry Haroutunian, MD, the physician director of the Betty Ford Center, a well-known alcohol and drug addiction treatment facility. "It has a cause and effect and an organ that's its target." That target organ is the brain.

Dr. Haroutunian goes on to define a disease as loss of function of an organ or organic system—the brain, in the disease of addiction. A disease produces the same set of symptoms in everyone who is affected. For addiction, those symptoms are loss of control when using the drug of choice, craving for that drug, and persistent use despite adverse consequences.

Dr. Haroutunian emphasizes that because addiction is a disease, people with this illness do not choose to act as they do. "When people have a disease, those things that are manifested by the disease are called symptoms, not behaviors," he says.

By Laurie Lewis. Reference: Haroutunian, Harry. *Disease of Addiction*. Betty Ford Center. DVD. Available from the Betty Ford Center; excerpts online at http://www.youtube.com/watch?v=d26eiTBRGjA&feature=reimfu and http:www.youtube.com/watch?v=sN3cAiHAzXl&feature=player_detailpage. Accessed October 18, 2012.

- **Genetics:** Genetic factors account for about half the likelihood that somebody will develop an addiction. Scientists are beginning to identify which genes are responsible.

- **Developmental Factors:** Adolescents are particularly prone to alcoholism because their brains are not yet fully developed. In particular, the areas of the brain that regulate judgment, impulsiveness, and delayed gratification are still developing. As a result, teens tend to have less self-control than adults.

- **Environmental Factors:** A stressful environment increases the likelihood of addiction. Social relationships also may play a role. For example, feeling like an outcast can lead a person to drink as a way to escape. A person is more likely to drink a lot when friends also drink heavily.

A Progressive Disease

For a drinker who develops tolerance to alcohol, there's only one way to get the feeling of pleasure: to drink more. Two alcoholic drinks may seem no more potent than two glasses of water. Four drinks don't produce a buzz either. Soon it's six, eight…then who's counting? The craving for alcohol, the memory of the high from alcohol, becomes so intense that it rules the drinker's life.

A heavy drinker who tries to stop "cold turkey" is likely to have symptoms of withdrawal. The symptoms include sweating, a rapidly beating heart, and anxiety. Many people who have experienced these troubling symptoms don't want to have them again, and they keep drinking to avoid withdrawal.

With more and more drinking, tolerance continues and the amount of alcohol needed to feel good keeps increasing. Addiction has developed. With it come changes in the way the drinker behaves. The addict loses self-control and makes bad decisions.

Meanwhile, more changes have been occurring in the brain. Neurotransmitters in addition to dopamine become off-balance. Now it's not only the reward system in the brain that is affected; it's also the system controlling the response to stress. The brain actually gets smaller because nerve cells are dying and not being replaced as quickly. Some areas of the brain are more affected than others. The frontal cortex of the brain, which inhibits impulsive behavior and controls decision making, problem solving, and other advanced thinking tasks, is particularly likely to get damaged from excessive alcohol use.

Why Adolescents Are So Vulnerable

The frontal cortex of an adolescent's brain is still developing. It continues to mature until about age 25. As a result, adolescents are more likely than adults to engage in risky behaviors, such as using alcohol to excess. The immature brain does not warn teens that they are acting recklessly and making bad decisions and doesn't put on the brakes to control their behavior.

In the adolescent brain, connections among cells that get used repeatedly become stronger, and those that don't get used weaken and disappear. A teenager on the road to alcohol addiction is strengthening the neural connections associated with drinking with every swig. At the same time, less used neural connections, such as those related to sound judgment, get weaker. After a while, a teenager may have no idea how much alcohol he is consuming, what he does when drunk, and why habitual drinking needs to stop.

Now consider what happens when an adolescent addicted to alcohol engages in relatively new activities. We'll use driving as an example, but the same reasoning applies to other activities not done as a child, such as having sex or holding down a job. The teen hasn't much experience behind the wheel, so responses and judgment are not as good as in more seasoned drivers. Add to that the weakened neural connections and still-developing frontal brain of the adolescent, and the result can be a dangerous situation not only for the teen but for anyone nearby.

How An Addict Behaves

The changes that occur in the brain with addiction are not visible to the naked eye, although scientists can see them using high-tech tools such as functional magnetic resonance imaging (fMRI) and positron emission tomography (PET). While the brain changes are not readily apparent, the abnormal behavior associated with the disease of addiction is clear to anyone.

The ABCs And D And E Of Addiction

The American Society of Addiction Medicine, a group of about 3000 physicians who work in the field of addiction, has come up with a list of five characteristics of addiction.

Abstaining inability; when you just can't say "no"

Behavior out of control

Craving, or increased desire for alcohol or the rewards associated with it

Decreased recognition of significant problems with one's behavior and interpersonal relationships

Emotional response abnormal

By Laurie Lewis. Reference: American Society of Addiction Medicine. Definition of Addiction (Chevy Chase, MD: ASAMD, April 19, 2011). http://www.asam.org/research-treatment/definition-of-addiction

---

Much of human behavior is based on cues from the environment and memories associated with those cues. Think about how most people start their day. When the alarm clock goes off, they get up not just because the sound awakens them but because it triggers a memory: Ignoring the alarm means being late. Half asleep, the riser stumbles into the bathroom and begins the morning routine, not really thinking about washing up and brushing teeth because these have become such routine behaviors that they can be done almost automatically.

In the same way, an addict responds to cues in the environment, acting on them without consciously thinking. Seeing a bottle of alcohol, the addict may get a sense of pleasure. The memory of the reward from alcohol makes the addict crave a drink, and then another and another. The environmental cue does not have to be as obvious as a bottle of alcohol. It could be a memory associated with drinking, such as a scent worn by a former girlfriend, boyfriend, or drinking partner.

Environmental cues are powerful triggers of cravings, which are an important feature of alcohol addiction. An alcoholic thinks about drinking all the time, until it practically becomes an obsession. Much of an addict's day may be spent in search of the next "fix" to satisfy the craving. One drink will not do the trick; more and more is necessary. Increasingly large amounts of time are lost to drinking and trying to recover from its effects.

Although addicts may try to hide their habit, tell-tale signs offer evidence of the problem. The user may begin to neglect his or her appearance. The drinker withdraws from friends and family, preferring to be alone with a bottle. Appointments, work, or school days may be missed. When confronted about the absence and not willing or able to tell the truth, the drinker creates a story. Every episode requires another made-up excuse, and before long the alcoholic is living a life of lies. Money that would have been spent on food and other necessities may be used instead to buy alcohol. When desperate for cash to buy another bottle, borrowing without asking—in other words, stealing—may seem to be the only solution in the irrational mind of the alcoholic.

The addict may recognize that this behavior is wrong and harmful and try to gain self-control. Easier said than done! The lure of alcohol is too great, and its continued use has already damaged normal self-control mechanisms in the brain. The drinker is no longer thinking clearly—remember, the part of the brain that controls rational thought is most affected by addiction. The addict behaves recklessly, perhaps driving while under the influence or gambling in hope of winning enough to feed the habit.

Because of changes in the stress response mechanisms in the brain, every little thing seems to create more stress and anxiety than usual. An environmental trigger that the addict might have ignored in pre-drinking days—a rude remark, say—now sets off a storm of inappropriate

231

behavior. Emotions may be abnormal or shift radically. The mood swings reflect the level of dopamine in the brain: feeling good when dopamine rises, depressed when it falls. The only way to avoid the low is to drink more.

Even as behavioral abnormalities increase, the addict may fail to make the connection with alcohol use. "It's not my fault," the addict may say. "The world is against me." Soon the addict is blaming everyone other than himself or herself. Relationships with friends and family suffer badly.

Summary: A Brain Disease That Affects Behavior

With such dramatic negative behavioral aspects, it's no wonder that alcohol addiction was once thought to be mainly a behavioral disorder with strong social effects. Now that scientists have been able to study what occurs in the brain of those with addiction, it has become clear that the abnormal behavior is the visible reflection of changes in a brain damaged by repeated and excessive alcohol use. Alcohol addiction is a brain disease with behavioral symptoms that affect social functioning.

The irrational, impulsive, deceptive behavior of the addict is both frustrating and painful to friends and family. They are hurt and angry. They wish the drinker would face reality, leave alcohol alone, and return to a more pleasant, pre-addiction frame of mind. That won't happen, because the abnormal behaviors of the alcoholic are not voluntary. They are symptoms of a disease called addiction. There is no cure for this disease, but there are ways to help keep it under control.

References

American Society of Addiction Medicine. Definition of Addiction (Chevy Chase, MD: ASAMD, April 19, 2011). http://www.asam.org/research-treatment/definition-of-addiction

Chartier KG, Hesselbrock MN, Hesselbrock VM. Development and vulnerability factors in adolescent alcohol use. *Child Adolesc Psych Clin N Am* 2010;19(3):493–504.

Enoch MA. The role of GABA(A) receptors in the development of alcoholism. *Pharmacol Biochem Behav* 2006;90(1):95–104.

Frederiksen L. Underage drinking: how teens can become alcoholics before age 21. Breaking TheCycles (blog), May 28, 2009. http://www.breakingthecycles.com/blog/2009/05/28/how-teens-can-become-alcoholics-before-age-21.

Gardner EL. Addiction and brain reward and antireward pathways. *Adv Psychosom Med* 2011;30:22–60.

Gilpin NW, Koob GF. Neurobiology and alcohol dependence. *Alcohol Research Health* 2008;31(3):185–195. http://pubs.niaaa.nih.gov/publications/arh313/185-195.htm

National Institute on Alcohol Abuse and Alcoholism. Neuroscience: pathways to alcohol dependence. *Alcohol Alert*. No. 77. April 2009. http://pubs.niaaa.nih.gov/publications/AA77/AA77.pdf

National Institute on Drug Abuse. Drugs, brains, and behavior: the science of addiction. August 2010. NIH Pub No. 10-5605. http://www.drugabuse.gov/publications/science-addiction

Chapter 29

Teen Dating Violence

Understanding Teen Dating Violence

Dating violence is a type of intimate partner violence. It occurs between two people in a close relationship. The nature of dating violence can be physical, emotional, or sexual.

- **Physical:** This occurs when a partner is pinched, hit, shoved, or kicked.

- **Emotional:** This means threatening a partner or harming his or her sense of self-worth. Examples include name calling, shaming, bullying, embarrassing on purpose, or keeping him/her away from friends and family.

- **Sexual:** This is forcing a partner to engage in a sex act when he or she does not or cannot consent.

- **Stalking:** This refers to a pattern of harassing or threatening tactics used by a perpetrator that is both unwanted and causes fear in the victim.

Dating violence can take place in person or electronically, such as repeated texting or posting sexual pictures of a partner online.

About This Chapter: This chapter begins with excerpts from "Understanding Teen Dating Violence," Centers for Disease Control and Prevention (CDC; www.cdc.gov), 2012. Text under the heading "Experiencing Teen Violence" is excerpted from "Teen Dating Violence," CDC, August 22, 2012. Text under the heading "Recognizing Teen Dating Violence" is excerpted from "Violence Against Women: Dating Violence," Office on Women's Health (www.womenshealth.gov), May 18, 2011. Text under the heading "Preventing Teen Dating Violence: is excerpted from "Teen Dating Violence: Help Prevent It," *The Sara Bellum Blog*, National Institute on Drug Abuse, February 14, 2012.

Why is dating violence a public health problem?

Dating violence is a serious problem in the United States. Many teens do not report it because they are afraid to tell friends and family.

- Among adult victims of rape, physical violence, and/or stalking by an intimate partner, 22.4% of women and 15.0% of men first experienced some form of partner violence between 11 and 17 years of age.

- Approximately 9% of high school students report being hit, slapped, or physically hurt on purpose by a boyfriend or girlfriend in the 12 months before surveyed.

Who is at risk for committing dating violence?

Studies show that people who harm their dating partners are more depressed and are more aggressive than peers. These are some other factors that increase risk for harming a dating partner:

- Trauma symptoms

- Alcohol use

- Having a friend involved in dating violence

- Having problem behaviors in other areas

- Belief that dating violence is acceptable

- Exposure to harsh parenting

- Exposure to inconsistent discipline

- Lack of parental supervision, monitoring, and warmth

How can we prevent dating violence?

The ultimate goal is to stop dating violence before it starts. Strategies that promote healthy relationships are vital. During the preteen and teen years, young people are learning skills they need to form positive relationships with others. This is an ideal time to promote healthy relationships and prevent patterns of dating violence that can last into adulthood.

Prevention programs change the attitudes and behaviors linked with dating violence. One example is Safe Dates, a school-based program that is designed to change social norms and improve problem solving skills.

Experiencing Teen Dating Violence

Unhealthy relationships can start early and last a lifetime. Dating violence often starts with teasing and name calling. These behaviors are often thought to be a "normal" part of a relationship. But these behaviors can set the stage for more serious violence like physical assault and rape.

What are the consequences of dating violence?

As teens develop emotionally, they are heavily influenced by their relationship experiences. Healthy relationship behaviors can have a positive effect on a teen's emotional development. Unhealthy, abusive or violent relationships can cause short-term and long-term negative effects, or consequences to the developing teen. Victims of teen dating violence are more likely to do poorly in school, and report binge drinking, suicide attempts, and physical fighting. Victims may also carry the patterns of violence into future relationships.

Learn More About Dating Violence

For a list of Centers for Disease Control and Prevention (CDC) activities, see www.cdc.gov/violenceprevention/pub/ipv_sv_guide.html. Other resources include the following:

CDC's Dating Matters:
Strategies to Promote Healthy Teen Relationships
www.cdc.gov/violenceprevention/datingmatters

National Dating Abuse Helpline
866-331-9474 or text 77054

National Domestic Violence Hotline
800-799-SAFE (7233)

National Sexual Assault Hotline
800-656-HOPE (4673)

National Sexual Violence Resource Center
www.nsvrc.org

Dating Matters: Understanding Teen Dating Violence Prevention
www.vetoviolence.org/datingmatters

Source: CDC, 2012.

Why does dating violence happen?

Communicating with your partner, managing uncomfortable emotions like anger and jealousy, and treating others with respect are a few ways to keep relationships healthy and nonviolent. Teens receive messages about how to behave in relationships from peers, adults in their lives, and the media. All too often these examples suggest violence in a relationship is ok. Violence is never acceptable. But there are reasons why it happens.

Violence is related to certain risk factors. Risks of having unhealthy relationships increase for teens who have these characteristics:

- Believe it's okay to use threats or violence to get their way or to express frustration or anger

- Use alcohol or drugs

- Can't manage anger or frustration

- Hang out with violent peers

- Have multiple sexual partners

- Have a friend involved in dating violence

- Are depressed or anxious

- Have learning difficulties and other problems at school

- Don't have parental supervision and support

- Witness violence at home or in the community

- Have a history of aggressive behavior or bullying

Dating violence can be prevented when teens, families, organizations, and communities work together to implement effective prevention strategies.

Recognizing Teen Dating Violence

If you haven't dated much, it can be hard to know when a relationship is unhealthy. Here are some signs of teen dating abuse:

- Constantly texting or sending instant messages (IMs) to monitor you

- Insisting on getting serious very quickly

- Acting very jealous or bossy

- Pressuring you to do sexual things

- Posting sexual photos of you online without permission

- Threatening to hurt you or themselves if you break up

- Blaming you for the abuse

Teenage girls in physically abusive relationships are much more likely than other girls to become pregnant. Abuse can get worse during pregnancy, and it can harm the baby growing inside you. Never get pregnant hoping that it will stop the abuse. You can ask your doctor about types of birth control that your partner doesn't have to know you are using.

If you are under 18, your partner could get arrested for having sex with you, even if you agreed to have sex. Laws covering this are different in each state.

No Excuses

It is never okay for someone to hit you or be cruel to you. You may think alcohol or drugs make a partner abusive. Those things may increase the chances of abuse, but they never make it right.

You also may think it is your fault that your partner has hurt you. But you don't control how your partner acts, and you can't make someone mistreat you.

Keep in mind that if you sometimes hit your partner first, you can get help learning how to stop. Talk to a mental health professional, like a school counselor, or a doctor or nurse.

Source: Office on Women's Health, May 18, 2012.

How can I leaving an abusive dating relationship?

If you think you are in an abusive relationship, learn more about getting help. See a doctor or nurse to take care of any physical problems. And reach out for support for your emotional pain. Friends, family, and mental health professionals all can help. If you're in immediate danger, dial 911.

If you are thinking about ending an abusive dating relationship, keep the following tips in mind:

- Create a safety plan, like where you can go if you are in danger.

- Make sure you have a working cell phone handy in case you need to call for help.

- Create a secret code with people you trust. That way, if you are with your partner, you can get help without having to say you need help.

- If you're breaking up with someone you see at your school, you can get help from a guidance counselor, advisor, teacher, school nurse, dean's office, or principal. You also might be able to change your class schedules or even transfer to another school.

- If you have a job, talk to someone you trust at work. Your human resources department or employee assistance program (EAP) may be able to help.

- Try to avoid walking or riding alone.

- Be smart about technology. Don't share your passwords. Don't post your schedule on Facebook, and keep your settings private.

Staying Safe When Meeting Someone New

If you are meeting someone you don't know or don't know well, you can take steps to stay safe:

- Meet your date in a public place
- Tell a friend or family member your date's name and where you are going
- Avoid parties where alcohol may be served
- Make sure you have a way to get home if you need to leave
- Have a cell phone handy in case you need to call for help

Source: Office on Women's Health, May 18, 2012.

Preventing Teen Dating Violence

Did you know that alcohol and drugs play a major role in increasing violence toward a partner in a relationship? One study found that, in junior high and high school, teens who drank alcohol before age 13 were more likely to be both victims and abusers when it comes to physical dating violence. Another study found that teenage girls in abusive relationships are more likely to abuse drugs and alcohol, have eating disorders, engage in unsafe sexual behaviors, and attempt suicide. Many of the factors that contribute to violence in relationships are preventable.

What are the warning signs?

Here are some signs that a partner might have abusive tendencies:

- Unable to control his or her anger or frustration

- Lack social skills

- Use drugs and/or alcohol

- Extremely jealous, insecure, or possessive

- Constantly put you down

- Check your personal e-mail or phone without asking permission

- Isolate you from your loved ones

Although some of these characteristics might sound common, they are extremely unhealthy. If you or someone you know is in a relationship where one person acts like this, there are places you or your friend can go for help.

A Program To Prevent Teen Dating Violence

Did you know that in the past 12 months, one in 10 teens report being hit or physically hurt on purpose by a boyfriend or girlfriend at least once? And nearly half of all teens in relationships say they know friends who have been verbally abused.

Before violence starts, a teen may experience controlling behavior and demands. One partner may tell another what to wear and who to hang out with. Over time, the unhealthy behavior may become violent.

Dating violence can have a negative effect on health throughout life. Victims of teen dating violence are more likely to do poorly in school, and report binge drinking, suicide attempts, physical fighting and current sexual activity. Teens who perpetrate dating violence may also carry these patterns of violence into future relationships.

The Centers for Disease Control and Prevention's Division of Violence Prevention is leading a new initiative, Dating Matters™: Strategies to Promote Healthy Teen Relationships. Dating Matters aims to promote respectful, nonviolent dating relationships among youth in high-risk, urban communities. The comprehensive approach will build upon current evidence-based practice and experience to reduce the burden of teen dating violence in these communities. The initiative will support communities as they implement prevention strategies in schools, with families, and in neighborhoods.

Over the next five years, Dating Matters™ will be implemented in middle schools and neighborhoods across Chicago, Illinois; Baltimore, Maryland; Ft. Lauderdale, Florida; and Oakland, California.

Source: "Prevent Teen Dating Violence," Centers for Disease Control and Prevention (www.cdc.gov), February 17, 2012.

What can I do to help?

Creating awareness about dating violence among teens can help prevent more teens from getting physically or emotionally abused in their relationships. For example, you might talk to your guidance counselor about hosting an event at your school. The Teen Dating Violence Awareness Month's website (http://www.teendvmonth.org) provides free materials to help get your event started.

Or, try talking to someone in your school's newspaper office to see if they'd be willing to publish an article about teen dating violence. Anything you do to help create awareness could have a positive impact on someone you know.

How can I (or someone I know) get help?

If you or someone you know is in an abusive relationship, please seek help. Many organizations are willing to provide a free, safe space, as well as counseling. You can call the 24-hour National Dating Abuse Helpline at 866-331-9474 or go to LoveIsRespect.org for live chat support. Help is only a text message away. Text "loveis" to 77054 to begin texting with an advocate who can help you.

Also, check out the Runaway and Homeless Youth and Relationship Violence Toolkit (available online at http://www.nrcdv.org/rhydvtoolkit).

The National Online Resource Center on Violence Against Women offers more detailed information on dating violence. (available online at http://www.vawnet.org/special -collections/TDV.php#200)

Chapter 30

Rape And Date Rape

Questions And Answers About Rape And Date Rape

What is rape and date rape?

Rape is sex you don't agree to, including forcing a body part or object into your vagina, rectum (bottom), or mouth. Date rape is when you are raped by someone you know, like a boyfriend. Both are crimes. Rape is not about sex—it is an act of power by the rapist and it is always wrong.

Date rape drugs, which often have no smell or taste, can be given to you without you knowing at parties or in a club—especially where alcohol is served. Alcohol can make you less aware of danger and make you less able to think clearly and resist sexual assault. If you are given date rape drugs, you may not be able to say "no" to unwanted sex and you may not be able to clearly remember what happened.

Remember: Even if you were drinking, it is NOT your fault.

What is sexual assault?

Sexual assault and abuse is any kind of sexual activity that you do not agree to, including inappropriate touching; vaginal, anal, or oral sex; sex that you say 'no' to; rape; attempted rape; and child molestation.

About This Chapter: This chapter begins with questions and answers excerpted from "What Is Rape and Date Rape?" Office on Women's Health (www.girlshealth.gov), September 22, 2009. Text under the heading "Additional Facts About Date Rape Drugs" is excerpted from "Date Rape Drugs Fact Sheet," Office on Women's Health (www.womenshealth.gov), December 5, 2008. Reviewed by David A. Cooke, MD, FACP, December 2012.

Sexual assault can be verbal, visual, or anything that forces a person to join in unwanted sexual contact or attention. Examples of this are voyeurism (when someone watches private sexual acts), exhibitionism (when someone exposes him/herself in public), incest (sexual contact between family members), and sexual harassment. It can happen in different situations, by a stranger in an isolated place, on a date, or in the home by someone you know.

What should I know about date rape drugs?

Date rape drugs are most commonly used to sexually assault a person. The drugs often have no color, smell, or taste and are easily added to drinks without the victim's knowledge. These drugs usually cause a person to become helpless—they can hardly move and are not able to protect themselves from being hurt. People who have been given date rape drugs say they felt paralyzed or couldn't see well, and had black-outs, problems talking, confusion, and dizziness. Date rape drugs can even cause death.

It's hard to know whether a party, club, or concert you plan to go to will be dangerous. Drugs may not be at every party you go to, but you should still have a plan for keeping yourself and your friends safe no matter what.

- Say "NO" to alcohol. Have water or soda instead.

- Open your own drinks.

- Don't let other people hand you drinks.

- Keep your drink with you at all times, even when you go to the bathroom.

- Don't share drinks.

- Don't drink from punch bowls or other large, common, open containers. They may already have drugs in them.

- Don't drink anything that tastes, looks, or smells strange. Sometimes, GHB tastes salty.

- Always go to a party, club, or concert with someone you trust, such as a friend or an older brother or sister.

- Stay away from "party drugs." They can be pills, liquids, or powders. These drugs can also leave you disoriented and vulnerable.

Here are some tips if you think that you or someone you know has been drugged and raped:

- Don't blame yourself. The rape was not your fault.

- Talk to an adult and go to the police station or hospital right away! If you don't have an adult to talk to first, just go to the police station or hospital.

- Don't urinate (pee) before getting help.

- Get a urine (pee) test as soon as possible. The drugs leave your system quickly. Rohypnol leaves your body 72 hours after you take it. GHB leaves the body in 12 hours.

- Don't douche, bathe, or change clothes before getting help. Doing these things can remove possible evidence of the rape, such as semen (fluid from a man) or hair belonging to the person who assaulted you.

- Get medical care right away. Tell the doctor or nurse if you think you were drugged. He or she will give you a urine test right away because date rape drugs leave your body quickly. You will also get a medical exam to make sure you don't have other injuries. The doctor or nurse will test you for sexually transmitted diseases (STDs), including HIV/AIDS, and offer you emergency contraception to prevent pregnancy. If the doctor or nurse does not mention testing for STDs or emergency contraception, ask for them.

- The counselor will help you figure out how to tell your parents/guardians. They may be angry or upset, but only because they care about you and don't want you to get hurt. Getting help and dealing with your emotions is the first step in healing.

- You can call a crisis center or a hotline to talk with a counselor. One national hotline is the 24-hour National Domestic Violence Hotline at 800-799-SAFE (800-799-7233) or 800-787-3224 (TDD). Feelings of shame, guilt, fear, and shock are normal. It is important to get counseling from a trusted professional.

Additional Facts About Date Rape Drugs

The three most common date rape drugs are Rohypnol, GHB, and ketamine. These drugs also are known as *club drugs* because they tend to be used at dance clubs, concerts, and raves. Rohypnol is the trade name for flunitrazepam. Abuse of two similar drugs appears to have

---

Get Help

National Sexual Assault Hotline: 800-656-4673

The hotline is free, private, and available 24 hours a day.

Source: Office on Women's Health, September 22, 2009.

---

replaced Rohypnol abuse in some parts of the United States. These are clonazepam (marketed as Klonopin in the U.S. and Rivotril in Mexico) and alprazolam (marketed as Xanax). GHB is short for gamma hydroxybutyric acid.

The term *date rape* is widely used. But most experts prefer the term *drug-facilitated sexual assault*. These drugs also are used to help people commit other crimes, like robbery and physical assault. They are used on both men and women. The term *date rape* also can be misleading because the person who commits the crime might not be dating the victim. Rather, it could be an acquaintance or stranger.

What do the drugs look like?

Rohypnol comes as a pill that dissolves in liquids. Some are small, round, and white. Newer pills are oval and green-gray in color. When slipped into a drink, a dye in these new pills makes clear liquids turn bright blue and dark drinks turn cloudy. But this color change might be hard to see in a dark drink, like cola or dark beer, or in a dark room. Also, the pills with no dye are still available. The pills may be ground up into a powder.

GHB has a few forms: A liquid with no odor or color, white powder, and pill. It might give your drink a slightly salty taste. Mixing it with a sweet drink, such as fruit juice, can mask the salty taste.

Ketamine comes as a liquid and a white powder.

What effects do these drugs have on the body?

These drugs are very powerful. They can affect you very quickly and without your knowing. The length of time that the effects last varies. It depends on how much of the drug is taken and if the drug is mixed with other drugs or alcohol. Alcohol makes the drugs even stronger and can cause serious health problems—even death.

Rohypnol: The effects of Rohypnol can be felt within 30 minutes of being drugged and can last for several hours. If you are drugged, you might look and act like someone who is drunk. You might have trouble standing. Your speech might be slurred. Or you might pass out. Rohypnol can cause these problems:

- Muscle relaxation or loss of muscle control

- Difficulty with motor movements

- Drunk feeling

- Problems talking

Slang Terms For Rohypnol

- Circles
- Forget Pill
- LA Rochas
- Lunch Money
- Mexican Valium
- Mind Erasers
- Poor Man's Quaalude
- R-2
- Rib
- Roach
- Roach-2
- Roches
- Roofies
- Roopies
- Rope
- Rophies
- Ruffies
- Trip-and-Fall
- Whiteys

Slang Terms For GHB

- Bedtime Scoop
- Cherry Meth
- Easy Lay
- Energy Drink
- G
- Gamma 10
- Georgia Home Boy
- G-Juice
- Gook
- Goop
- Great Hormones
- Grievous Bodily Harm (GBH)
- Liquid E
- Liquid Ecstasy
- Liquid X
- PM
- Salt Water
- Soap
- Somatomax
- Vita-G

Slang Terms For Ketamine

- Black Hole
- Bump
- Cat Valium
- Green
- Jet
- K
- K-Hole
- Kit Kat
- Psychedelic Heroin
- Purple
- Special K
- Super Acid

Source: Office on Women's Health, December 2008.

- Nausea
- Can't remember what happened while drugged
- Loss of consciousness (black out)
- Confusion
- Problems seeing
- Dizziness
- Sleepiness
- Lower blood pressure
- Stomach problems
- Death

GHB: GHB takes effect in about 15 minutes and can last three or four hours. It is very potent: A very small amount can have a big effect. So it's easy to overdose on GHB. Most GHB is made by people in home or street "labs." So, you don't know what's in it or how it will affect you. GHB can cause these problems:

- Relaxation

- Drowsiness

- Dizziness

- Nausea

- Problems seeing

- Loss of consciousness (black out)

- Seizures

- Can't remember what happened while drugged

- Problems breathing

- Tremors

- Sweating

- Vomiting

- Slow heart rate

- Dream-like feeling

- Coma

- Death

Ketamine: Ketamine is very fast-acting. You might be aware of what is happening to you, but unable to move. It also causes memory problems. Later, you might not be able to remember what happened while you were drugged. Ketamine can cause these problems:

- Distorted perceptions of sight and sound

- Lost sense of time and identity

- Out of body experiences

- Dream-like feeling

- Feeling out of control

- Impaired motor function

- Problems breathing

- Convulsions

- Vomiting

- Memory problems

- Numbness

- Loss of coordination

- Aggressive or violent behavior

- Depression

- High blood pressure

- Slurred speech

Is alcohol a date rape drug? What about other drugs?

Any drug that can affect judgment and behavior can put a person at risk for unwanted or risky sexual activity. Alcohol is one such drug. In fact, alcohol is the drug most commonly used to help commit sexual assault. When a person drinks too much alcohol, these consequences occur:

- It's harder to think clearly.

- It's harder to set limits and make good choices.

- It's harder to tell when a situation could be dangerous.

- It's harder to say "no" to sexual advances.

- It's harder to fight back if a sexual assault occurs.

- It's possible to blackout and to have memory loss.

The club drug "ecstasy" (MDMA) has been used to commit sexual assault. It can be slipped into someone's drink without the person's knowledge. Also, a person who willingly takes ecstasy is at greater risk of sexual assault. It can lower a person's ability to give reasoned consent. Once under the drug's influence, a person is less able to sense danger or to resist a sexual assault.

Even if a victim of sexual assault drank alcohol or willingly took drugs, the victim is not at fault for being assaulted. You cannot "ask for it" or cause it to happen.

Chapter 31

Sexual Risk Behaviors And Sexually Transmitted Infections

You probably have heard of sexually transmitted infections (STIs)—also called sexually transmitted diseases, or STDs. But if you are like many people, you might not know that much about how STIs could impact your health. You might not think you need to worry about STIs. Yet STIs are a major public health concern in the United States, where an estimated 19 million new infections occur each year. STIs affect people of all backgrounds and economic levels. Thankfully, most STIs are preventable. Taking a few protective steps can lower your risk of getting an STI.

What is a sexually transmitted infection (STI)?

A sexually transmitted infection (STI) is an infection you can get by having intimate sexual contact with someone who already has the infection. STIs can be caused by viruses, bacteria, and parasites. You can have an STI and not even know it.

How are STIs spread?

STIs are spread during vaginal or anal intercourse, oral sex, and genital touching. It is possible to get some STIs without having intercourse. You can't tell if a person has an STI by the way he or she looks. Talking about sex is awkward for some people. They may not bring up safe sex or STIs with their partners. If you have unprotected sex, you may be exposed to the STIs that your partner's past and present partners have had. This is true even if you have been sexually active with only one person.

About This Chapter: This chapter includes excerpts from "Chapter 11: Sexually Transmitted Infections," *The Healthy Woman: A Complete Guide for All Ages*, Office on Women's Health (www.womenshealth.gov), November 1, 2008. Revised by David A. Cooke, MD, FACP, December 2012.

Alcohol And HIV/AIDS

Each year in the United States, between 55,000 and 60,000 people become infected with the human immunodeficiency virus (HIV), for a total of more than 1.1 million now infected. The population that once was primarily made up of homosexual white men is now composed increasingly of people of color, women, and young people. Also, as more young women are becoming infected, there is growing concern that the virus will be transmitted to their children, either during pregnancy or after birth.

One of the main reasons for this shift in the HIV population is that heterosexual sex is now a primary route for HIV transmission. Alcohol use is one of the factors that increases the risk of HIV transmission among heterosexuals. Particularly among women, a strong association has been seen between alcohol and other drug abuse, infection with HIV, and progression to acquired immune deficiency syndrome (AIDS). Although additional studies are needed to further define alcohol use patterns among infected and at-risk people, it is clear that alcohol use is closely intertwined with the spread of HIV.

Source: Excerpted from "Alcohol and HIV/AIDS: Intertwining Stories," National Institute on Alcohol Abuse and Alcoholism (www.niaaa.nih.gov), *Alcohol Alert*, No. 80, 2010.

What are some common types of STIs?

Bacterial Vaginosis (BV): BV is the most common vaginal infection in women of childbearing age. With BV, the normal balance of bacteria in the vagina is changed so that there are more "harmful" bacteria and fewer "good" bacteria. BV is not always a STI, and it can occur without sex. However, it can also be sexually transmitted. Antibiotics are used to treat and cure BV.

Chlamydia: Chlamydia is the most frequently reported STI caused by bacteria. It is a "silent" disease because 75 percent of infected women and at least half of infected men have no symptoms. Severe complications can result from untreated chlamydia. Antibiotics are used to treat and cure chlamydia.

Genital Herpes: Genital herpes is caused by the herpes simplex viruses type 1 (HSV-1) and type 2 (HSV-2). Most genital herpes is caused by HSV-2. About one in four women in the United States have had HSV-2 infection. The virus will stay in the body forever. But outbreaks, for people who have them, tend to be less severe and occur less often over time. Also, antiviral therapy can shorten outbreaks and make them less severe, or keep them from happening.

Gonorrhea: Gonorrhea is caused by a type of bacteria that thrives in warm, moist areas of the reproductive tract. It also can grow in the mouth, throat, eyes, and anus. Most women who have gonorrhea have no symptoms. Untreated gonorrhea can lead to serious health problems.

Antibiotics are used to cure gonorrhea. But gonorrhea has become more and more resistant to antibiotics, which means the drugs do not work as well or at all. Still, it's important to get tested and treated by a doctor.

Hepatitis B: Hepatitis B (HBV) is one type of viral hepatitis. With hepatitis, the liver does not work well. In most people, HBV gets better on its own. Long-lasting hepatitis (chronic) can lead to scarring of the liver, liver failure, and liver cancer. Chronic HBV can be suppressed with some antiviral drugs. But these drugs don't work for all people. Vaccines are available for hepatitis A and B.

HIV/AIDS: HIV stands for human immunodeficiency virus. When you are infected with a virus, it first invades a few cells in the body and makes many copies of itself. The new viruses then leave these cells and seek out more cells to invade. Viruses often kill the cells they invade. HIV invades cells of the immune system, which protects the body from disease. HIV primarily invades immune cells called CD4 positive (CD4+) T cells. These cells tell other immune cells when they are needed to fight a specific infection. Usually, a healthy, uninfected person has about 1000 CD4+ T cells per microliter (millionth of a liter) of blood. This is known as your CD4 count. If you become HIV-infected, your CD4 count may stay normal for several years. This is because your body is able to replace the CD4+ T cells that HIV destroys, at least for a while. Without treatment, your CD4 count will eventually drop. When it drops below 200, you have developed AIDS (which stands for acquired immune deficiency syndrome). You can also develop AIDS if your CD4 count is above 200 and you have certain infections or cancers.

Pubic Lice: Also called "crabs," pubic lice are parasites found in the genital area on pubic hair and sometimes on other coarse body hairs. Pubic lice are common. They are different from head lice. Special shampoos and medicines are used to kill pubic lice.

Human Papillomavirus (HPV) And Genital Warts: There are more than 100 types of HPV, 30 of which are passed through sexual contact. The types of HPV that infect the genital area are called genital HPV. HPV is very common. Most sexually active people will have it at some point in their lives.

Some types of genital HPV are "high risk," which means they put a woman at greater risk of getting cervical cancer. "High risk" does not have to do with the risk of getting HPV. Low-risk types of HPV do not cause cervical cancer. But low-risk types of HPV may cause genital warts.

There is no treatment or cure for HPV. However, two new HPV vaccines protect against some HPV types that cause cancer or warts, and these vaccines are now recommended for men and women between the ages of 9 and 26 years old to reduce risk of infection and spread of the virus.

Syphilis: Syphilis is caused by a type of bacteria. It progresses in stages. Without treatment, the infection will continue to progress, possibly leading to death. Syphilis can be cured with an antibiotic. Penicillin is the preferred drug to treat syphilis at all stages. Doctors can use other medicines for people who cannot take penicillin.

Trichomoniasis: This infection, also called "trich," is caused by a parasite. It usually is passed through sexual contact. But it also can be picked up from contact with damp, moist objects. Antibiotics are used to treat and cure trichomoniasis.

How are STIs treated?

The treatment depends on the type of STI. For some STIs, treatment may involve using medicine or getting a shot. For STIs that cannot be cured, like genital herpes, treatment can ease symptoms. During treatment, follow all of your doctor's orders and avoid sex during treatment or an outbreak. And be sure to finish all the medicine your doctor gives you, even if your symptoms go away. With most STIs, your sexual partner(s) should be treated, too. This can keep you from getting the STI again or your partner from passing it to other people. Remember, the sooner an STI is found, the easier it is to treat and the less likely you will have health complications.

Sexual Risks And Health Consequences

Many young people engage in sexual risk behaviors that can result in unintended health outcomes. For example, these statistics pertain to U.S. high school students surveyed in 2011:

- 47.4% had ever had sexual intercourse

- 33.7% had had sexual intercourse during the previous three months, and, of these 39.8% did not use a condom the last time they had sex

- 76.7% did not use birth control pills or Depo-Provera to prevent pregnancy the last time they had sex

- 15.3% had had sex with four or more people during their life

To reduce sexual risk behaviors and related health problems among youth, schools and other youth-serving organizations can help young people adopt lifelong attitudes and behaviors that support their health and well-being—including behaviors that reduce their risk for HIV, other STDs, and unintended pregnancy.

Source: From "Sexual Risk Behavior: HIV, STD, and Teen Pregnancy Prevention," Centers for Disease Control and Prevention (www.cdc.gov), July 24, 2012.

How can untreated STI's affect a person's health?

You might be too shy to talk to your doctor about your risk of STIs or any symptoms you might be having. But not talking to your doctor could be far worse than any embarrassment you might feel. Untreated STIs can cause severe health problems especially for women, such as pelvic inflammatory disease, infertility, ectopic pregnancy, widespread infection to other parts of the body, caner, organ damage, and even death.

STIs can cause additional health problems for pregnant women. STIs during pregnancy can cause early labor, cause the water to break early, and cause infection in the uterus after the birth. STIs also can cause problems for the unborn baby. Some STIs can cross the placenta and infect the baby while it is in the uterus. Others can be passed from a pregnant woman to the baby during delivery. The harmful effects to babies range from low birth weight, to chronic liver disease, to stillbirth. Some of these problems can be prevented if the mother has routine prenatal care, which includes screening tests for STIs at various points during the pregnancy. Other problems can be treated if the infection is found at birth or within a few days after birth. Some STIs can also be passed to a baby through breastfeeding. And some medicines used to treat STIs can pass to a baby through breast milk.

What is pelvic inflammatory disease (PID)?

Pelvic inflammatory disease, or PID, is a broad term used to describe an infection of a woman's pelvic organs. Many types of bacteria can cause PID. Often, PID is a complication of untreated STIs—mainly chlamydia and gonorrhea. Damage from PID can cause a woman to become infertile (not able to become pregnant). In fact, about one in every five women with PID becomes infertile. PID also can cause chronic pelvic pain and ectopic pregnancy (pregnancy in the fallopian tube, which can be life threatening). It can be hard to tell if a woman has PID because there are no specific tests for PID and she might have mild or no symptoms. Women who have symptoms might have pain in the lower belly area, fever, or an unusual vaginal discharge, which may smell bad. They may also have pain during sex, bleeding between periods, or pain during pelvic exam.

Once found, PID can be cured with antibiotics—but any damage already done to a woman's reproductive organs before treatment cannot be reversed, so early treatment of PID is important. A woman should see her doctor right away if she thinks she might have an STI or PID.

How can a person be protected from STIs?

Even though STIs pass easily from person to person, there are steps you can take to lower your risk of getting an STI. The following steps work best when used together—no single strategy can protect you from every single type of STI.

Don't have sex. The surest way to avoid getting any STI is to practice abstinence, which means not having vaginal, oral, or anal sex. Keep in mind that some STIs, such as genital herpes, can be spread without having intercourse.

Be faithful. Having sex with one uninfected partner who only has sex with you will keep you safe from STIs. Both partners must be faithful all the time to avoid STI exposure. This means that you have sex only with each other and no one else. The fewer sex partners you have, the lower your risk of being exposed to an STI.

Use condoms correctly and EVERY time you have sex. Use condoms for all types of sexual contact, even if penetration does not take place. Condoms work by keeping blood, a man's semen, and a woman's vaginal fluid—all of which can carry STIs—from passing from one person to another. Use protection from the very beginning to the very end of each sex act, and with every sex partner. And be prepared: Don't rely on your partner to have protection.

Know that certain birth control methods—and other methods—don't protect against STIs. Birth control methods including the pill, shots, implants, intrauterine devices (IUDs), diaphragms, and spermicides will not protect you from STIs. They only can help keep you from getting pregnant. Still, many women who use these forms of birth control don't use condoms. If you use one of these birth control methods, make sure to also use a condom with every sex act. Also, don't use contraceptives that contain the spermicide nonoxynol-9 (N-9). N-9 can irritate the vagina, which might make it easier for an STI—including HIV—to get into your body. Keep in mind that women who are unable to become pregnant can still get STIs

You might have heard of other ways to keep from getting STIs—such as washing genitals before sex, passing urine after sex, douching after sex, or washing the genital area with vinegar after sex. These methods DO NOT prevent the spread of STIs.

Talk with your sex partner(s) about using condoms before having sex. This way, you can set the ground rules and avoid misunderstandings during a moment of passion. Hopefully, you and your partner will agree to use condoms all the time. But know this: You can control their use by making it clear that you will not have any type of sex at any time without a condom. Remember, it's your body, and it's up to you to make sure you are protected.

Don't assume you're at low risk for STIs if you have sex only with women. Some common STIs are spread easily by skin-to-skin contact. Also, most women who have sex with women have had sex with men, too. So a woman can get an STI from a male partner, and then pass it to a female partner.

Don't abuse drugs or alcohol. Drinking and drug use can put you at greater risk of STIs. Drinking too much and using drugs are linked to sexual risk-taking, such as having sex with more than one partner and not using condoms. Drug users who share needles risk exposure to blood-borne infections that also can be passed sexually, such as HIV and hepatitis B. Drinking too much alcohol or using drugs puts you at risk of sexual assault and possible exposure to an STI.

HIV Among Youth

All young people should know how to protect themselves from infection with the human immunodeficiency virus (HIV). Too many young people in the United States are at risk for HIV infection. This risk is especially notable for young gay, bisexual, and other men who have sex with men (MSM), especially young African American or Latino MSM, and all youth of minority races and ethnicities.

In 2009, young persons accounted for 39% of all new HIV infections in the U.S. For comparison's sake, persons aged 15–29 comprised 21% of the U.S. population in 2010. Young MSM, especially those of minority races and ethnicities, are at increased risk for HIV infection. In 2009, young MSM accounted for 27% of new HIV infections in the U.S. and 69% of new HIV infections among persons aged 13–29. Among young black MSM, new HIV infections increased 48% from 2006 through 2009.

The Added Problem Of Substance Use

Young people in the U.S. use alcohol, tobacco, and other drugs at high rates. The 2009 National Youth Risk Behavior Survey conducted by the Centers for Disease Control and Prevention (CDC) found that 24.2% of high school students had had five or more drinks of alcohol in a row on at least one day during the 30 days before the survey, and 20.8% had used marijuana at least one time during the 30 days before the survey. Both casual and chronic substance users are more likely to engage in high-risk behaviors, such as unprotected sex, when they are under the influence of drugs or alcohol. Runaways, homeless young people, and young persons who have become dependent on drugs are at high risk for HIV infection if they exchange sex for drugs, money, or shelter.

Lack Of Awareness

Research has shown that a large proportion of young people are not concerned about becoming infected with HIV. This lack of awareness can translate into not taking measures that could protect their health.

Abstaining from sex and drug use is the most effective way to avoid HIV infection, but adolescents need accurate, age-appropriate information about HIV and acquired immune deficiency syndrome (AIDS), how to reduce or eliminate risk factors, how to talk with a potential partner about risk factors and how to negotiate safer sex, where to get tested for HIV, and how to use a condom correctly.

Source: Excerpted from "HIV among Youth," Centers for Disease Control and Prevention (www.cdc.gov), December 2, 2011.

Get tested for STIs. If either you or your partner has had other sexual partners in the past, get tested for STIs before becoming sexually active. Don't wait for your doctor to ask you about getting tested—ask your doctor! Many tests for STIs can be done at the same time as your regular pelvic exam.

Have regular checkups and pelvic exams—even if you think you're healthy. During the checkup, your doctor will ask you a lot of questions about your lifestyle, including your sex life. This might seem too personal to share. But answering honestly is the only way your doctor is sure to give you the care you need. Your doctor might also do a Pap test or HPV testing to check for signs of cancer in your cervix. Ask your doctor how often you need a Pap test. Also, ask your doctor if the HPV vaccine is right for you.

Chapter 32

Impaired Driving

Facts About Teen Drivers

Motor vehicle crashes are the leading cause of death for U.S. teens. In 2010, seven teens ages 16 to 19 died every day from motor vehicle injuries. Per mile driven, teen drivers ages 16 to 19 are three times more likely than drivers aged 20 and older to be in a fatal crash. Fortunately, teen motor vehicle crashes are preventable, and proven strategies can improve the safety of young drivers on the road.

Among teen drivers, these are the groups at especially high risk for motor vehicle crashes:

- **Males:** In 2010, the motor vehicle death rate for male drivers and passengers ages 16 to 19 was almost two times that of their female counterparts.

- **Teens Driving With Teen Passengers:** The presence of teen passengers increases the crash risk of unsupervised teen drivers. This risk increases with the number of teen passengers.

- **Newly Licensed Teens:** Crash risk is particularly high during the first months of licensure.

Teens are more likely than older drivers to underestimate dangerous situations or not be able to recognize hazardous situations. Teens are also more likely than older drivers to speed and allow shorter headways (the distance from the front of one vehicle to the front of the next). The presence of male teenage passengers increases the likelihood of this risky driving behavior.

About This Chapter: This chapter begins with excerpts from "Teen Drivers: Fact Sheet," Centers for Disease Control and Prevention (CDC; www.cdc.gov), October 2, 2012. It continues with excerpts from "Impaired Driving: Get the Facts," CDC, October 2, 2012; "Impaired Driving: Research and Activities," CDC, February 17, 2011; and "Drinking and Driving: A Threat to Everyone," CDC, October 4, 2011.

Among male drivers between 15 and 20 years of age who were involved in fatal crashes in 2010, 39% were speeding at the time of the crash and 25% had been drinking. Furthermore, compared with other age groups, teens have the lowest rate of seat belt use. In 2011, only 54% of high school students reported they always wear seat belts when riding with someone else.

Alcohol is also a concern. At all levels of blood alcohol concentration (BAC), the risk of involvement in a motor vehicle crash is greater for teens than for older drivers. Here are some statistics:

- In 2010, 22% of drivers aged 15 to 20 involved in fatal motor vehicle crashes were drinking.

- In a national survey conducted in 2011, 24% of teens reported that, within the previous month, they had ridden with a driver who had been drinking alcohol and 8% reported having driven after drinking alcohol within the same one-month period.

- In 2010, 56% of drivers aged 15 to 20 were killed in motor vehicle crashes after drinking and driving were not wearing a seat belt.

- In 2010, half of teen deaths from motor vehicle crashes occurred between 3:00 p.m. and midnight and 55% occurred on Friday, Saturday, or Sunday.

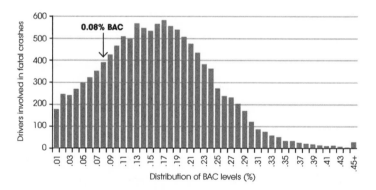

Figure 32.1. Impaired drivers involved in fatal crashes are often well over the illegal threshold of 0.08% BAC (Source: "Policy Impact: Alcohol Impaired Driving," Centers for Disease Control and Prevention, February 2011).

Impaired Driving: Get The Facts

Every day, almost 30 people in the United States die in motor vehicle crashes that involve an alcohol-impaired driver. This amounts to one death every 48 minutes. The annual cost of alcohol-related crashes totals more than $51 billion.

- In 2010, 10,228 people were killed in alcohol-impaired driving crashes, accounting for nearly one-third (31%) of all traffic-related deaths in the United States.

- Of the 1,210 traffic deaths among children ages 0 to 14 years in 2010, 211 (17%) involved an alcohol-impaired driver.

- Of the 211 child passengers ages 14 and younger who died in alcohol-impaired driving crashes in 2010, over half (131) were riding in the vehicle with the alcohol-impaired driver.

- In 2010, over 1.4 million drivers were arrested for driving under the influence of alcohol or narcotics. That's one percent of the 112 million self-reported episodes of alcohol-impaired driving among U.S. adults each year.

- Drugs other than alcohol (for example, marijuana and cocaine) are involved in about 18% of motor vehicle driver deaths. These other drugs are often used in combination with alcohol.

Preventing Deaths And Injuries From Alcohol-Impaired Drivers

The following are effective measures for preventing deaths and injuries from alcohol-impaired drivers:

- Actively enforcing existing 0.08% BAC laws, minimum legal drinking age laws, and zero tolerance laws for drivers younger than 21 years old in all states

- Promptly taking away the driver's licenses of people who drive while intoxicated

- Using sobriety checkpoints

- Putting health promotion efforts into practice that influence economic, organizational, policy, and school/community action

- Using community-based approaches to alcohol control and DWI (driving while intoxicated) prevention

- Requiring mandatory substance abuse assessment and treatment, if needed, for DWI offenders

Sobriety Checkpoints

Sobriety checkpoints are traffic stops where law enforcement officers assess drivers' level of alcohol impairment; these checkpoints consistently reduce alcohol-related crashes, typically by 9%.

Source: "Impaired Driving: Get the Facts," CDC, October 2, 2012.

Impaired Driving: Prevention Research

A systematic review conducted by researchers from the Centers for Disease Control and Prevention (CDC) on behalf of the Task Force on Community Preventive Services concluded that well-executed multi-component interventions with community mobilization are effective in reducing alcohol-related crashes. The interventions included most or all of following: responsible beverage service training, other efforts to limit alcohol access, sobriety checkpoints, and a strong local media component. Based on these findings, the Task Force recommended that multi-component interventions with community mobilization be widely implemented.

Ignition Interlock Programs: Ignition interlocks are installed in vehicles to prevent operation by anyone with a blood alcohol concentration (BAC) above a specified level (usually 0.02%–0.04%). CDC reviewed the effectiveness of ignition interlocks programs to reduce alcohol-impaired driving recidivism and alcohol-related crashes. The review concluded that ignition interlocks are associated with a median 67% reduction in re-arrest rates for alcohol-impaired driving. Based on strong evidence of the effectiveness of interlocks in reducing re-arrest rates while they are on the vehicle, the Task Force recommended that ignition interlock programs be more widely implemented. They also noted that the public health benefits of the intervention are currently limited by the small proportion of offenders who install interlocks in their vehicles. More widespread and sustained use of interlocks among this population could have a substantial impact on alcohol-related crashes.

Minimum Legal Drinking Age (MLDA) Laws: Some college administrators have suggested that minimum legal drinking age (MLDA) laws contribute to the problem of underage alcohol use and that lowering the MLDA could reduce binge drinking among underage students. Two systematic reviews conducted on behalf of the Task Force on Community Preventive Services provide evidence to refute such claims.

One review assessed the effect of both raising and lowering the MLDA on fatal and nonfatal crashes. Raising the MLDA reduced crashes among 18-20 year old drivers by a median of 16%, while lowering the MLDA increased crashes among the targeted group by a median of 10%.

The other review assessed the effect of programs to enforce laws prohibiting retail sale of alcohol to minors through the use of retailer compliance checks. These enhanced enforcement programs reduced sales to underage or youthful-looking decoys by a median of 42%. The programs were effective in on-premises (for example, bars) and off-premises (for example, liquor stores) establishments, as well as in rural and urban communities, and among different ethnic and socioeconomic groups.

Sobriety Checkpoints: A systematic review conducted by CDC researchers on behalf of the Task Force on Community Preventive Services concluded that sobriety checkpoints reduce alcohol-related crashes. Sobriety checkpoints are traffic stops where law enforcement officers systematically select drivers to assess their level of alcohol impairment. The goal of sobriety checkpoints is to deter alcohol-impaired driving by increasing drivers' perceived risk of arrest. Results indicated that sobriety checkpoints consistently reduced alcohol-related crashes, typically by about 20 percent. The results were similar regardless of how the checkpoints were conducted, for short-term "blitzes," or when checkpoints were used continuously for several years. This suggests that the effectiveness of checkpoints does not diminish over time.

Drinking And Driving: A Threat To Everyone

U.S. drivers got behind the wheel after drinking about 112 million times in 2010. Whenever anyone drives drunk, they put everyone on the road in danger. Choose not to drink and drive and help others do the same.

Though episodes of drinking and driving have gone down by 30% during the past five years, it remains a serious problem. Alcohol-impaired drivers are involved in about one in three crash deaths.

Certain groups are more likely to drink and drive than others:

- Men were responsible for four in five episodes (81%) of drinking and driving in 2010.

- Young men ages 21–34 made up only 11% of the U.S. population in 2010, yet were responsible for 32% of all instances of drinking and driving.

- 85% of drinking and driving episodes were reported by people who also reported binge drinking. Binge drinking means five or more drinks for men or four or more drinks for women during a short period of time.

Everyone Can Help

- Choose to not drink and drive and help others do the same. If drinking occurs, designate a nondrinking driver when with a group; otherwise, get a ride home or call a taxi. Don't let friends drink and drive.

- Choose not to binge drink and help others not to do it.

- Talk with a doctor or nurse about drinking and driving and request counseling if drinking is causing health, school, or social problems.

Ignition Interlocks Reduce Alcohol-Impaired Driving

Ignition interlocks are devices that can be installed in vehicles to prevent someone from operating a vehicle with a blood alcohol concentration (BAC) above a specified level. This level is usually 0.02 to 0.04 grams per deciliter (g/dL); the minimum illegal BAC level is 0.08 g/dL in every state. The devices work by sampling the driver's breath before the vehicle can be started and periodically while it is operating.

Interlocks are most often used to prevent impaired driving by people who have already been convicted of driving while intoxicated (DWI). They may be mandated through the court system or offered as an alternative to a suspended driver's license. The Task Force on Community Preventive Services, an independent nonfederal body of public health experts, recommends the use of ignition interlocks for people convicted of alcohol-impaired driving on the basis of strong evidence of their effectiveness in reducing re-arrest rates.

As of December 2010, 13 states required interlocks for all convicted offenders, including a first conviction. More than half of all states require some offenders—such as those with multiple convictions, or an extremely high BAC at the time of arrest—to install ignition interlocks. Nonetheless, only a small proportion of DWI offenders participate in interlock programs.

The Centers for Disease Control and Prevention (CDC) recommends more widespread use of interlocks and ignition interlocks for everyone convicted of DWI, even for first convictions.

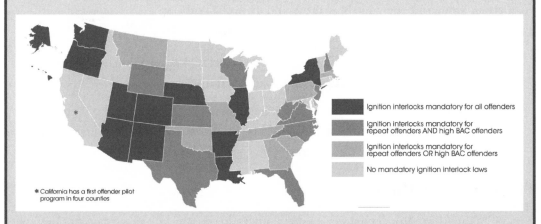

* California has a first offender pilot program in four counties

Ignition interlocks mandatory for all offenders

Ignition interlocks mandatory for repeat offenders AND high BAC offenders

Ignition interlocks mandatory for repeat offenders OR high BAC offenders

No mandatory ignition interlock laws

Figure 32.2. How state ignition interlock laws measure up (Source: "Policy Impact: Alcohol Impaired Driving," Centers for Disease Control and Prevention, February 2011).

Source: Excerpted from "Ignition Interlocks Reduce Alcohol-Impaired Driving," Centers for Disease Control and Prevention (CDC), February 22, 2011.

- Never ride with a person who has been drinking, but whenever you ride in a car—even with a sober driver—buckle up every time, no matter how short the trip. Encourage passengers in the car to buckle up, including those in the back seat. Seat belts help keep everyone safe on the road. Seat belts can protect every passenger on every trip. Just by buckling up, you reduce your risk of serious injuries and deaths from crashes by about 50%.

Part Five
Alcoholism Treatment
And Recovery

Chapter 33

Rethinking Drinking

How Much Do You Drink?

Do you think you may drink too much at times? Do you think "everyone" drinks a lot? See Figure 33.1 for results from a nationwide survey of 43,000 adults by the National Institutes of Health on alcohol use and its consequences.

Can You "Hold Your Liquor"?

If so, you may be at greater risk. For some people, it takes quite a few drinks to get a buzz or feel relaxed. Often they are unaware that being able to "hold your liquor" isn't protection from alcohol problems, but instead a reason for caution. They tend to drink more, socialize with people who drink a lot, and develop a tolerance to alcohol. As a result, they have an increased risk for developing alcoholism. The higher alcohol levels can also cause liver, heart, and brain damage that can go unnoticed until it's too late. And all drinkers need to be aware that even moderate amounts of alcohol can significantly impair driving performance, even when they don't feel a buzz from drinking.

Thinking About A Change?

It's up to you as to whether and when to change your drinking. Other people may be able to help, but in the end it's your decision. Weighing your pros and cons can help.

Pros: What are some reasons why you might want to make a change? Here are some examples:

About This Chapter: Excerpted and adapted from "Rethinking Drinking," National Institute on Alcohol Abuse and Alcoholism (www.niaaa.nih.gov), April 2010.

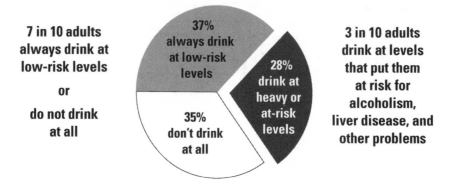

7 in 10 adults always drink at low-risk levels

or

do not drink at all

3 in 10 adults drink at levels that put them at risk for alcoholism, liver disease, and other problems

Figure 33.1. Alcohol use by adults* in the United States (*Although the minimum legal drinking age in the U.S. is 21, this survey included people aged 18 or older.)

- To improve my health
- To improve my relationships
- To avoid hangovers
- To do better at school
- To lose weight or get fit
- To save money
- To avoid more serious problems
- To meet my own personal standards

Cons: What are some possible reasons why you might not want to change?

Compare: Compare your pros and cons. Is there a difference between where you are and where you want to be?

Ready?

Are you ready to change your drinking? Don't be surprised if you continue to have mixed feelings. You may need to re-make your decision several times before becoming comfortable with it.

If you're not ready to change yet, consider these suggestions in the meantime:

- Keep track of how often and how much you're drinking.

- Notice how drinking affects you.

- Make or re-make a list of pros and cons about changing.

- Deal with other priorities that may be in the way of changing.

- Ask for support from your doctor, a friend, or someone else you trust.

Don't wait for a crisis or to "hit bottom." When someone is drinking too much, making a change earlier is likely to be more successful and less destructive to individuals and their families.

To Cut Down Or To Quit?

If you're considering changing your drinking, you'll need to decide whether to cut down or to quit. It's a good idea to discuss different options with a doctor, a parent, or someone else you trust. For teens, quitting completely is strongly advised because there are serious health-related consequences associated with underage drinking—and it is illegal. For adults, quitting is strongly advised if they have tried cutting down but cannot stay within the limits they set. Other indicators that quitting is the best option include people who have had an alcohol use disorder or now have symptoms; people who have a physical or mental condition that is caused or worsened by drinking; people who are taking a medication that interacts with alcohol; or women who are or may become pregnant.

Adults who do not have any of these conditions, can talk with their healthcare providers to determine whether they should cut down or quit based on factors such as family history of alcohol problems, age, drinking-related injuries, and symptoms such as sleep disorders and sexual dysfunction.

Planning For Change

Even when you have committed to change, you still may have mixed feelings at times. Making a written "change plan" will help you to solidify your goals, why you want to reach them, and how you plan to do it. A sample form is provided in Figure 33.2.

Reinforce Your Decision With Reminders

Enlist technology to help. Change can be hard, so it helps to have concrete reminders of why and how you've decided to do it. Some standard options include carrying a change plan in your wallet or posting sticky notes at home. If you have a computer or mobile phone, consider these high-tech ideas:

Change plan

Goal:

- ☐ I want to drink no more than ____ drink(s) on any day and no more than ____ drink(s) per week
- ☐ I want to stop drinking (Remember: Teens are strongly advised to quit.)

Timing: I will start on this date: _____

Reasons: My most important reasons to make these changes are:

_____

_____

_____

Strategies: I will use these strategies:

_____

_____

_____

People: The people who can help me are (names and how they can help):

_____

_____

_____

Signs of success: I will know my plan is working if:

_____

_____

_____

Possible roadblocks: Some things that might interfere **and how I'll handle them**:

_____

_____

_____

Figure 33.2. Ready to begin? If so, start by filling out a change plan.

- Fill out a "change plan" online at the Rethinking Drinking website (http://rethinkingdrinking .niaaa.nih.gov), email it to yourself (be sure to use a private account), and review it weekly.

- Store your goals, reasons, or strategies in your mobile phone in short text messages or notepad entries that you can retrieve easily when an urge hits.

- Set up automated mobile phone or e-mail calendar alerts that deliver reminders when you choose, such as a few hours before you usually go out.

- Create passwords that are motivating phrases in code, which you'll type each time you log in, such as 1Day@aTime, 1stThings1st!, or 0Pain=0Gain.

If You Want To Quit Drinking

The four strategies described here are especially helpful if you want to quit drinking. But if you think you may be dependent on alcohol and decide to stop drinking completely, don't go it alone. Sudden withdrawal from heavy drinking can be life threatening. Seek medical help to plan a safe recovery.

Find Alternatives: If drinking has occupied a lot of your time, then fill free time by developing new, healthy activities, hobbies, and relationships or renewing ones you've missed. If you have counted on alcohol to be more comfortable in social situations, manage moods, or cope with problems, then seek other, healthy ways to deal with those areas of your life.

Avoid "Triggers": What triggers your urge to drink? If certain people or places make you drink even when you don't want to, try to avoid them. If certain activities, times of day, or feelings trigger the urge, plan something else to do instead of drinking. If drinking at home is a problem, keep no alcohol there.

Plan To Handle Urges: When you cannot avoid a trigger and an urge hits, consider these options: Remind yourself of your reasons for changing (it can help to carry them in writing or store them in an electronic message you can access easily). Or, talk things through with someone you trust. Or, get involved with a healthy, distracting activity, such as physical exercise or a hobby that doesn't involve drinking. Or, instead of fighting the feeling, accept it and ride it out without giving in, knowing that it will soon crest like a wave and pass.

Know Your "No": You're likely to be offered a drink at times when you don't want one. Have a polite, convincing "no, thanks" ready. The faster you can say no to these offers, the less likely you are to give in. If you hesitate, it allows you time to think of excuses to go along. Tools to help you manage urges to drink and build drink refusal skills are available on the Rethinking Drinking website (http://rethinkingdrinking.niaaa.nih.gov).

Support For Quitting

The suggestions in this section will be most useful for people who have become dependent on alcohol, and thus may find it difficult to quit without some help. Several proven treatment approaches are available. One size doesn't it all, however. It's a good idea to do some homework on the internet or at the library to find social and professional support options that appeal to you, as you are more likely to stick with them. Chances are excellent that you'll pull together an approach that works for you.

Social Support: One potential challenge when people stop drinking is rebuilding a life without alcohol. It may be important to educate family and friends, develop new interests and

---

A Message To Teens Who Already Use Drugs, Alcohol, Or Tobacco

Maybe you tried drinking, drugs, or smoking because you were curious. Or because you felt stressed. Or because you just felt like breaking the rules. Whatever your reasons, though, there are even better reasons to stop these nasty habits. Want some? How about your future, your health, your safety — even your good looks! That's right. Drugs, alcohol, and cigarettes put all of those at risk.

It's definitely worth it to try to quit. And with the strength, courage, and smarts you've got inside you, you can do it!

If you need a little inspiration, check out some of the reasons to quit below. Then read on for ways to beat the habit before it beats you.

Some good reasons to quit alcohol and drugs:

- Even if you feel like you're doing fine now, things can get out of control pretty fast. You can get sick or addicted before you know it.
- Drugs and alcohol can make it more likely you will do something you wouldn't usually do, like have unsafe sex.
- Drugs and alcohol will change the way your brain works.
- Drugs are illegal, and it's against the law to buy alcohol if you're under 21. You can fail an alcohol breath test after just one drink.

Some good reasons to quit smoking:

- The benefits of quitting kick in fast. For example, just 12 hours after quitting, the level of carbon monoxide in your blood drops to normal. Two weeks to three months after

---

social groups, find rewarding ways to spend your time that don't involve alcohol, and ask for help from others. When asking for support from friends or significant others, be specific. This could include asking them to not offer you alcohol or not use alcohol around you. You may need to ask them to give words of support and withhold criticism. It may be helpful if they not ask you to take on new demands right away. Perhaps they can support you by going to a group like Al-Anon.

For yourself, consider joining Alcoholics Anonymous or another mutual support group. Recovering people who attend groups regularly do better than those who do not. Groups can vary widely, so shop around for one that's comfortable. You'll get more out of it if you become actively involved by having a sponsor and reaching out to other members for assistance.

---

quitting, your heart and lungs begin to work better. A year after, your risk of heart disease goes down.

- Smoking gives you wrinkles and stains your teeth. It stinks up your breath and hair, and you may not even notice since you get used to the smell.
- Most teens would rather date someone who doesn't smoke.
- Many buildings won't let you smoke inside anymore, so smoking can be pretty lonely—and cold.

Whether you've used a lot or a little, it's never too late to stop smoking, drinking, and using drugs. Of course, it can be tough. You may even have physical feelings of withdrawal, like headaches. But you probably can think of other times you had to do something difficult—and succeeded. Don't give up!

These ideas can help you make a plan to quit and stick with it.

- Ask for help from a trusted adult, friends, and family.
- Think of ways to say "no." Check out some tips for turning down drugs, alcohol, and smoking online at http://www.girlshealth.gov/substance/index.cfm.
- Come up with a specific plan for quitting. Then steer clear of situations where you might be tempted.
- Try other ways to deal with stress, like exercising.
- Find out about support groups. It's great to connect with other people who know how you feel.
- Consider going to a program or treatment center for help.

For more tips on how to quit and other helpful information, check out the resources at the end of this book.

Source: Excerpted from "If You Already Use Drugs, Alcohol, or Tobacco," Office on Women's Health (www.girlshealth .gov), May 18, 2010.

It's common for people with alcohol problems to feel depressed or anxious. Mild symptoms may go away if you cut down or stop drinking. See a doctor or mental health professional if symptoms persist or get worse. If you're having suicidal thoughts, call your health care provider or go to the nearest emergency room right away. Effective treatment is available to help you through this difficult time.

Professional Support: Advances in the treatment of alcoholism mean that patients now have more choices and health professionals have more tools to help.

Newer medications can make it easier to quit drinking by offsetting changes in the brain caused by alcoholism. These options (naltrexone, topiramate, and acamprosate) don't make you sick if you drink, as does an older medication (disulfiram). None of these medications are addictive, so it's fine to combine them with support groups or alcohol counseling.

A major clinical trial recently showed that patients can now receive effective alcohol treatment from their primary care doctors or mental health practitioners by combining the newer medications with a series of brief office visits for support.

Alcohol counseling (talk therapy) also works well. There are several counseling approaches that are about equally effective—12 step, cognitive-behavioral, motivational enhancement, or a combination. Getting help in itself appears to be more important than the particular approach used, as long as it offers empathy, avoids heavy confrontation, strengthens motivation, and provides concrete ways to change drinking behavior.

Some people will need more intensive programs. If you need a referral to a specialized, intensive treatment program, ask your doctor.

Don't Give Up

Changing habits such as smoking, overeating, or drinking too much can take a lot of effort, and you may not succeed with the first try. Setbacks are common, but you learn more each time. Each try brings you closer to your goal.

Whatever course you choose, give it a fair trial. If one approach doesn't work, try something else. And if a setback happens, get back on track as quickly as possible.

In the long run, your chances for success are good. Research shows that most heavy drinkers, even those with alcoholism, either cut back significantly or quit.

Chapter 34

Alcoholism Treatment Principles

Treating Alcoholism

An alcoholic will rarely stop drinking and stay sober without outside help. Also, he or she usually will not stop drinking without some kind of outside pressure. This pressure may come from family, friends, clergy, health care professionals, or law enforcement or judicial authorities.

There was at one time a widespread belief that alcoholics would not get help until they had "hit bottom." This theory has generally been discredited as many early and middle stage alcoholics have quit drinking when faced with consequences or a convincing warning from a physician regarding the potentially fatal consequences of continued drinking.

There are obvious advantages to getting the alcoholic into treatment earlier rather than later. One advantage is that, the earlier treatment is begun, the probability of having less expensive treatment, such as outpatient care, is increased. There is also a greater likelihood of success in treatment with an individual who has not yet lost everything and still has a supportive environment to return to, including an intact family and good health. If an alcoholic doesn't get help until very late in the disease, there may have been irreparable harm done relationships.

The alcoholic does not initially have to want to get help to go into treatment. Many people go into treatment because of some kind of threat such as possible incarceration. However, even the individual that is forced will eventually have to personally accept the need for treatment for it to be effective.

About This Chapter: Excerpted and adapted from *Alcoholism In The Workplace: A Handbook for Supervisors*, Office of Personnel Management (www.opm.gov), 2006. Reviewed by David A. Cooke, MD, FACP, December 2012.

There are various kinds of treatment and programs for alcoholism. Though some alcoholics do stop drinking on their own, this is rare. Most alcoholics require some type of treatment or help. The following are some common types of programs and approaches to treatment:

Alcoholics Anonymous (AA): AA is what is called a 12-step program and involves a spiritual component (not affiliated with any particular religion) and a supportive group of fellow alcoholics to provide a network for total abstinence from alcohol. There are AA meetings where alcoholics can gather to learn about the disease, hear talks from recovering alcoholics, and enjoy the support of fellow alcoholics who are learning, or have learned, how to stay sober. AA is not really a formal organization as it has no leaders. It is a loose confederation of groups formed by recovering alcoholics operating on common principles spelled out in the book *Alcoholics Anonymous* (it is also known as the "Big Book") which spells out the Twelve Steps and the principles of AA.

There are other support groups such as Rational Recovery which have a different focus than AA. Some individuals find approaches other than AA to be more useful in their treatment.

Detoxification: Detoxification, also known as "detox," is a process whereby the alcoholic undergoes a supervised withdrawal. The body can begin to recover from the toxic effects of alcohol and the patient can become sober. This is something that is best done in a medical setting where the patient can be closely monitored and have his or her medical condition evaluated. Detoxification can last anywhere from two to seven days.

Inpatient Treatment: This consists of a formal, residential program which may include detox at the beginning. Typically an inpatient program would include education about the disease; medical treatment for related medical conditions and nutritional stabilization; counseling, including individual and group therapy sessions; an introduction to a 12-step program; and monitoring of the patient including drug and/or alcohol testing to ensure compliance with the program. Inpatient programs last anywhere from one to six weeks, although they are typically three to four weeks. Some are connected with hospitals while others are not. There are some programs called *day treatment* in which patients spend the entire day at the treatment center but go home at night or on weekends. Inpatient treatment is very expensive and can easily cost $5,000 to $10,000.

Outpatient Treatment: This consists of counseling and treatment on a daily or weekly basis in an office or clinic setting. Outpatient treatment is often a follow-up to an inpatient or detox program. In some cases, the severity of the addiction is such that inpatient care is not needed, and the client undergoes only outpatient treatment. It may include education about the disease, individual or group therapy, or follow-up counseling. Outpatient treatment is not as expensive as inpatient treatment and may last anywhere from one month to a year.

Combination Treatment: Quite often, treatment will consist of a combination of all of the above, depending on such factors as the severity of the problem, the individual's insurance coverage, whether detox is needed, and the availability of programs.

Post Treatment

After the initial treatment program, the recovering alcoholic may be in follow-up counseling and treatment for an extended period of time, possibly up to a year. This may include outpatient counseling and AA meetings.

Relapse

An important and frustrating facet of treating alcoholism is relapse or a return to drinking. An alcoholic often relapses due to a variety of factors including: inadequate treatment or follow-up, cravings for alcohol that are difficult to control, failure by the alcoholic to follow treatment instructions, failure to change lifestyle, use of other mood altering drugs, and other untreated mental or physical illnesses. Relapses are not always a return to constant drinking and may only be a one-time occurrence. However, relapses must be dealt with and seen as a sign to the alcoholic that there are areas of his or her treatment and recovery that need work. Relapse prevention is an area in the treatment field that is receiving increased attention and research. A basic part of any effective treatment program will include relapse prevention activities.

Chapter 35

Alcohol Withdrawal And Delirium Tremens

What is alcohol withdrawal?

Alcohol withdrawal is a brain disorder that occurs when alcohol use is suddenly stopped after a prolonged period of heavy use. It can cause a variety of physical and neurological symptoms.

In the normal brain, there is a complex balance between nerves that should be active and nerves that should be inactive. For example, you don't want the portion of your brain that controls your right leg to be active when you're sitting in a chair.

Alcohol has a generalized depressant effect on the brain, and it reduces nerve activity. When high levels of alcohol are present for a long time, the brain adapts by stepping up nerve activity to compensate for the alcohol effects. When alcohol levels drop abruptly, nerve activity rebounds.

Imagine two teams pulling on a rope in a tug-of-war. One team suddenly drops their end of the rope, and the other team goes flying backwards. This is, in effect, what happens in the brain when alcohol is suddenly stopped. Nerves throughout the brain become go into overdrive when the alcohol is removed.

The brain imbalances set off by withdrawal can cause a variety of symptoms. They can range from tremor and irritability, to severely high blood pressure and hallucinations, to seizures, brain damage, and death.

Who is at risk for alcohol withdrawal?

By definition, alcohol withdrawal requires consuming a substantial amount of alcohol for a sustained period of time. Therefore, it is seen exclusively in alcoholics, whether or not they

---

About This Chapter: The text in this chapter was written by David A. Cooke, MD, FACP. © 2013 Omnigraphics, Inc.

recognize their addiction. Generally speaking, the risk of withdrawal directly relates to the amount of alcohol used and the duration of use.

Alcohol withdrawal is not completely predictable, however. There are individual differences in susceptibility to withdrawal, and genetic factors are probably involved. Some people will experience withdrawal with levels of alcohol use that do not trigger it in others.

While it is not an absolute rule, withdrawal is unlikely if a person has been drinking for less than three days, and has been drinking less than six standard drinks per day (for women) or eight standard drinks per day (for men). As the number of drinks per day, and the number of days of drinking increase, odds of withdrawal increase rapidly.

Prior alcohol withdrawal is one of the strongest risk factors for future alcohol withdrawal. Prior withdrawal severity also tends to predict future withdrawal severity. People who have previously suffered alcohol withdrawal seizures or delirium tremens are at especially high risk of suffering withdrawal again if they suddenly stop drinking.

What triggers alcohol withdrawal?

By definition, alcohol withdrawal occurs when alcohol intake is abruptly stopped or decreased. This usually happens in one of two settings.

First, an alcoholic may decide to stop drinking. This might be due to feeling ill, recognition of the harm alcohol is causing, or pressure from friends or family.

Second, an alcoholic may be prevented from drinking alcohol. For example, a heavy drinker might run out of money to purchase alcohol. Alternatively, an alcoholic might be in a situation where they don't have access to alcohol. It is quite common for hospitalized patients to suffer withdrawal, as they may not have disclosed their alcohol use to their doctor. Withdrawal is also common among people who have been recently arrested and held in jails.

It is worth knowing that alcohol withdrawal can occur even when there are still significant amounts of alcohol in the blood stream. Some alcoholics drink so heavily that they can withdraw even with blood levels above legal definitions of intoxication.

What are the signs of alcohol withdrawal?

Depending upon the person and their degree of alcohol dependence, withdrawal symptoms may appear within a few hours, and almost always within 24 hours, of the last drink. Early symptoms include anxiety, irritability, poor sleep, vivid dreams, loss of appetite, nausea, vomiting, and headache. Rapid heartbeat, elevated blood pressure, tremor, and sweating may be noted.

In some cases, hallucinations can occur, in which the person may see, hear, or feel things that are not really present. These are usually brief and fleeting, and don't usually result in confusion. Less commonly, seizures can occur, usually within 8–24 hours of the last drink.

For the majority of people experiencing withdrawal, symptoms are mild to moderate, peaking within 24–72 hours of onset, and disappearing within a few days to a week. More severe or prolonged symptoms may warn of the onset of DTs (delirium tremens).

Are DTs (delirium tremens) the same thing as alcohol withdrawal?

DTs are a particularly dangerous form of withdrawal. Not everyone who suffers withdrawal develops DTs, but anyone who has DTs is undergoing withdrawal.

Delirium tremens is distinguished from ordinary withdrawal by the presence of altered mental status (*delirium*) and prominent signs of central nervous system hyperactivity (the *tremens*). Additionally, symptoms of DTs typically occur somewhat later than those of uncomplicated withdrawal, usually about 48 hours after the last drink.

Hallucinations are not unusual in mild alcohol withdrawal. However, in DTs, hallucinations are intense, and connections to reality are lost. People having DTs suffer severe confusion, and it is very difficult for them to perceive the real world.

Along with an altered mental state, a person with DTs may develop dangerously high heart rate, blood pressure, and fevers. Uncontrollable tremors and twitches are common, and may progress to seizures. In the most severe cases, strings of intense seizures may occur, and this is likely to result in death unless there is prompt medical intervention.

In the past, DTs had a significant fatality rate. However, death is rare today for those who receive medical treatment.

What can be done to treat alcohol withdrawal?

The best way to treat alcohol withdrawal is to prevent it in the first place. Avoiding stopping alcohol abruptly will usually prevent withdrawal, and some heavy drinkers will taper down their alcohol use over a period of days to weeks to achieve this.

A heavy drinker should seek medical evaluation first, before the alcohol is stopped. Prediction formulas based on the drinker's history help estimate the odds of severe withdrawal, and the potential impact of any other medical conditions can be weighed. Depending on the degree of risk, a medical professional may treat the person as an outpatient, or arrange for admission to a medical facility for more intensive monitoring.

Alcohol withdrawal is usually treated with a class of sedative medications called benzodiazepines. Diazepam (Valium®), lorazepam (Ativan®), and chlordiazepoxide (Librium®) are most commonly used for this purpose. Benzodiazepines affect the brain differently than alcohol, but have sufficient similarities to tame the frenzied neural activity that occurs during withdrawal. Typically, the medication is tapered over a period of a few days to a week or two, and then stopped. This allows for the brain to adapt to the removal of alcohol in a more controlled manner. There are also several other types of medication that can be used if benzodiazepines are not felt to be best for the patient.

If a person is judged to be at low risk, they may remain at home and be monitored by friends or family, checking in frequently with a physician. Usually, the physician will prescribe a benzodiazepine taper as a prophylactic measure. If symptoms become severe, or seizures occur, the person will be admitted to the hospital.

For higher risk individuals, they may be referred to a local detoxification facility, where they can be closely watched for signs of withdrawal. If signs of serious withdrawal develop while at the detox facility, or if the person is judged to be at very high risk, they will be admitted to the hospital for more intensive medical supervision and treatment.

In a medical setting, the patient is assessed hourly for the presence and severity of withdrawal symptoms. A number of alcohol severity rating scales have been developed for this kind of use. Usually, medications are given based on severity scores, to limit the severity of the withdrawal, and to prevent the most dangerous symptoms from appearing. Once the most dangerous phases are past, the person can be discharged with close followup as an outpatient.

Chapter 36

Sobriety: The First 30 Days

Introduction

This chapter is not a substitute for treatment. It will give you an idea of what to expect when you leave detox. It has suggestions to help you stay off illicit drugs and alcohol. Not all of the suggestions will apply to you. Just do what works for you.

Your next step is to go to substance abuse treatment. Treatment will help you recover and also help you with other needs. Ask the detox staff about treatment. Beginning treatment as soon as you leave detox is best, but there is sometimes a waiting period. The treatment staff can help you until your treatment begins.

You may not be able to go to treatment. You should still get help staying off drugs and alcohol. Find a self-help or other community group for people in recovery, such as Alcoholics Anonymous (AA) or Narcotics Anonymous (NA) or other group. If a spiritually oriented program is important to you, try a faith-based organization (such as a church) that welcomes people in recovery. Going it alone is the most difficult way to stay away from drugs and alcohol. Get help.

Before you went to detox your drug or alcohol problem was in the driver's seat. Even after you finish detox, the factors that "drive" your substance use are still in place. Your substance use disorder is still there. The challenge you face now is to take back the steering wheel and begin to recover.

About This Chapter: This chapter includes excerpts from "Chapter 1: The First 30 Days," *The Next Step... Toward a Better Life*, Substance Abuse and Mental Health Services Administration (www.samhsa.gov), HHS Pub. No. (SMA) 10-4474, 2011.

Recovery happens in stages. The first stage is the very big adjustment while your body and brain get used to not having drugs or alcohol. This stage is a very bumpy road to travel and can take four weeks or longer, depending on your habit. (Methamphetamine and crack users may need several months to adjust.)

This chapter helps you avoid drugs and alcohol while you make this adjustment. When you have adjusted to being sober, and the road feels less bumpy, you will start longer-term recovery. You will set new goals, make better decisions, and plan your time.

Remember: YOU CAN DO THIS.

Detox Is Not A "Cure"

Going through detox means you have taken a big first step in getting free of drugs or alcohol. However, detox is only the beginning. The drugs or alcohol may be gone from your body, but the people, places, and problems that led you to drug and alcohol abuse are still there.

Leaving Detoxification: Now What?

Perhaps you have been through detox before and you have doubts about staying sober and off drugs. You can do it. Many people go through detox more than once.

Maybe you tried to go it alone last time. This time, get help. Counselors can help you if you are struggling to stay sober or have other specific needs.

Go to self-help group meetings. These groups are a no-lose situation. They cost nothing, are available almost everywhere and any time, and you can find one that meets your ethnic and gender preferences. There is no waiting list. They know what you are going through. They know about resources in your community. You have more choices and opportunities than you realize.

People, Places, Things: Steps To Take Now

There is no right way and no wrong way to stay sober and off drugs. Whatever works, works. The things that work best are those that help you deal with triggers. A trigger is anything that leads to using or drinking.

Many self-help groups use the acronym H.A.L.T. to describe certain triggers. You are more likely to use or drink when you are Hungry, Angry, Lonely, or Tired.

You are also more likely to use or drink when you are around the people, places, and things that were part of your old drug or drinking life.

What Happens In Substance Abuse Treatment?

Not all treatment programs are alike, but most follow this general idea:

First, the counselor will ask you questions about your drinking or drug use, your physical health, and other issues in your life. This is called assessment. The counselor will use the answers to your questions to determine how to help you. Many counselors are in recovery and know what you are going through.

Together, you and the counselor will make a treatment plan. The treatment plan is a written outline of your goals and anti-drink/drug activities. It will also contain the "tools" you will need to help you stay sober. These can include the following:

- Help in identifying triggers (a trigger is anything that makes you crave alcohol or drugs)
- Relapse prevention training
- Stress management
- Self-help groups in which you are comfortable
- Medicine for pain, cravings, or depression
- Time or money management skills
- Job skills

Treatment has two goals. One goal is to help you stop using. The other goal is to help you relearn how to live without drugs or alcohol. It can take a long time for substance abuse to develop, and it can take a long time to relearn how to live without using.

Source: SAMHSA, 2011.

Before you walk out of detox, plan now to stay away from anyone, any place, and anything that will cause you to relapse. For instance, consider the following suggestions:

- Delete the names of the people you drank or used with from your cell phone, e-mail, and other devices. Avoid the old crowd as much as you can.

- As much as you can, avoid the people who get you angry.

- Find good company. Ask your friends or family to help you stay sober.

- Ask detox staff about AA, NA, or other local self-help groups.

- Go to 90 meetings in 90 days.

- Map out different routes to avoid dealers and bars.

- Don't visit or meet someone if you know he or she has alcohol or drugs.

- Fill your refrigerator so you will always have something good to eat.

- Have someone who doesn't use clear the alcohol, drugs, and equipment from your home, car, and other places.

- Put away your cash, ATM, or credit cards if having money is one of your triggers. Shop with non-using friends or family.

- As much as you can, rest, relax, and sleep.

- Make a list of the bad effects alcohol or drugs had on your life, friends, and family. Be honest.

- Make a list of the benefits of staying off drugs and alcohol. Add to this list every day—new people you have met, ways you are proud of yourself.

Drugs Used To Treat Alcohol Addiction

Naltrexone

Naltrexone blocks opioid receptors that are involved in the rewarding effects of drinking and the craving for alcohol. It reduces relapse to heavy drinking, defined as four or more drinks per day for women and five or more for men. Naltrexone cuts relapse risk during the first three months by about 36 percent but is less effective in helping patients maintain abstinence.

Acamprosate

Acamprosate (Campral®) acts on the gamma-aminobutyric acid (GABA) and glutamate neurotransmitter systems and is thought to reduce symptoms of protracted withdrawal, such as insomnia, anxiety, restlessness, and dysphoria. Acamprosate has been shown to help dependent drinkers maintain abstinence for several weeks to months, and it may be more effective in patients with severe dependence.

Disulfiram

Disulfiram (Antabuse®) interferes with degradation of alcohol, resulting in the accumulation of acetaldehyde, which, in turn, produces a very unpleasant reaction that includes flushing, nausea, and palpitations if the patient drinks alcohol. The utility and effectiveness of disulfiram are considered limited because compliance is generally poor. However, among patients who are highly motivated, disulfiram can be effective, and some patients use it episodically for high-risk situations, such as social occasions where alcohol is present. It can also be administered in a monitored fashion, such as in a clinic or by a spouse, improving its efficacy.

- Talk to a counselor if your living conditions are a concern. Having drugs in the neighborhood or house is a powerful trigger to relapse. So is an abusive living situation. If you cannot change your living situation, it is even more important to have lots of anti-drug skills to rely on.

Potholes Ahead

The biggest mistake you can make is to think you can simply go back to your life and not use drugs and alcohol. Staying sober takes a lot of hard work. The road ahead is full of potholes that can knock you off course.

Remember that your substance abuse is something that you once learned to do. Now that you have been through detox, you need to "unlearn" substance use and "relearn" how to live sober. You may be drug-free, but you are still on "automatic pilot." You could drink or use drugs without thinking about it.

Topiramate

Topiramate is thought to work by increasing inhibitory (GABA) neurotransmission and reducing stimulatory (glutamate) neurotransmission. Its precise mechanism of action in treating alcohol addiction is not known, and it has not yet received approval from the U.S. Food and Drug Administration (FDA). Topiramate has been shown in two randomized, controlled trials to significantly improve multiple drinking outcomes, compared with a placebo. Over the course of a 14-week trial, topiramate significantly increased the proportion of patients with 28 consecutive days of abstinence or non-heavy drinking. In both studies, the differences between topiramate and placebo groups were still diverging at the end of the trial, suggesting that the maximum effect may not have yet been reached. Importantly, efficacy was established in volunteers who were drinking upon starting the medication.

Combined With Behavioral Treatment

While a number of behavioral treatments have been shown to be effective in the treatment of alcohol addiction, it does not appear that an additive effect exists between behavioral treatments and pharmacotherapy. Studies have shown that getting help is one of the most important factors in treating alcohol addiction, compared to getting a particular type of treatment.

Source: From *Alcohol Addiction, Principles of Drug Addiction and Treatment: A Research-Based Guide, Second Edition*, National Institute on Drug Abuse, April 2009.

To stay away from drugs and alcohol during this period, you have to take action:

- Use your anti-drugs/anti-drinks (explained in the next section).

- Practice new thinking, especially the reminder "I am a substance abuser and I must work to recover."

- Take small steps in simple, everyday matters.

Taking action will help you get through this phase in several ways. It gives you a growing sense of control over your life. Best of all, instead of trying to not do something, which is difficult, you can do something else, which is easier. The something else is your anti-drug or anti-drink.

Your "Anti-Drugs" And "Anti-Drinks"

An "anti-drug" or "anti-drink" is anything that helps you stay away from drugs or alcohol. It can be simple, like the following ideas:

- Chewing gum or eating candy when you crave a drink

- Calling your self-help group sponsor or a friend instead of going to places where you might use

- Watching movies

- Shooting baskets

- Reading

- Keeping pictures of your family in your pocket as motivation to stay away from alcohol and drugs

- Joining a faith organization that supports recovery

- Finding a new hobby that keeps you busy and away from others who use

The more anti-drugs you have, the better. By doing your anti-drugs/anti-drinks, you can gradually shut off that automatic pilot and get back in the driver's seat. The people who are most successful in staying sober do two anti-drugs/drinks in particular: go to counseling and join a self-help group.

Practicing anti-drug activities doesn't mean you have to be busy. It can also mean mental activity such as prayer and meditation. There are many forms of meditation, including mindfulness training. Mindfulness training is taught in hospitals for stress and pain control. These mental exercises can help get you out of "automatic pilot."

Just like exercising a muscle, these anti-drug activities feel more natural with use. Use the form in Figure 36.1 to make a list of your own anti-drinks/anti-drugs. Copy it and keep it with you. Unless you are ready with a list of ideas to avoid alcohol and drugs, it will be too easy for you to start drinking or using again.

You may have a fear of falling into your old patterns, but this will not last. For now, your focus is on the next four weeks or so, and on avoiding the people, places, and things that are connected to using. Your impulses will feel less and less overwhelming over time.

What's Wrong With This Picture?

You may think that being sober means that everything will now be fine. Actually, the early days of abstinence can look and feel pretty bad.

Change, even good change, can be frightening. Because getting sober is a big change, it can also be a time of crisis. The changes of new abstinence are sometimes called the "trauma of recovery." Your life and the lives of the people around you were probably organized around your substance use. The sudden absence of your use can disorganize your life in a painful way.

The change you made by becoming sober also has a ripple effect on your family and friends. Getting sober creates chaos, just like the chaos created by substance use. Remember that the people around you are affected too:

- They need your attention, especially your family members.

- They could think or say that they prefer you "on drugs."

- They might not understand the adjustments you are going through.

- They might have invested a lot of energy in taking care of you. Now that you are abstinent, they have to find other ways to relate to you.

- They might not understand all the things you need to do to stay sober and off drugs.

- They might try to control you to keep from relapsing.

- They might resent the upheaval the drugs and alcohol caused.

- They might resent that you often leave for sobriety activities.

- They might find your unstable feelings difficult to deal with.

Your job is to stay focused on your anti-drugs/anti-drinks strategies. Here are some tips where others are concerned:

When I am confronted with drugs or alcohol, I will do this:

1)_____

2)_____

3)_____

4)_____

5)_____

6)_____

7)_____

8)_____

9)_____

10)_____

11)_____

12)_____

13)_____

14)_____

15)_____

16)_____

17)_____

18)_____

19)_____

20)_____

Figure 36.1. List Your Anti-Drinks/Anti-Drugs

- Let friends and family focus on their own adjustments.

- Stay positive. Even small changes toward positive thinking help yourself and others. Negative thinking helps no one.

- Go to AA or similar group meetings for encouragement from people who understand.

Drugs or alcohol caused many of your problems, but not all of them. Getting sober will not cure all of them. Now that you are sober, you are suddenly faced with problems in a new way. Let the bigger issues wait until you are feeling better. Stick to the daily problems so the most important things are taken care of.

More About The First 30 Days

Drug and alcohol use mixed up your thinking patterns. Now that you are detoxified, your brain needs time to adjust to life without chemicals. As this happens, you can have feelings that don't make any sense. Here are some examples:

- Feeling like you've been asleep for years and can't handle the simplest situation without "using."

- Feeling grief in letting go of your use.

- Feeling "stranded" and wonder "what now?"

- Feeling like you lost the friends or family who are still using.

- Feeling that sobriety is like punishment or being deprived.

- Feeling strange during ordinary activities because you have forgotten how to do things sober.

- Pain from other problems can suddenly resurface.

- You can have trouble thinking clearly.

- You might struggle with anxiety or depression.

- You might feel overwhelmed.

- You might "space out."

- Impulsive behaviors can pose a challenge.

- Your emotions can run to extremes with anger, self-pity, hopelessness, or defensiveness.

- It might be difficult to remember things.

Why Meds Work For Some People, But Not For Others

You can add alcoholism to the growing list of conditions that may be addressed with medication, depending on a patient's genetic characteristics. That was the message delivered recently in a lecture by National Institute on Alcohol Abuse and Alcoholism (NIAAA) clinical director Dr. Markus Heilig, who studied the effect—or lack thereof—of the drug naltrexone (an opioid antagonist commonly used in the treatment of drug addiction) on a person's wired desire to reach for a drink. It appears as though people struggling with alcoholism for whom naltrexone is an effective treatment possess a particular genetic variant. That variant is worked on by the drug to stymie its push to make the body want alcohol.

Heilig, who studies alcoholism and anxiety disorders as chief of the Laboratory of Clinical and Translational Studies, felt compelled to unravel this mysterious disparity in effectiveness. He started with a simple theory: "If patients respond differently," he said, "maybe they are different [physiologically]. In the age of the mapped genome and personalized medicine, this is not difficult to imagine."

Research shows that in the early phases of alcoholism, people drink because it is pleasurable—the body tells the mind that drinking is rewarding. Heilig wanted to determine why the medicinal blunting of the circuitry that rewards intake of alcohol worked for some patients but not for others.

Heilig found that in people who possess a specific genetic variant, this chemical pleasure reward is much more pronounced because when alcohol is consumed, their bodies release a swell of dopamine that heightens the physical connection to drinking. This intense reward only prompts the body to want more alcohol, continuing the cycle and strengthening the chemical connection. In people without the variant, their bodies' dopamine release was nonexistent.

In cases of people with the mutation, naltrexone works to block the reward cascade of dopamine following the consumption of alcohol. With no dopamine reward, the body has less reason to want a drink, so the patient can more easily walk away from alcohol. In people without this genetic switch flipped on, naltrexone is not an effective intervention tool.

Unfortunately, this finding is only one part of the puzzle. While naltrexone can help many people in the early stages of addiction when the body still believes it's being rewarded for drinking, it isn't nearly as effective once the brain has turned a corner in its addiction.

"Over time, the addicted brain transitions from 'reward craving' to 'relief craving,'" Heilig said. Instead of the body wanting alcohol because it feels good, it wants it because not having alcohol will make the body feel bad. That's what scientists call a "negatively reinforced drug craving"—the body must have the chemical fix or it will suffer withdrawal symptoms.

In tests, naltrexone isn't particularly effective in helping with the relief stage, nor is it able to help curb the sense of anxiety that is felt by all alcoholics when placed under stress. This anxiousness often causes people to relapse into drinking to relieve anxiety.

Heilig said there are currently several stress-related mechanisms that seem promising for inclusion in treatment strategies, though none is quite ready for prime time. He said that like human beings themselves, each treatment plan will be as individual as the patient.

Source: Excerpted from "Why Meds Work for Some People, but Not for Others," by Valerie Lambros, *NIH Record*, National Institutes of Health, Vol. LXII, No. 10, May 14, 2010.

- It can be difficult to commit to things.

- Your physical coordination might not work as well.

- You might have trouble sleeping.

- You might constantly stress about every aspect of life.

- You might feel numb or "drugged" with emotions—depression, anger, helplessness—just like when you were using.

These emotions mean your brain is recovering now that the alcohol or drugs are gone. Here are some suggestions for helping cope during this time:

- Don't expect too much of yourself. Your physical coordination and ability to concentrate won't work as well for a while.

- Try to avoid doing things that could make you feel worse, like eating junk food or drinking coffee.

- Find humor in situations instead of feeling sorry for yourself.

- Remind yourself that your emotional state will get better soon if you stay sober.

- Get as much sleep as possible. Don't worry too much about sleep disturbances. You will sleep better soon.

- Eat well, including healthy snacks if you are hungry.

- Take vitamins to restore needed nutrition.

Cravings can occur at any time and are often triggered by events (such as New Year's Eve) or sensations (the smell of alcohol or cigarette smoke). Like your other symptoms, cravings will fade as the days and weeks go by.

You might dream that you are drinking or using drugs and wake up feeling high, or frustrated at not being high.

Feeling anxious or depressed for a short time can be a part of this bumpy road. However, if it lasts too long, you should get treatment.

Moving On

When does this adjustment period end? Give yourself at least a month. (People who use heroin or crack may need six months.)

As time goes by, you may notice that your head is clearer. Instead of fighting your impulses, you can relax and just go through your day. You can think about the weeks ahead, instead of just today. You are moving into longer-term recovery.

Remember: YOU CAN DO THIS.

Chapter 37

Long-Term Addiction Recovery

As your brain and body get used to being without drugs and alcohol, you'll find that life feels better and you no longer feel overwhelmed. Instead of worrying about things that don't happen, you deal with problems as they come up.

You are getting along better with the people close to you, and you can be more open and honest. You have a better sense of what issues belong to you, and what issues belong to other people. You are enjoying yourself a little more and doing fun things.

It is time to adopt a long-term recovery plan that involves the following components:

• Setting new goals and the steps to get there

• Improving your relationships

• Learning more ways to handle situations without substance use

• Learning to manage your time

• Identifying your triggers and ways to handle them

Your Recovery Plan

Why do you need a recovery plan? To be in recovery, you need to be moving forward. If you stop moving forward, the old patterns are waiting to take over again, ready to grab the steering wheel.

About This Chapter: This chapter includes excerpts from "Chapter 2: Long-Term Recovery," *The Next Step… Toward a Better Life*, Substance Abuse and Mental Health Services Administration (www.samhsa.gov), HHS Pub. No. (SMA) 10-4474, 2011.

12-Step Programs

After detoxification, almost every addict will need a combination of professional (group or individual) counseling plus attendance at a self-help group to maintain sobriety. The self-help support approach to treatment of alcohol and drug dependence began in 1935 with the development of Alcoholics Anonymous (AA), the first and largest 12-step group. Millions of people believe they have maintained sobriety and health through these programs. Narcotics Anonymous (NA), Cocaine Anonymous (CA) and other offshoots of AA use the same 12-step model.

In general, any person who has continued alcohol or drug use despite significant consequences (for example, family and health problems) may benefit from a 12-step approach. The main message of these programs is that addiction is a chronic relapsing disorder with no cure, and recovery is an ongoing process that needs continual work.

12-step programs are not religious organizations. References to God and the Higher Power are generic spiritual terms that do not refer to a particular religion. The higher power may be conceptualized as nothing more than the group itself.

For those who still are unable to resonate with the spiritual approach of AA or NA, other self-help groups are available such as Rational Recovery (RR), which emphasizes a self-actualizing cognitive-behavioral approach.

Source: Excerpted from *Diagnosis and Treatment of Drug Abuse in Family Practice—American Family Physician Monograph*, National Institute on Drug Abuse (www.nida.nih.gov), 2003. Reviewed by David A. Cooke, MD, FACP, December 2012.

The point of a recovery plan is always to stay off drugs and sober. It does not have to be very detailed.

Getting help as part of your plan is a good idea. You might be carrying a heavy load of feelings that you have stuffed away all your life. If you have been "doctoring" your emotions with drugs or alcohol, then going without counseling, sponsor, or a group of peers will make it hard for you to stay sober.

Be sure to include medical and dental care in your plan. It will be easier for you to stay off drugs and alcohol if you are not in pain. Make sure your doctor, dentist, and other providers know about your recovery. It will help them care for you, especially if you need medicine for pain. If you need a doctor or dentist, ask your alcohol or drug abuse counselor how to find one.

1. Setting Goals

After years of substance abuse, many people forget what some of their goals and joys once were. Others never had any goals. Your goals should be clear and rewarding. They shouldn't be too hard or too easy. Ordinary, everyday goals keep your life moving forward and keep the old patterns from taking over. They can include elements such as these:

- A job or educational/vocational program

- Social time with substance-free co-workers, friends, and family

- Hobbies and recreation to organize free time

- Completing parole requirements, if necessary

Each goal should be broken down into steps. You should also have a timetable. Here are some examples of ineffective goals and some examples of practical goals:

Ineffective Goals

- Just be strong when I am offered drugs or alcohol

- Make more money

- Don't get arrested for driving without a license

- Show other people that they are wrong

Practical goals

- Find a basketball, soccer, or softball team to join

- Get involved with school activities

- Open a savings account

Goals can be of any size, including jogging or taking young siblings to the playground twice a week. The important thing is that your goals are rewarding and help you stay away from alcohol and drugs.

2. Making Good Decisions

At this point, you have been off drugs for a while. Your head feels better, but you could still be thinking in old ways. To stay in recovery, you need new ways of thinking, and better ways to make decisions.

Friends and family can help you with ideas for different ways to handle tough situations. So can counselors and members of your self-help group.

You can also think situations through on paper by making a kind of decision map. To do this, take a situation you often face, such as "teacher yells at me for being late." Write it in the middle of a piece of paper. Draw a circle around it. Around the circle, add all the reactions you can think of. Here are some examples:

- "I get mad and yell back.
- "I apologize and sit quietly until I calm down."
- "I leave and get drunk."

Draw a circle around each of these reactions, and connect them with a line to the first circle.

Each of these reactions leads to other things, such as these potential consequences:

- "I get mad and yell back" leads to "I get suspended."
- "I leave and get drunk" leads to "I get arrested for DUI."
- "I apologize and sit quietly" leads to "my friends feel better toward me and I get better grades."

Draw a circle around these and connect them to the cause. Making this type of map allows you to see where your decisions take you. Making a map of events and your responses can help you see what leads to drug or alcohol use. Better decisions can help keep you away from alcohol and off drugs.

3. Managing Time

Being in recovery means always moving forward. To move forward, you need to think differently about time. This involves two things.

First, learn to mark time by the clock and the calendar, not by drug-using or drinking events. If you often say things like "that was the time I got drunk and…" then you are using drinking event to mark time.

Divide the day by the clock, not "before I start drinking" and "after I start drinking." Telling time with drinking or drug-using events is part of your substance use disorder. You need to change that pattern. When you talk about the past or any other subject, mention dates or times instead of alcohol or drug use.

Second, you used to spend most of your time and energy on drinking or using. You need to fill that time with other things, and not just do nothing. Get a small calendar or notebook. Fill it with your goals and ways to use your free time. Fill your days with a school, a job, and other activities that will keep you sober, and keep drugs and alcohol from taking over again.

Using your time wisely also helps you avoid anger and other emotions that lead to drinking and drug use. Good use of time helps you fulfill your responsibilities. You can avoid trouble with the people around you by being reliable.

Buy an appointment book or a calendar. Even a pad of paper is okay, as long as you stick to your schedule. Look at your goals and the steps you need to take to get there. Fill in the steps in your calendar or appointment book. Be sure to schedule relaxing times. You do not need to be busy every minute. You should not feel controlled by the clock. But you should use your time in ways that help you with your goals and avoid substance use.

Here are some helpful schedule suggestions:

- Go to meetings. Attending face-to-face or even online self-help groups will help you fill time, stay sober, and meet people who are in recovery.

- Go to religious services. Recovery can have a spiritual side, and it can be helpful to find a religious group with whom you are comfortable.

- Overworking is not a good way to stay sober or stay off drugs. If you overwork to fill up time, you may get so tired that you use drugs or alcohol to relax. Or you may be lonely when work is over. The extra money can be a trigger to "treat yourself" to drugs or alcohol.

- Remember the activities and practices you used at first to help you stay away from drugs or alcohol—your "anti-drugs" and "anti-drinks" (see the previous chapter for more information). They can help you fill your time by giving you positive things to do.

- Your calendar/appointment book can also help you track your progress. After a while, you can flip through earlier pages and see yourself growing a new alcohol-free and drug-free life.

4. Relationships

While you have been getting used to being sober, others have been getting used to the new you. Your relationships will show this ripple effect.

People You May Have Hurt: People may think you can't be trusted. This attitude can be discouraging. You might say to yourself, "If everyone thinks I'm going to get drunk, then I might as well get drunk." Don't let other people's attitudes offend you. Pay attention to your own work on staying sober. Their attitudes will change with time.

If people are angry with you, then you can feel anger, too, or some other emotion that you are not ready to handle. If you used to turn to alcohol or other drugs when you were angry or upset, then you need a plan for these situations. If possible, walk away and do something else until you calm down. Look at your anti-drug/anti-drink list. Don't let the situation trigger a relapse. Use a decision map to think about how to react in a better way.

As you get more stable, others will have more confidence in you. This can have a surprising side effect. As others trust you more, they might get more honest with you. They might be more open with their feelings. This can be hard to deal with. Let these conflicts provoke a change for the better in your relationships.

Consider going to assertiveness training, anger management, or other classes. Encourage your family to get help for themselves, such as a self-help group or a counselor.

People You Drank Or Used With: Others who are still using might not like the changes in you. They can feel rejected or guilty about their own behavior. Dealers don't want to lose your business. A third of people in recovery relapse because of pressure from others.

- Remember that those who offer you drugs or alcohol, even friends or family, are not doing what's best for you.

- Say no immediately, in a way that is convincing.

- Practice saying no with another person, such as "No, thank you, but I'll have a cup of coffee" or "No, I'm not using any more, it's causing me too many problems."

- Don't say something that suggests they can ask again, like "maybe later" or "I'm on medication."

- Suggest something else to do, such as a movie or a walk.

- Do not allow the conversation to remain on drugs. Change the subject. Counselors call this "drug refusal training," and you might want to get help if saying no is a problem for you.

5. Spotting And Stopping A Relapse

It takes a long time for new skills and patterns to take hold. Don't let your guard down. You are in a battle for your life, and you must beware of an ambush.

A slip is a single episode of use. Think of a slip as information, a signal that something is not working. Think about what happened, and figure out what changes are needed.

A relapse, on the other hand, is a return to more-than-once use. If you relapse, it is important to get back on track again. The sooner you stop a relapse, the better. You will eventually succeed. Don't discourage yourself, "I blew it so why should I continue trying?" All-or-nothing thinking, self-blame, and other negative reactions will not help you get back on track. Negative thinking only makes relapse easier and abstinence harder.

Here are some signs of a possible relapse:

- A dream in which you drink or use can be a warning. Think about what you are doing and how you might be drifting toward use.

- People often relapse when they feel better and more in control: they think that moderate use is okay. This thinking often leads to relapse.

- Daydreaming about the "fun" you had while using is a sign of relapse.

- Finding yourself talking about old times (sharing "war stories") can also signal a relapse about to happen.

Here are some suggestions to prevent a relapse:

- Call a counselor or sober friends.

- Leave the situation and walk or jog around the block a few times.

- Eat or distract yourself with a book or movie.

- Tell your friends and family to stop you when you talk about the fun you had while drinking or using.

- Make a list of the good things about your new life, such as better relationships, success at school, looking better, or time and money for hobbies.

- Stop yourself from daydreaming about the fun of drug and alcohol use, and think about the downside.

- If you have already relapsed at least once, think of how it happened. What can you do differently this time?

"Just be strong and say no" is not enough to handle the situations you will face. Write down the ways you could relapse, and come up with a strategy to handle them. Make a copy to keep with you.

6. Knowing The Stumbling Blocks

The "Looking Good" Trap: The "looking good" trap refers to the fact that you are getting healthier. You look much better. No one would guess by your appearance that you have a substance use problem. Other people can tempt you to slip or relapse. You might also begin to doubt that you have a drug or drinking problem. Don't let the mirror fool you. Remind yourself that your looks improve faster than your ability to stay sober.

Money: Paydays can be a big stumbling block. Some people binge when they get their paycheck, especially if it is the first paycheck they have had for a while. As paydays approach, you must plan how to get your paycheck deposited and pay for necessities without spending the money on drugs or alcohol. If money is one of your triggers, don't carry any until you are stable in your abstinence. Arrange for direct deposit of your paycheck if possible. If you need to, take a friend or family member with you when you go shopping.

Dealers and other users know when checks arrive and might come looking for you. Plan ways to avoid them.

Thinking Patterns: To keep recovery going, it is important not to trick yourself. Don't romanticize your past life. Don't expect your desire for drugs or alcohol to go away quickly. When you have cravings, use "healthy thinking" to help yourself through the moment. For example, stop and remind yourself of the pain that drugs caused you. Review the good things about being sober.

Don't talk about the fun of substance use. Ask your friends to interrupt you when this happens. Don't listen when others talk about the fun of use. Change the subject or walk away for a moment.

You might even find yourself doubting you have a drug problem. If that happens, put it to a test: Go to an AA or similar meeting and listen to their stories. If they sound like yours, you will be reminded how sneaky your addiction is.

Other Substances: Stay away from drugs you didn't have a problem with. Your chosen drug may have been alcohol, but you should also stay away from ice, marijuana, crack, and anything else that can trick you into using again.

Triggers And Cravings: Cravings can suddenly come back after three or six months. However, they may quickly fade to a low level again. Practice your anti-drugs/anti-drinks until they do. Even without cravings, your triggers can still ambush you. You always need to be aware of the people, places, and things that can cause you to relapse.

Emotional Issues: Some people experience severe depression and anxiety in the months after detox. If depression or anxiety gets in the way of your recovery, you should get treatment.

Anger often leads to relapse. Situations that can cause anger, especially giving or receiving criticism, need careful handling. Take a class in anger management or assertiveness training, and plan time to avoid conflict.

If you have experienced physical or emotional abuse, staying away from drugs and alcohol will be even more difficult. Find a counselor trained in treating trauma. If you are in an abusive relationship, it will be very difficult for you to stay sober. Abuse and drug use go hand in hand. Get help.

Getting Help: Remember, "detox" is not "cure." Before you leave detox, enroll in substance abuse treatment or another source of help as a way to start your new life. Help for staying sober can come from many different sources:

- Substance abuse counselors

- Case managers

- Vocational counselors

- Housing advocates

- Mental health counselors

- Trauma/abuse specialists

- Outreach workers

- Psychiatrists, psychologists, or social workers

There is overlap in these job types. Detox staff may or may not provide substance abuse counseling. Many counselors also do case management. Some mental health counselors can help you get over abuse.

Outreach workers and case managers provide referrals, and most case managers can also help you escape an abusive relationship. Take advantage of everything you can to stay away from alcohol and drugs.

Four Signs Of Recovery

- I can address problems as they happen, without using drugs or alcohol, and without getting stressed out.

- I have at least one person I can be completely honest with.

- I have personal boundaries and know which issues are mine and which ones belong to other people.

- I take the time to restore my energy—physical and emotional—when I am tired.

Source: SAMHSA, 2011.

Legal Issues

Your drug or alcohol use may have gotten you into trouble with the police. If you stay off alcohol and drugs and stay in treatment, the law gives you some protection to help you recover. But that help is limited, and you have to do your part.

If you are on parole, it is important that you finish your term of supervision in the community. One of the goals of parole is to change old drinking and drug-using patterns. Parole also adds structure to a person's life with work and other requirements. This structure helps prevent relapse. Most people in recovery who violate parole also relapse.

Part Six
Alcoholism In The Family

Chapter 38

Children Of Alcoholics

More Than 7 Million Children Live With A Parent With Alcohol Problems

An annual average of 7.5 million children younger than the age of 18 (10.5 percent of all children; see Figure 38.1) live with a parent who had an alcohol use disorder in the past year. These children are at a greater risk for depression, anxiety disorders, problems with cognitive and verbal skills, and parental abuse or neglect. Furthermore, they are four times more likely than other children to develop alcohol problems themselves.

Children may be exposed to family alcohol problems regardless of their household composition. According to the 2005 to 2010 National Surveys on Drug Use and Health (NSDUHs), of the 7.5 million children living with a parent with an alcohol use disorder, most of these children (6.1 million) lived with two parents and either one or both of these parents had an alcohol problem. However, 1.4 million children lived in households with single parents who had alcohol use disorders. In these households, 1.1 million children lived with a mother, and 0.3 million lived with a father.

About This Chapter: This chapter includes information from "More than 7 Million Children Live with a Parent with Alcohol Problems," *Data Spotlight*, National Survey on Drug Use and Health, Center for Behavioral Health Statistics and Quality, Substance Abuse and Mental Health Services Administration (www.samhsa.gov), February 16, 2012. The National Survey on Drug Use and Health (NSDUH) is an annual survey sponsored by the Substance Abuse and Mental Health Services Administration (SAMHSA). The survey collects data by administering questionnaires to a representative sample of the population through face-to-face interviews at their places of residence. The chapter also includes excerpts from "Protecting Children in Families Affected by Substance Use Disorders," Child Welfare Information Gateway (www.childwelfare.gov), a service of the Children's Bureau, Administration for Children and Families, 2009.

There are many resources to help children when a parent has an alcohol problem. The National Association for Children of Alcoholics (http://www.nacoa.org/) provides information and resources for professionals who work with these families. For additional resources, visit http://www.samhsa.gov/treatment/.

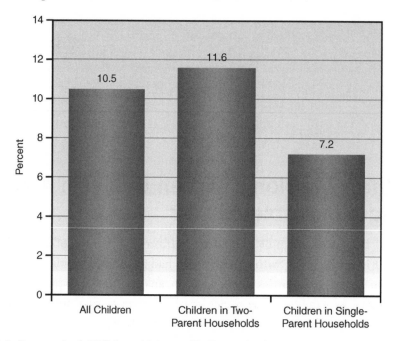

Figure 38.1. Percent of Children Living with Parent with a Past Year Alcohol Use Disorder, by Household Composition: 2005 to 2010

How Parental Substance Use Disorders Affect Children

A predictable, consistent environment, coupled with positive caregiver relationships, is critical for normal emotional development of children. Parental substance abuse and dependence have a negative impact on the physical and emotional well-being of children and can cause home environments to become chaotic and unpredictable, leading to child maltreatment. The children's physical and emotional needs often take a back seat to their parents' activities related to obtaining, using, or recovering from the use of drugs and alcohol.

The Impact On Childhood Development

Exposure to parental substance use disorders (SUDs) during childhood also can have dire consequences for children. Compared to children of parents who do not abuse alcohol or drugs, children of parents who do, and who also are in the child welfare system, are more likely to experience physical, intellectual, social, and emotional problems. Among the difficulties in providing services to these children is that problems affected or compounded by their parents' SUDs might not emerge until later in their lives.

Disruption Of The Bonding Process

When mothers or fathers abuse substances after delivery, their ability to bond with their child—so important during the early stages of life—may be weakened. In order for an attachment to form, it is necessary that caregivers pay attention to and notice their children's attempts to communicate. Parents who use marijuana, for example, may have difficulty picking up their babies' cues because marijuana dulls response time and alters perceptions. When parents repeatedly miss their babies' cues, the babies eventually stop providing them. The result is disengaged parents with disengaged babies. These parents and babies then have difficulty forming a healthy, appropriate relationship.

Neglected children who are unable to form secure attachments with their primary caregivers may have these characteristics:

- Become more mistrustful of others and may be less willing to learn from adults

- Have difficulty understanding the emotions of others, regulating their own emotions, or forming and maintaining relationships with others

- Have a limited ability to feel remorse or empathy, which may mean that they could hurt others without feeling their actions were wrong

- Demonstrate a lack of confidence or social skills that could hinder them from being successful in school, work, and relationships

- Demonstrate impaired social cognition, which is awareness of oneself in relation to others as well as of others' emotions. Impaired social cognition can lead a person to view many social interactions as stressful.

Emotional, Academic, And Developmental Problems

Children who experience either prenatal or postnatal drug exposure are at risk for a range of emotional, academic, and developmental problems. For example, they are more likely to experience symptoms of depression and anxiety, suffer from psychiatric disorders, exhibit behavior problems, score lower on school achievement tests, and demonstrate other difficulties in school.

These children may behave in ways that are challenging for biological or foster parents to manage, which can lead to inconsistent caregiving and multiple alternative care placements.

Positive social and emotional child development generally has been linked to nurturing family settings in which caregivers are predictable, daily routines are respected, and everyone recognizes clear boundaries for acceptable behaviors. Such circumstances often are missing in the homes of parents with SUDs. As a result, extra supports and interventions are needed to help children draw upon their strengths and maximize their natural potential despite their home environments. Protective factors, such as the involvement of other supportive adults (for example, extended family members, mentors, clergy, teachers, neighbors), may help mitigate the impact of parental SUDs.

Lack Of Supervision

The search for drugs or alcohol, the use of scarce resources to pay for them, the time spent in illegal activities to raise money for them, or the time spent recovering from hangovers or withdrawal symptoms can leave parents with little time or energy to care properly for their children. These children frequently do not have their basic needs met and often do not receive appropriate supervision. In addition, rules about curfews and potentially dangerous activities may not be enforced or are enforced haphazardly. As a result, SUDs are often a factor in neglect cases.

Parentification

As children grow older, they may become increasingly aware that their parents cannot care for them. To compensate, the children become the caregivers of the family, often extending their caregiving behavior to their parents as well as younger siblings. This process is labeled *parentification.*

Parentified children carry a great deal of anxiety and sometimes go to great lengths to control or to eliminate their parents' use of drugs or alcohol. They feel responsible for running the family. These feelings are reinforced by messages from the parents that the children cause the parents' SUDs or are at fault in some way if the family comes to the attention of authorities. Sometimes these children must contact medical personnel in the case of a parent's overdose, or they may be left supervising and caring for younger children when their parents are absent while obtaining or abusing substances.

Social Stigma

Adults with SUDs may engage in behaviors that embarrass their children and may appear disinterested in their children's activities or school performance. Children may separate themselves from their parents by not wanting to go home after school, by not bringing friends to the house, or by not asking for help with homework. These children may feel a social stigma attached to certain aspects of their parents' lives, such as unemployment, homelessness, an involvement with the criminal justice system, or SUD treatment.

Adolescent Substance Use And Delinquency

Adolescents whose parents have SUDs are more likely to develop SUDs themselves. Some adolescents mimic behaviors they see in their families, including ineffective coping behaviors such as using drugs and alcohol. Many of these children also witness or are victims of violence. It is hypothesized that substance abuse is a coping mechanism for such traumatic events. Moreover, adolescents who use substances are more likely to have poor academic performance and to be involved in criminal activities. The longer children are exposed to parental SUD, the more serious the negative consequences may be for their overall development and well-being.

Child Abuse As A Precursor to Substance Use Disorders

Many people view SUDs as a phenomenon that leads to or exacerbates the abuse or neglect of children. Research also suggests, however, that being victimized by child abuse, particularly sexual abuse, is a common precursor of SUDs. Sometimes, victims of abuse or neglect "self-medicate" (that is, drink or use drugs to escape the unresolved trauma of the maltreatment). One study found that women with a history of childhood physical or sexual abuse were nearly five times more likely to use street drugs and more than twice as likely to abuse alcohol as women who were not maltreated. In another study, childhood abuse predicted a wide range of problems, including lower self-esteem, more victimization, more depression, and chronic homelessness, and indirectly predicted drug and alcohol problems.

Source: Child Welfare Information Gateway, 2009.

Chapter 39

The Dynamics Of An Alcoholic Family

Alcoholism affects many people in addition to the drinker. It also affects the people with whom the drinker interacts, especially the family. Many experts call alcoholism a family disease.

All families have their own ways of doing things, and most have their own secrets. The biggest secret of a family where someone has a drinking problem is the very fact that it is a family plagued by alcoholism. To hide this secret, family members may take on responsibilities that would ordinarily be assumed by the alcoholic person. They may neglect their own needs and feelings. The family may isolate themselves from others so nobody finds out their secret. They don't want anyone to know that alcohol is as much a part of the family as the parents, children, and other relatives.

Living With An Alcoholic

Home should be a safe place where each and every person can be themselves. The parents should provide a nurturing, protective, predictable environment for their youngsters. Children should be allowed to be children and to mature under the guidance of trustworthy adults.

An alcoholic family falls far short of this ideal. The drinker's behavior is unpredictable, and it determines the way other family members act. Suppose the father is the alcoholic, for example. Sometimes he is a funny, loving dad, and the family enjoys being together. But when under the influence of alcohol, this same father may fly into a rage, shouting, throwing things around, even hitting his wife or children. The mother might try to protect her children by sending them outside to play or to another part of the house to watch television or study. Knowing how

About This Chapter: "The Dynamics Of An Alcoholic Family," by Laurie Lewis, reviewed by David A. Cooke, MD, FACP, December 2012. © 2013 Omnigraphics, Inc.

their father is acting, the kids can't concentrate on their homework. Maybe the result will be a bad grade on a test the next day. The student worries not just about the poor grade but about how dad will react if he finds out. Will he drink even more or lash out again in anger?

Besides behaving unpredictably and sometimes violently, an alcoholic may not be able to function like a responsible adult. Maybe drinking will become so serious that a parent is unable to keep a job or care for the family. The non-drinking parent may have to work extra-long hours to bring in enough money to support the family. The children may have to look after themselves. Often the burden falls on the oldest children, who have to babysit their younger brothers and sisters, get them dinner, and wash their clothes. No wonder the older kids have little time for their own schoolwork and friends! When they do take time to be with friends, they don't want to bring them home. They'd be too embarrassed if the alcoholic parent lost control and the family's shameful secret got out.

Shame is only one emotion that the family of an alcoholic feels. Family members may be angry or disappointed with the alcoholic, especially if that person has made promises that are not met. The family of the alcoholic lives in fear of the next outburst. Nobody feels safe. Children may feel neglected, unloved, and worthless. Everyone is stressed. The frustration level in the family is high because the non-alcoholics don't know what to do to help the drinker quit.

It's Not Your Fault

Alcoholics have difficulty taking responsibility for their drinking problem. They blame others for their behavior. Maybe an alcoholic parent, for example, will scream at the children, "You're driving me crazy!" and reach for a drink.

Even without parents pointing the finger of blame, children and adolescents often think they are responsible. "If only I did better in school, my mom wouldn't drink so much," a youngster might say. "I'm always getting in trouble. I upset dad and he needs to drink to get calmer," another might think.

It's simply not true. People don't drink too much because somebody else makes them. Alcoholism is a disease. Nobody can cause this disease in another person, just like nothing a person does to a loved one can cause cancer.

Family members often feel they have failed when they cannot convince the alcoholic to stop drinking. Again, it's nobody's fault. The alcoholic must be ready and willing to give up drinking and stay sober. It's hard work, and people often fail several times before they finally are able to avoid alcohol forever.

New Family Roles

By trying to help the alcoholic, family and friends often become trapped in a codependent or enabling relationship. The enabler makes it possible for the alcoholic to continue drinking, for example, by making excuses for alcohol-related absences and by handling tasks the drinker fails to complete. The alcoholic depends on the enabler, who in turn needs the drinker's dependence to feel valuable. Many codependent enablers have low self-esteem but feel they can look after the alcoholic's best interests better than the drinker can. They think they are helping but are actually making the situation worse for both themselves and the alcoholic. The enabler's needs become secondary to the drinker's, and the alcoholic does not have to take responsibility for inappropriate behavior and addiction.

To keep the family together, members may take on other specific roles. The non-drinking parent may become a super-parent, assuming all adult responsibilities for the household. Sometimes that role falls to the older children, especially in single-parent households. Whether an adult or an adolescent, the super-parent looks after everyone's needs except his or her own.

Rather than becoming the family's caretaker, some children become super-achievers. They escape from family troubles by excelling in school, sports, music, chess, or some other activity. Their accomplishments make the family proud and wipe away, at least in part, the shame of the family's drinking problem. Healthy though it may seem to rise above the stress of an alcoholic family, the super-achieving child carries the burden of always having to excel and is at risk for great disappointment if he or she fails to remain a star.

In contrast to the super-achiever, some youngsters hold the alcoholic family together by playing the role of bad child. These kids are always in trouble, and their misbehaving takes the family's attention away from the alcoholic. Instead of focusing on the problem drinker, the family and their social contacts try to find ways to help the problem child. With attention on the youngster, it may be easy to overlook the real cause of the family's stress.

Other children become neither super-achievers nor bad kids. They almost seem to fade into the woodwork. These youngsters may spend most of their time at home in their own room or sit glazed for hours in front of television. They don't want to make waves and seldom express their feelings. Other family members can easily overlook the needs of the quiet child who makes few demands, causing the youngster to feel ignored, neglected, and unimportant.

A Problem For All Ages

In an alcoholic family, a parent usually is the one with a drinking problem. But anyone could become an alcoholic. It could be a child, a grandparent, or a member of the extended family. Regardless of who is the drinker, family dynamics can be affected.

Parents are the most important role models in children's lives. When children see their parents use alcohol, they may think it's okay to follow the example. Alternatively, they may reject alcohol because of the negative effects they have witnessed firsthand. But parental drinking alone doesn't determine whether a child will become an alcoholic. Several studies have demonstrated that the drinking habits of younger adolescents are influenced less by their parents' example than by the limits their parents set and other parenting behaviors.

Having a sibling who drinks can lead a child to risky behavior. Parents tend to focus their attention on a child with a substance abuse problem, often ignoring the needs of the abusers' brothers and sisters. Sometimes these siblings begin to act out to get their parents' attention.

Some families have a history of alcoholism in multiple generations. Children might witness the abnormal family dynamics between their parents and grandparents, and perhaps aunts and uncles, and think this is normal adult behavior. The family might also assume that the youngest generation will follow in the path of alcoholism.

Long-Term Effects

Children of alcoholics are four times more likely than others to develop drinking problems. But more than half of children of alcoholics do not become alcoholics themselves. Both genetics and the way a child is raised help determine the future.

Help Is Just a Meeting Away At Al-Anon Or Alateen

You may think nobody could possibly understand the stress you go through living in an alcoholic family. You are so wrong! Millions of people know just how you feel because they are living with the same problem. And they're not hard to find. Just go to http://www.al-anon.alateen.org to locate a nearby meeting of people like you.

That website describes Al-Anon and Alateen. Al-Anon is a group for family and friends of alcoholics, and Alateen is a subgroup specifically for adolescents. Both groups have meetings where people with a loved one who has a drinking problem can talk about their situation with others in the same boat. Attendees don't share their full names, but they do share their experiences and coping strategies. And best of all, they support each other as only someone going through the same tough time can do.

You can attend an Al-Anon or Alateen meeting even if the drinker in your family doesn't admit that he or she has an alcohol problem. If your relative's drinking worries you, it is a problem for you. Going to a meeting where you can be in a comfortable, safe place to talk about the situation at home is one of the best things you can do for yourself.

A child whose parents have not been reliable, supportive nurturers may have difficulty developing trusting, healthy relationships in later life. Sometimes a bond with another adult, who provides the nurturing that the family cannot, is enough to reverse the negative influence and help the youngster mature into a trusting, caring adult.

Despite their difficult home life, many children of alcoholics become strong, capable adults. Those who have confronted alcoholism head-on, with their family, through counseling or support groups like Al-Anon, or by their own inner strength, may have the best chance of rising above their dysfunctional family roots. Without a doubt, it is possible to overcome the negative influences of an alcoholic family.

References

Al-Anon. Media interview questions. Accessed October 24, 2012. http://www.al-anon.alateen.org/media-interview-questions.

Gossrau-Breen D, Kuntsche E, Gmel G. My older sibling was drunk: younger siblings' drunkenness in relation to parental monitoring and the parent-adolescent relationship. *J Adolesc* 2010;33(5):643-652.

Hills Treatment Center. Family article series. Accessed October 24, 2012. http://www.thehillscenter.com/family.

National Institute on Alcohol Abuse and Alcoholism. A family history of alcoholism: are you at risk? NIH Pub No. 03-5340. September 2007.

Querin DS, Querin KB. Substance abuse as a family disease: Part I: impact on the family. Accessed October 24, 2012. http://or.americanmentalhealth.com/family.trust.

University of Notre Dame. Family history of alcoholism. 2008. http://oade.nd.edu/support-for-students/family-history-of-alcoholism.

U.S. Department of Health and Human Services. Chapter 2: Impact of substance abuse on families. In: *Substance abuse treatment and family therapy: a treatment improvement protocol* TIP 39. 2005. DHHS Pub No. (SMA) 05-4006.

van der Zwaluw CS, Scholte RHJ, Vermulst AA, Buitelaar JK, Verkes RJ, Engels RCME. Parental problem drinking, parenting, and adolescent alcohol use. *J Behav Med* 2008;31:189–200.

Yu J. The association between parental alcohol-related behaviors and children's drinking. *Drug Alcohol Depend* 2003;69(3): 253–262.

Chapter 40

A Family History Of Alcoholism: Are You At Risk?

If you are among the millions of people in this country who have a parent, grandparent, or other close relative with alcoholism, you may have wondered what your family's history of alcoholism means for you. Are problems with alcohol a part of your future? Is your risk for becoming an alcoholic greater than for people who do not have a family history of alcoholism? If so, what can you do to lower your risk?

Many scientific studies, including research conducted among twins and children of alcoholics, have shown that genetic factors influence alcoholism. These findings show that children of alcoholics are about four times more likely than the general population to develop alcohol problems. Children of alcoholics also have a higher risk for many other behavioral and emotional problems. But alcoholism is not determined only by the genes you inherit from your parents. In fact, more than one-half of all children of alcoholics do not become alcoholic. Research shows that many factors influence your risk of developing alcoholism. Some factors raise the risk while others lower it.

Genes are not the only things children inherit from their parents. How parents act and how they treat each other and their children has an influence on children growing up in the family. These aspects of family life also affect the risk for alcoholism. Researchers believe a person's risk increases if he or she is in a family with the following difficulties:

- An alcoholic parent is depressed or has other psychological problems
- Both parents abuse alcohol and other drugs

About This Chapter: This chapter begins with excerpts from "A Family History of Alcoholism: Are You at Risk?" National Institute on Alcohol Abuse and Alcoholism (NIAAA; www.niaaa.nih.gov), September 2007. It continues with an excerpt from "The Genetics of Alcoholism," NIAAAA, *Alcohol Alert*, No. 60, July 2003. Reviewed by David A. Cooke, MD, FACP, December 2012.

- The parents' alcohol abuse is severe

- Conflicts lead to aggression and violence in the family

The good news is that many children of alcoholics from even the most troubled families do not develop drinking problems. Just as a family history of alcoholism does not guarantee that you will become an alcoholic, neither does growing up in a very troubled household with alcoholic parents. Just because alcoholism tends to run in families does not mean that a child of an alcoholic parent will automatically become an alcoholic too. The risk is higher but it does not have to happen.

If you are worried that your family's history of alcohol problems or your troubled family life puts you at risk for becoming alcoholic, here is some common-sense advice to help you:

- **Avoid Underage Drinking:** First, underage drinking is illegal. Second, research shows that the risk for alcoholism is higher among people who begin to drink at an early age, perhaps as a result of both environmental and genetic factors.

- **Drink Moderately As An Adult:** Even if they do not have a family history of alcoholism, adults who choose to drink alcohol should do so in moderation—no more than one drink a day for most women, and no more than two drinks a day for most men, according to guidelines from the U.S. Department of Agriculture and the U.S. Department of Health and Human Services. Some people should not drink at all, including women who are pregnant or who are trying to become pregnant, recovering alcoholics, people who plan to drive or engage in other activities that require attention or skill, people taking certain medications, and people with certain medical conditions.

What is alcoholism?

Alcoholism, or alcohol dependence, is a disease that includes four symptoms:

- **Craving:** A strong need, or urge, to drink.

- **Loss Of Control:** Not being able to stop drinking once drinking has begun.

- **Physical Dependence:** Withdrawal symptoms, such as upset stomach, sweating, shakiness, and anxiety after stopping drinking.

- **Tolerance:** The need to drink greater amounts of alcohol to get "high."

Source: NIAAA, September 2007. Reviewed by David A. Cooke, MD, FACP, December 2012.

- **Consider Your Family History:** People with a family history of alcoholism, who have a higher risk for becoming dependent on alcohol, should approach moderate drinking carefully. Maintaining moderate drinking habits may be harder for them than for people without a family history of drinking problems. Once a person moves from moderate to heavier drinking, the risks of social problems (for example, drinking and driving, violence, and trauma) and medical problems (for example, liver disease, brain damage, and cancer) increase greatly.

- **Talk To A Health Care Professional:** Discuss your concerns with a doctor, nurse, nurse practitioner, or other health care provider. They can recommend groups or organizations that could help you avoid alcohol problems.

The Genetics Of Alcoholism

Research has shown conclusively that familial transmission of alcoholism risk is at least in part genetic and not just the result of family environment. The task of current science is to identify what a person inherits that increases vulnerability to alcoholism and how inherited factors interact with the environment to cause disease. This information will provide the basis for identifying people at risk and for developing behavioral and pharmacologic (medicine-use) approaches to prevent and treat alcohol problems. The advances being made now are built on the discovery 50 years ago of the role in inheritance of DNA, the genetic material in cells that serves as a blueprint for the proteins that direct life processes. Alcoholism research, like other fields, is capitalizing on the scientific spinoffs of this milestone, among them the Human Genome Project and related efforts to sequence the genomes, the complete DNA sequences, of selected animals.

A Complex Genetic Disease

Studies in recent years have confirmed that identical twins, who share the same genes, are about twice as likely as fraternal twins, who share on average 50 percent of their genes, to resemble each other in terms of the presence of alcoholism. Recent research also reports that 50 to 60 percent of the risk for alcoholism is genetically determined, for both men and women. Genes alone do not preordain that someone will be alcoholic; features in the environment along with gene–environment interactions account for the remainder of the risk.

Research suggests that many genes play a role in shaping alcoholism risk. Like diabetes and heart disease, alcoholism is considered genetically complex, distinguishing it from genetic diseases, such as cystic fibrosis, that result primarily from the action of one or two copies of a single gene and in which the environment plays a much smaller role, if any. The methods used to search for genes in complex diseases have to account for the fact that the effects of any one gene may be subtle and a different array of genes underlies risk in different people.

One well-characterized relationship between genes and alcoholism is the result of variation in the liver enzymes that metabolize (break down) alcohol. By speeding up the metabolism of alcohol to a toxic intermediate, acetaldehyde, or slowing down the conversion of acetaldehyde to acetate, genetic variants in the enzymes alcohol dehydrogenase (ADH) or aldehyde dehydrogenase (ALDH) raise the level of acetaldehyde after drinking, causing symptoms that include flushing, nausea, and rapid heartbeat. The genes for these enzymes and the alleles (gene variants) that alter alcohol metabolism have been identified. Genes associated with flushing are more common among Asian populations than other ethnic groups, and the rates of drinking and alcoholism are correspondingly lower among Asian populations.

Chapter 41

The Link Between Paternal Alcohol Use And Adolescent Substance Abuse

Alcohol dependence or abuse—and even moderate alcohol use—among fathers living with adolescents (youths aged 12 to 17) may increase the risk of substance use among those children. Increasing public awareness of the association between paternal alcohol use and adolescent substance use may help to focus attention on providing treatment for affected fathers and support for their children to prevent or reduce adolescent substance use. The National Survey on Drug Use and Health (NSDUH) gathers information that can help to provide a better understanding of the relationship between paternal alcohol use and adolescent substance use.

The NSDUH sample includes a subsample of parents and children who live in the same household. The survey annually collects data on the use of alcohol and illicit drugs,[1] including questions about symptoms of dependence or abuse. Dependence or abuse is defined using criteria specified in the *Diagnostic and Statistical Manual of Mental Disorders (DSM-IV)*,[2] which include symptoms such as withdrawal, tolerance, use in dangerous situations, trouble with the law, and interference in major obligations at work, school, or home during the past year.

This report examines rates of adolescent substance use and substance use disorders (dependence on or abuse of alcohol or illicit drugs) by level of alcohol use in the past year among fathers (that is, no alcohol use, alcohol use but no alcohol use disorder, and alcohol use disorder). It focuses on biological, step-, adoptive, and foster children aged 12 to 17 who were living with their fathers at the time of the survey interview.[3] All findings are based on annual averages from combined 2002 to 2007 NSDUH data.

About This Chapter: From "Fathers' Alcohol Use and Substance Use among Adolescents," The NSDUH Report, National Survey on Drug Use and Health, Substance Abuse and Mental Health Services Administration (www .samhsa.gov), June 18, 2009.

Fathers' Alcohol Use

Almost one in twelve (7.9 percent) fathers living with adolescents aged 12 to 17 had an alcohol use disorder, while 68.1 percent used alcohol in the past year but did not have an alcohol use disorder; 24.1 percent did not use alcohol in the past year. Nearly one third (31.2 percent) of fathers living with adolescents indicated binge alcohol use in the past month.[4]

Adolescent Alcohol Use And Alcohol Use Disorder

The rate of past year alcohol use among adolescents was lower for those who lived with a father who did not use alcohol in the past year than for those who lived with a father who used alcohol but did not have an alcohol use disorder and for those who lived with a father with an alcohol use disorder (21.1 vs. 33.2 and 38.8 percent, respectively). Adolescents' past year alcohol use rates did not differ significantly between those who lived with fathers who had an alcohol use disorder and those who lived with fathers who used alcohol but who did not have an alcohol use disorder.

Table 41.1. Level of Past Year Alcohol Use among Fathers Living with Adolescents*: 2002 to 2007

Alcohol Use	Percent
Alcohol Use, but No Alcohol Use Disorder	68.1%
No Alcohol Use	24.1%
Alcohol Use Disorder	7.9%

* Percentages do not add to 100% due to rounding.

Source: 2002 to 2007 SAMHSA National Surveys on Drug Use and Health (NSDUHs).

Table 41.2. Alcohol Use and Alcohol Use Disorder among Adolescents (Living with a Father), by the Father's Level of Alcohol Use in the Past Year: 2002 to 2007

Adolescent Outcomes	Father Did Not Use Alcohol	Father Used Alcohol, but Did Not Have an Alcohol Use Disorder	Father Had an Alcohol Use Disorder
Past Year Alcohol Use	21.1%	33.2%	38.8%
Past Month Binge Alcohol Use*	5.7%	9.2%	13.1%
Past Year Alcohol Use Disorder	3.0%	4.7%	10.3%

* Binge alcohol use is defined as drinking five or more drinks on the same occasion (i.e., at the same time or within a couple of hours of each other) on at least one day in the past 30 days.

Source: 2002 to 2007 SAMHSA National Surveys on Drug Use and Health (NSDUHs).

The rates of past month binge alcohol use and past year alcohol use disorder among adolescents increased with the level of paternal alcohol use. For example, the rate of alcohol use disorder among adolescents who lived with a father who did not use alcohol in the past year was lower than the rate among those who lived with a father who used alcohol in the past year but did not have an alcohol use disorder (3.0 vs. 4.7 percent), which in turn was lower than the rate among those who lived with a father with an alcohol use disorder (10.3 percent).

Adolescent Illicit Drug Use And Drug Use Disorder

Paternal alcohol use also was related to adolescent illicit drug use. The percentage of adolescents using illicit drugs in the past year increased with the level of paternal alcohol use, with illicit drug use reported by 14.0 percent of adolescents who lived with a father who did not use alcohol in the past year, 18.4 percent of those who lived with a father who used alcohol but did not have an alcohol use disorder, and 24.2 percent of those who lived with a father with an alcohol use disorder. The rate of past year illicit drug use disorder among adolescents was 2.6 percent among those who lived with a father who did not use alcohol in the past year, 3.9 percent among those who lived with a father who used alcohol but did not have an alcohol use disorder, and 4.2 percent among those who lived with a father with an alcohol use disorder.

Table 41.3. Illicit Drug Use and Drug Use Disorder among Adolescents (Living with a Father), by the Father's Level of Alcohol Use in the Past Year: 2002 to 2007

Adolescent Outcomes	Father Did Not Use Alcohol	Father Used Alcohol, but Did Not Have an Alcohol Use Disorder	Father Had an Alcohol Use Disorder
Past Year Illicit Drug Use	14.0%	18.4%	24.2%
Past Year Illicit Drug Use Disorder	2.6%	3.9%	4.2%

Source: 2002 to 2007 SAMHSA National Surveys on Drug Use and Health (NSDUHs).

Discussion

Alcohol use among fathers, even at levels not sufficient to warrant a diagnosis of an alcohol use disorder, is associated with several substance use behaviors and disorders among the adolescent children who live with them. These findings highlight the continuing need to educate fathers, mothers, and family support systems professionals about the potential impact of paternal alcohol use on adolescent substance use. In addition, these findings suggest the importance of providing treatment for fathers with alcohol use disorders and family support services for children of these fathers.

End Notes

1. NSDUH defines illicit drugs as marijuana/hashish, cocaine (including crack), inhalants, hallucinogens, heroin, or prescription-type drugs used nonmedically.

2. American Psychiatric Association. (1994). *Diagnostic and statistical manual of mental disorders (4th ed.)*. Washington, DC: Author.

3. An estimated 72.4 percent of adolescents aged 12 to 17 lived with a father. See U.S. Census Bureau, Population Division, Fertility & Family Statistics Branch. (2008, August 27). *America's families and living arrangements: 2004. Table C2. Household relationships and living arrangements of children under 18 years, by age, sex, race, and Hispanic origin: 2004*. Retrieved April 14, 2009, from http://www.census.gov/population/www/socdemo/hh-fam/cps2004.html

4. Binge alcohol use is defined as drinking five or more drinks on the same occasion (that is., at the same time or within a couple of hours of each other) on at least one day in the past 30 days.

Chapter 42

What To Do If A Family Member Abuses Alcohol

In the United States, about 7.5 million people under age 18 live with at least one alcoholic parent. It's hard for teens trapped in this situation. Some feel guilty that they can't save their parent. They may carry a parent's alcoholism as a shameful secret and feel isolated and alone.

Living with an alcoholic means walking on eggshells, always wondering what will happen next. Some teens are forced to take on the parent's responsibilities, like getting younger siblings ready for school in the morning because a parent is passed out or already drinking.

When a family revolves around a parent's drinking problem, teens' friendships, schoolwork, and plans for the future can suffer. But parents' alcoholism should not ruin children's lives. There *are* ways to cope and help is available so teens can move forward, succeed, and *be* teens.

Coping With A Family Member's Drinking

It's tough to admit that somebody you love and look up to cannot control their drinking. Going through certain questions can help teens realize their concerns are valid.

According to Alateen, being worried about how much someone drinks is a key sign that you are being affected by their drinking habits. If you find yourself secretly trying to smell the drinker's breath or if you sometimes tell lies to cover up for the drinker, those are also signs that you're being affected. Alateen notes that being hurt or embarrassed by a drinker's behavior can also signal that there's a problem. If you search for a person's hidden alcohol, that's another strong indication that their drinking is cause for concern.[1]

About This Chapter: "What To Do If A Family Member Abuses Alcohol," by Lisa Esposito, reviewed by David A. Cooke, MD, FACP, December 2012. © 2013 Omnigraphics, Inc.

Alcoholism is a disease. Alcoholics can't control their drinking or stop on their own. Teens are not responsible for a friend's or family member's drinking. They didn't cause the problem, and it's not their fault. Teens can't make another person stop drinking, either. That's a choice only the alcoholic can make.

Alcoholism is never considered fully cured. Instead, people who quit are known as recovering alcoholics. It's a lifelong process. Teens *can* show love and support as a family member or friend goes through recovery.

When A Sibling Or Friend Drinks

Certain signs can alert teens that a brother, sister, or friend has a problem with alcohol. Drinking regularly and drunk driving are clear signs. But when friends drop out of all activities or act like a different person when they drink, that also points to a problem.

A teen might be reluctant to tell parents or other adults about another teen's problem. But if a young person talks about suicide plans or hurting themselves, an adult needs to know. When a person drinks to the point of passing out and can't be wakened, it's called alcohol poisoning. If this happens, the teen should call 911. Alcohol poisoning is a medical emergency that can result in coma and even death.

Some parents host parties in their home where minors are allowed to drink. Parents may think this is a safer environment, but it just encourages underage drinking. In fact, they may be breaking the law. In certain states, if an adult—including an older sibling—provides liquor to a minor who then gets hurt or killed in an accident, that adult can go to jail.[2]

Teens who drink influence younger brothers and sisters to drink. Boys are more likely to drink if older brothers do so, and girls are more likely to drink if their older sisters do.[3] By choosing not to abuse alcohol, teens not only help themselves but also act as good role models for younger siblings who look up to them.

What Teens Can Do To Help A Problem Drinker

Learning about alcoholism can help teens understand what a family member or friend is dealing with. Local libraries and the internet provide a wealth of information. Speaking up is one step to improving the situation. Teens can talk to the person about their concerns, offer support, and volunteer to go along when the person seeks help. They can let their family member or friend know that they care.

Approaching a problem drinker isn't easy. The person may make get angry or make excuses. People who abuse alcohol are often in denial. They may lie to themselves and others and refuse to face unpleasant facts. Teens should be ready to give specific examples of how the drinker has changed and of things they do that cause concern.

What Works

Here are some suggestions for having a conversation about problem drinking with someone you care about.[4]

- Think about what you're going to say in advance.

- Choose a time when your family member or friend is sober and calm.

- Talk in a place with privacy.

- Talk about specific behaviors and how you feel when they occur.

- Listen without judging.

- Be prepared to have more than one talk before your parent, friend, brother, or sister *really* listens.

What Doesn't Work

While it's important to speak up, some approaches work better than others. It's best to be calm and straightforward, not dramatic or emotional.

- Preaching at an alcohol abuser will push him or her away. Lecturing, threatening, or bribing won't work. Begging someone not to drink or trying to make them feel guilty won't work.

- It's no use trying to argue or reason with the person while they're drinking. They can't carry on a real conversation.

- Pouring out or watering down someone's supply of alcohol doesn't work. They will just replace it.

- Enabling means mean making it easier for an alcoholic to continue drinking and protecting them from consequences. For instance, teens may feel forced to lie or make excuses for a parent who is late to work or fails to show up for a teacher conference. Enabling only makes things worse in the long run.

- Giving money to a friend with a drinking problem is another kind of enabling.

It may take a long time before the person admits to having a problem and is willing to seek help. Some alcoholics never do so. Others try but suffer relapses and start drinking again. People may relapse and recover more than once. Teens can continue to show their concern and express their support.

Not Just Parents

When a teen's extended family members—grandparents, aunts, uncles, and cousins—abuse alcohol, it also can be painful and difficult. These drinkers can create awkward situations and ruin family get-togethers. They may urge young relatives to have a drink to keep them company. Sometimes it's enough to say no and walk away. If that doesn't work, one strategy is for the teen to blame their parents, as in, "Sorry, my mother (or father) would be furious if you gave me alcohol."

Saying No To Drinking With Friends

At parties and other teen gatherings, friends and acquaintances sometimes pressure others to drink. There are ways to say "no" without making a big deal of it. A simple "no thanks, I don't drink" or "I'll just have a soda" are low-key ways of refusing. Changing the subject or making an excuse like "I have a test tomorrow" can also work. "Broken record" is a refusal technique that means repeating a response over and over until people finally back off.

If friends don't let up on the pressure to drink, it's probably time to find other friends who respect teens' choices. There's strength in numbers. Hanging out with non-drinkers makes it easier for teens not to drink.

Getting Teens' Lives Back On Track

Parents whose own lives are out of control from drinking can't properly guide and support their children. So teens need to look out for themselves. They have their own physical and mental health to consider. They have school responsibilities and outside activities. Teen years should be a time to become more independent and have fun with friends.

The following strategies can help teens avoid isolation and find strength to manage their own lives:

- Find a trustworthy person to talk to. It could be a non-alcoholic relative or a reliable neighbor. It could be a friend's parent. It could be a teacher, school counselor, coach, activity leader, minister, or rabbi.

- Separate yourself from a parent's drinking. Don't see it as *your* problem.

- Look to yourself and others who care about you for comfort and approval.

- Distance yourself and become more independent. This is a gradual process and a big adjustment for any teen. But for teens with alcoholic parents, it can be the groundwork for a better future. Children who learn to remove themselves do better as adults than those who remain entangled in their parents' problems.[5] It's possible to be aware and supportive without being dragged down.

- Concentrate on your own talents, skills, and abilities. Do things that you enjoy. Join a team, play in the school band, volunteer on the yearbook staff. If you already have activities or hobbies, keep up with them.

- Stay in touch with your friends. Keep texting, calling, and spending time with them.

- Keep a journal or write about your feelings if that helps.

- Education is as important as ever. Children of alcoholics who stay involved with school do better than those who fall behind or drop out.[6] Ask for help if you have trouble completing assignments or concentrating in class.

- Be aware of your own mental health. If you have signs of an eating disorder or cutting or you're always sad or angry, seek outside help. You can talk to a school counselor or call a crisis hotline.

Things To Remember

Alcoholism is a disease.

You can't stop someone else from drinking

It's not your fault.

You didn't cause the problem.

Talk to others. You're not alone.

Make healthy choices.

Take care of yourself.

You have your own life ahead of you.

The first priority is staying safe. Teens with alcoholic parents are at higher risk for neglect, verbal abuse, and physical abuse.[7] Alcohol makes some parents more likely to lose control and burst out in anger. A teen in immediate danger should leave at once or call 911. Teens exposed to physical harm can call the National Domestic Violence Hotline at 800-799-SAFE (7233).

Children of abusive or neglectful alcoholics are sometimes removed to the care of grandparents or other relatives.

Drinking And Driving

Teens should never get in a car with a person who has been drinking, even if the person is trying to sober up. Alcohol stays in a person's body for hours after they drink. Drinking coffee, taking a cold shower, and getting fresh air are folk-remedy strategies that don't help.[8]

Rather than riding along, teens should make arrangements with non-alcoholic parents or reliable friends to pick them up when they need a ride. It helps to carry cash in case a taxi is needed.

If teens cannot avoid being passengers with drinking drivers, they should sit in the middle of the back seat and wear a seatbelt.[9]

Getting Help

Talking to trusted adults, friends, or professionals can help teens feel less isolated and alone. Getting help is not a sign of weakness: It's a sign of strength.

School Counseling Centers

Most schools have guidance counselors who help students keep up with their schoolwork and catch academic problems early. Some centers have social workers on staff who know about local services for troubled families. Some schools have support groups for teens or can connect teens to outside programs.

Addictions Counselors

These professionals work with people who are addicted to alcohol or drugs. They also help family members understand what causes the addiction and why alcoholics behave in certain ways.

Family Doctors And Pediatricians

Doctors who teens see for their routine medical care are also interested in their emotional health. Teens can tell doctors when they're concerned about a parent's drinking. Doctors can make sure the teen is not being harmed, recommend sources of help, and tactfully ask parents about their drinking. This could be the first step to getting an alcoholic parent into treatment.

Mental Health Professionals

Face-to-face counseling with a therapist can help undo the emotional damage of living with an alcoholic. Teens have a chance to talk about feelings they've kept bottled up inside. Therapists work with teens' symptoms of depression, eating disorders, self-harm, or anxiety. Teens learn not to blame themselves for someone else's drinking.

Self-Help Groups

The groups listed below help teens affected by someone else's problem drinking. They provide a safe environment and help participants recognize that they are not alone and deserve better. Teens can talk to others in their situation and see that progress and success are possible.

- **Alateen** is a part of Al-Anon Family Groups. Teens with stepparents, grandparents, siblings, friends, or others with drinking problems provide mutual support and share tips for coping.

- **Hazelden Sibling Group** is for brothers and sisters being treated or in recovery for alcohol or drug addiction. Teens can talk with peers in similar situations. They learn how alcoholism affects both people with the disease and their families from videos and talks with addiction professionals.

- **National Association For Children Of** Alcoholics builds public awareness and offers prevention services.

- **Local and online help:** States, cities, and communities offer a variety of services for people whose lives are affected by alcohol. School counselors can refer and recommend suitable area programs for teens. Internet searching can also uncover resources such as online support groups or special camps to give youths a break from chaotic home lives.

Breaking The Cycle Of Alcoholism

For several reasons, children of alcoholics are at higher risk of having drinking problems themselves someday. But many children of alcoholics overcome that risk. Resilient teens can grow up to lead healthy, productive lives.[10] They can break the cycle of family alcoholism.

Notes

1. Alateen. "How Do You Know If You Are Affected By Someone's Drinking?" Accessed October 28, 2012. http://www.al-anon.alateen.org/affected-by-someones-drinking.

2. Join Together/Partnership at Drugfree.org. "Liability Laws Make Parents Responsible For Underage Drinking In Their Home." January 3, 2012. http://www.drugfree.org/join-together/alcohol/liability-laws-make-parents-responsible-for-underage-drinking-in-their-home.

3. George Washington University Medical Center. "The Alcohol Cost Calculator For Kids: Teens' Alcohol Problems." Accessed November 3, 2012. http://www.alcohol costcalculator.org/kids/teens/print-teens.php.

4. Mothers Against Drunk Driving (MADD). "The Power To Take A Stand." October 2012. http://www.madd.org/underage-drinking/power-of-youth.

5. Health Canada. "Resilient Children Of Alcohol-Dependent Parents." May 7, 2007. http://www.hc-sc.gc.ca/hc-ps/pubs/adp-apd/child-resilient-enfant/alcohol-alcooliques-eng.php.

6. Marylou Mylant, et al. "Adolescent Children Of Alcoholics: Vulnerable Or Resilient?" *Journal of the American Psychiatric Nurses Association* 8. 2002. http://jap.sagepub.com/cgi/content/abstract/8/2/57.

7. American Academy of Pediatrics. "Child Abuse: What Every Parent Should Know" March 5, 2012.

8. See note 4 above.

9. National Council on Alcoholism and Drug Dependence, Inc. "Concerned About Someone?" Accessed October 28, 2012. http://www.ncadd.org/index.php/for-youth/concerned-about-someone.

10. See note 5 above.

Chapter 43

If Your Sibling Has A Fetal Alcohol Spectrum Disorder

Having a brother or sister can be fun. It can also be tough. They don't always do what you'd like. Or say what you'd like. Sometimes they embarrass you. If your sibling is different from everyone else, it's even harder.

If your sibling has a fetal alcohol spectrum disorder (FASD), it can be hard to understand and scary to think about. This chapter can help answer some questions you may have. It tells you about FASD and helps you explore your feelings.

Fetal Alcohol Spectrum Disorders

Fetal alcohol spectrum disorders (FASDs), can happen to kids whose moms drink alcohol when they're pregnant. The alcohol gets into the baby's body and hurts the brain. It can also hurt the bones and other organs.

There are different types of fetal alcohol spectrum disorders, like fetal alcohol syndrome (FAS). Kids with FAS look different. They are small for their age. They have small eyes and thin upper lips. The area between their nose and upper lip is smooth. Most people have a ridge there called a *philtrum*.

Other kids with an FASD look like you and me. But they have trouble learning and getting along. They also might have problems seeing, hearing, talking, or paying attention. Some kids with an FASD have problems with math. Many kids can't tell time or count money. They may not understand what you're saying and may not laugh at your jokes. Some have trouble sitting still or waiting in line. Having an FASD makes life very hard.

About This Chapter: From "My Sibling Has a Fetal Alcohol Spectrum Disorder: Can I Catch It?" DHHS Pub. No. (SMA) 06-4247. Rockville, MD: Center for Substance Abuse Prevention, Substance Abuse and Mental Health Services Administration, 2006. Reviewed by David A. Cooke, MD, FACP, December 2012.

For More Information

Want to know more about fatal alcohol spectrum disorders (FASDs)? You can check your local library or your school library. There's also a lot of information on the internet. You can visit the website of the Substance Abuse and Mental Health Service Administration's Fetal Alcohol Spectrum Disorders Center for Excellence at fasdcenter.samhsa.gov. You can also call 866-STOPFAS (866-786-7327). Or you can e-mail the Center at fasdcenter@samhsa.gov. Two other resources are The Arc (www.thearc.org) and the National Organization on Fetal Alcohol Syndrome (www.nofas.org).

Remember, you are not alone.

All kids are special. Kids with an FASD have good things about them, just like other kids. They can be very friendly and cheerful. They can have lots of energy and work hard. They're often kind to younger kids and animals.

Kids with an FASD like to help out and want to be liked. And they tend to play fair. You and your siblings with an FASD can teach each other and learn from each other.

Sometimes My Sibling Is A Pain

It's OK to have all kinds of feelings, such as being mad sometimes. Just remember that your brother or sister can't help it. Kids with an FASD can't always control how they act or what they say. They might walk up to strangers and say, "Hi." You might get mad at them or be embarrassed. Talking to an adult or friend can help.

Some kids feel guilty that they are OK while their sibling has an FASD. Remember, you didn't cause your sibling's disability and you can't make it go away. If your brother or sister does something wrong, it's OK to say so. You might have to say it over and over. Kids with an FASD don't always remember the rules. And if your sibling never gets it, just walk away. Fighting won't help.

Can I Catch an FASD?

No. You can't catch it. Kids are born with an FASD. FASD is only caused when a mom drinks alcohol while she is pregnant.

Moms don't hurt their babies on purpose. Some moms drink alcohol before they know they are pregnant. Others need help to stop drinking alcohol. So don't blame your mom or your sibling's mom, because she didn't hurt your siblings on purpose. Blaming her won't help your sibling.

If you think your mom is drinking too much, you might want to call Al-Anon/Alateen at 888-4AL-ANON (888-425-2666) or the National Association for Children of Alcoholics (888-55-4COAS 301-468-0985). Talking to a teacher, counselor, or adult friend or relative may also help.

Accepting kids with an FASD can help them a lot. They often feel left out and get ignored because other kids are afraid or think they're weird. You can help your sibling by letting your friends know about FASD.

Mom And Dad Are So Busy

Many kids whose siblings have an FASD feel jealous of all the attention their siblings get. It doesn't seem fair. You still need and deserve attention.

Tell your parents how you feel. Set aside time alone with one or both of them. Making your time with Mom or Dad part of the schedule might help.

Finding Others With Siblings Affected By FASD

You might feel all alone and think no one else has the same feelings or experiences. But you're not alone. Sadly, many women drink alcohol when they're pregnant, so a lot of kids have an FASD. Some places have groups for siblings to share their feelings and help each other. One place that you or your parents can call is The Arc (800-433-5255 or 202-534-3700) or visit their website at www.thearc.org.

Therapy Sessions Are Boring

Some kids with an FASD need help learning how to do things. This is called therapy. There are many kinds of therapy. Physical therapy helps kids move around. Occupational therapy can help with everyday tasks, like brushing your teeth. Some kids need speech therapy to help them talk. And some need counseling to help them deal with their feelings about FASD and other problems.

You might need to go to your sibling's therapy sessions. Being stuck in a waiting room can be boring, so bring a book or some games to keep you busy. It might be important to participate in therapy like counseling to share your thoughts and feelings. If not, ask about what your sibling does in therapy. You can learn ways to help and you might find it interesting.

Taking Care Of My Sibling

Taking care of your sibling is nice, but it's not your job. Talk to your parents if you feel like they're asking you to do too much. And if your sibling has a tantrum or might get hurt, get your parents right away. Don't try to handle it yourself.

Do help when you can. Your sibling may watch to see how you do things. Teaching him or her can make you feel better about yourself. It can also help you understand what your sibling is going through.

I Don't Know How To Help

You have a special role in teaching your sibling. You can help by nicely reminding him or her to do things. You can repeat things if he or she doesn't understand or forgets. You can help your sibling with homework or chores. You can play games or sing or listen to music. Look for things your sibling likes that you can do together. Also be careful about what you say. Slang is fun with your friends, but kids with an FASD don't always understand it. If you ask, "What's up?" your sibling might look up to see what's there. So try to say exactly what you mean, like, "What are you doing?" or "How are you feeling?"

I Have To Be "Super Kid"

Some siblings feel like they have to do extra well to make up for their brother or sister's FASD. You might think getting straight A's or winning at sports will make your parents feel better. You don't have to do that. Just be yourself. Do your best because it makes *you* happy.

Your sibling may not be able to do all the things you can, but he or she can do other things. Remember, your parents can be proud of you and your sibling for whatever you each can do.

Remember the "Seven Cs" (from the National Association for Children of Alcoholics):

- I didn't **C**ause it.

- I can't **C**ure it.

- I can't **C**ontrol it.

- I can take better **C**are of myself by **C**ommunicating my feelings and making healthy **C**hoices, and **C**elebrating myself.

Part Seven
If You Need More Information

Chapter 44

Alcohol Treatment And Recovery Resources

Substance Abuse And Crisis Hotlines

Adcare Hospital Alcohol Hotline
800-ALCOHOL (800-252-6465)

Al-Anon/Alateen Information Line
800-344-2666

American Council on Alcoholism
800-527-5344

Center for Substance Abuse Treatment
800-662-HELP (800-662-4357)
800-487-4889 (TDD)

Girls and Boys Town National Hotline
800-448-3000

Marijuana Anonymous
800-766-6779

Narconon International Help Line
800-775-8750

National Child Abuse Hot Line
800-4-A-CHILD (800-422-4453)

National Council on Alcoholism and Drug Dependence
800-622-2255

National Drug and Alcohol Treatment Referral Service
800-662-HELP (800-662-4357)

About This Chapter: Information in this chapter was compiled from many sources deemed reliable. Inclusion does not constitute endorsement, and there is no implication associated with omission. All contact information was verified in December 2012.

National Runaway Switchboard

800-RUNAWAY (800-786-2929)

National Sexual Assault Hotline

800-656-HOPE (800-656-4673)

National Suicide Hopeline

800-442-HOPE (800-442-4673)

800-SUICIDA (800-784-2432) (Spanish)

7 days a week, 24 hours a day

National Suicide Prevention Lifeline

800-273-TALK (800-273-8255)

To Locate Treatment Facilities In Your Area

To find alcohol and drug abuse treatment or mental health treatment facilities and programs around the country, use the Substance Abuse Treatment Services Locator:

Substance Abuse Treatment Facility Locator

Substance Abuse And Mental Health Services Administration
5600 Fishers Lane
Rockville, MD 20857
Website: http://www.findtreatment.samhsa.gov

Through this website you can search more than 11,000 alcohol and drug abuse/addiction treatment facilities and programs.

If you prefer, you can call the SAMHSA Treatment Referral Helpline:

- 800-662-HELP (4357)
- 800-487-4889 (TDD)

Treatment Facility Locator services are free and confidential. Information is available in English and Spanish for individuals and family members facing substance abuse and mental health issues, 24 hours a day, seven days a week.

You can also locate contact information for State Substance Abuse Agencies through the Substance Abuse Treatment Facility Locator website: Click on Substance Abuse Treatment Services Locator. Then, under "Other Links" click on State Substance Abuse Agencies, and select your state's name from the pull-down menu.

Mutual Help Groups For Alcoholics And Children Of Alcoholics

AddictionsAndRecovery.org

160 Eglinton Avenue East
Suite 601
Toronto, ON M4P 3B5
Canada
Phone: 416-920-2982
Website:
http://www.addictionsandrecovery.org

Adult Children Of Alcoholics World Service Organization, Inc.

1400 East 33rd Street
Signal Hill, CA 90755
Phone: 562-595-7831 (message only)
Fax: 562-595-7822
Website: http://www.adultchildren.org
E-mail: info@adultchildren.org

Al-Anon/Alateen Family Groups

Al-Anon Family
Group Headquarters, Inc.
Al-Anon Family Group
Headquarters (Canada), Inc.
1600 Corporate Landing Parkway
Virginia Beach, VA 23454-5617
Toll-Free: 888-4AL-ANON
(888-425-2666)
Phone: 757-563-1600
Fax: 757-563-1655
Website: http://www.al-anon.alateen.org
E-mail: wso@al-anon.org

Alcoholics Anonymous

A.A. World Services, Inc.
P.O. Box 459, Grand Central Station
New York, NY 10163
Phone: 212-870-3400
Fax: 212-870-3003
Website: http://www.aa.org

Alcoholics For Christ

1316 North Campbell Road
Royal Oak, MI 48067
Phone: 248-399-9955
Website:
http://www.alcoholicsforchrist.com
E-mail: office@alcoholicsforchrist.com

Alcoholics Victorious

P.O. Box 4422
Tequesta, FL 33469
Fax: 561-598-9079
Website:
http://www.alcoholicsvictorious.org

Calix Society

International Office
3881 Highland Avenue, Suite 201
White Bear Lake, MN 55110
Toll-Free: 800-398-0524
Phone: 651-773-3117
Website: http://www.calixsociety.org

Celebrate Recovery

Website: http://www.celebraterecovery.com
E-mail: info@celebraterecovery.com

Centre For Addiction And Mental Health

33 Russell Street
Toronto, ON M5S 2S1
Canada
Toll Free: 800-463-6273
Phone: 416-595-6111
Website: http://www.camh.net

Chemically Dependent Anonymous

General Service Office
P.O. Box 423
Severna Park, MD 21146
Toll-Free: 888-CDA-HOPE
(888-232-4673)
Website: http://www.cdaweb.org

Children Of Alcoholics Foundation

50 Jay Street
Brooklyn, NY 11201
Toll Free: 800-DRUG-HELP
(800-378-4435)
Website: http://www.phoenixhouse.org
E-mail: coaf@phoenixhouse.org

Co-Anon Family Groups World Services

P.O. Box 12722
Tucson, AZ 85732-2722
Toll-Free National Referral Line:
800-347-8998
Toll-Free: 800-898-9985 (Voice Recorder)
Phone: 520-513-5028 (Voice Recorder)
Website: http://www.co-anon.org
E-mail: info@co-anon.org

Dual Recovery Anonymous

World Services Central Office
P.O. Box 8107
Prairie Village, KS 66208
Phone: 913-991-2703
(9:00–5:00 CT)
Website:
http://draonline.org
E-mail:
draws@draonline.org

Faces and Voices of Recovery

1010 Vermont Avenue, #618
Washington, DC 20005
Phone: 202-737-0690
Fax: 202-737-0695
Website:
http://www.facesandvoicesofrecovery.org

Families Anonymous

701 Lee Street
Suite 670
Des Plaines, IL 60016
Toll-Free: 800-736-9805
Phone: 847-294-5877
Fax: 847-294-5837
Website:
http://www.familiesanonymous.org
E-mail:
famanon@FamiliesAnonymous.org

Hopelinks

Toll-Free: 866-806-2821
Website:
http://www.hopelinks.net

Jewish Alcoholics, Chemically Dependent Persons, and Significant Others

135 West 50th Street, 6th Floor
New York, NY 10020
Toll-Free: 888-523-2769
Phone: 212-632-4600
Fax: 212-399-3525
Website: http:// www.jbfcs.org/JACS

LifeRing Secular Recovery

LifeRing Service Center
1440 Broadway, Suite 312
Oakland CA 94612-2023
Toll-Free: 800-811-4142
Phone: 510-763-0779
Fax 510-763-1513
Website: http://lifering.org
E-mail: service@lifering.org

Men For Sobriety

P.O. Box 618
Quakertown, PA 18951-0618
Phone: 215-536-8026
Fax: 215-538-9026
E-mail: NewLife@nni.com

Nar-Anon Family Group Headquarters, Inc.

22527 Crenshaw Boulevard
Suite 200B
Torrance, CA 90505
Toll-Free: 800-477-6291
Phone: 310-534-8188
Fax: 310-534-8688
Website: http://www.nar-anon.org
E-mail: WSO@nar-anon.org

Narcotics Anonymous

P.O. Box 9999
Van Nuys, CA 91409
Phone: 818-773-9999
Fax: 818-700-0700
Website: http://www.na.org
E-mail: fsmail@na.org

National Asian Pacific American Families Against Drug Abuse

340 East 2nd Street, Suite 409
Los Angeles, CA 90012
Phone: 213-625-5795
Fax: 213-625-5796
Website: http://www.napafasa.org
E-mail: napafasa@napafasa.org

National Treatment Referral Center

Toll-Free: 800-662-HELP (800-662-4357)

OneHealth Solutions, Inc.

(Formerly Known As Sober Circle)
420 Stevens Avenue, Suite 200
Solana Beach, CA 92075
Phone: 858-947-6333
Fax: 858-481-4332
Website: http://onehealth.com
E-mail: support@onehealth.com

Overcomers Outreach, Inc.

12828 Acheson Drive
Whittier, CA 90601
Toll-Free: 800-310-3001
Phone: 562-698-9000; Fax: 562-698-2211
Website: http://www.overcomersoutreach.org
E-mail: info@overcomersoutreach.org

Recoveries Anonymous

R.A. Universal Services
P.O. Box 1212
East Northport, NY 11731
Website: http://www.r-a.org
E-mail: raus@r-a.org

Recovery International

105 West Adams
Suite 2940
Chicago, IL 60603
Toll-Free: 866-221-0302
Phone: 312-337-5661
Fax: 312-726-4446
Website:
http://www.lowselfhelpsystems.org
E-mail:
info@lowselfhelpsystems.org

Salvation Army

National Headquarters
615 Slaters Lane
P.O. Box 269
Alexandria, VA 22313
Website: http://www.
salvationarmyusa.org

Secular Organizations For Sobriety (Save Ourselves)

4773 Hollywood Boulevard
Hollywood, CA 90027
Phone: 323-666-4295
Fax: 323-666-4271
Website:
http://www.cfiwest.org/sos
E-mail: SOS@CFIWest.org

SMART Recovery

Self Help For Substance Abuse
and Addiction
7304 Mentor Avenue
Suite F
Mentor, OH 44060
Toll-Free: 866-951-5357
Phone: 440-951-5357
Fax: 440-951-5358
Website:
http://www.smartrecovery.org
E-mail: info@smartrecovery.org

Streetcats

A Service of Streetcats
Foundation for Youth And
National Children's Coalition
Phone: 415-671-6670
(1:00–4:00 PT)
Website: http://streetcats.org
E-mail: helpingyouth@yahoo.com

Teen-Anon

1550 NE 137
Portland, OR 97230
Website:
http://www.teen-anon.com/home.htm
E-mail: teenanon@yahoo.com

Women For Sobriety, Inc.

P.O. Box 618
Quakertown, PA 18951-0618
Phone: 215-536-8026
Fax: 215-538-9026
Website: http://
www.womenforsobriety.org

Chapter 45

Organizations Providing Information About Alcohol And Substance Abuse

African American Family Services, Inc.

2616 Nicollet Avenue South
Minneapolis, MN 55408
Phone: 612-871-7878
Fax: 612-871-2567
Website: http://www.aafs.net
E-mail: contact@aafs.net

Al-Anon

1600 Corporate Landing Parkway
Virginia Beach, VA 23454
Phone: 757-563-1600
Fax: 757-563-1655
Website:
http://www.al-anon.alateen.org
E-mail: wso@al-anon.org

Alcoholics Anonymous (AA)

AA World Services, Inc.
P.O. Box 459, Grand Central Station
New York, NY 10163
Phone: 212-870-3400
Website: http://www.aa.org

Alcohol Justice

(Formerly Known As Marin Institute)
24 Belvedere Street
San Rafael, CA 94901
Phone: 415-456-5692
Fax: 415-456-0491
Website: http://alcoholjustice.org

About This Chapter: Information in this chapter was compiled from many sources deemed reliable. Inclusion does not constitute endorsement, and there is no implication associated with omission. All contact information was verified in December 2012.

American Liver Foundation

39 Broadway
Suite 2700
New York, NY 10006
Toll-Free: 800-GO-LIVER
(800-465-4837)
Phone: 212-668-1000
Fax: 212-483-8179
Website: http://www
.liverfoundation.org

Center of Alcohol Studies

Rutgers, the State
University of New Jersey
607 Allison Road
Piscataway, NJ 08854
Phone: 732-445-2190
Fax: 732-445-5300
Website: http://www
.alcoholstudies.rutgers.edu

Center for Substance Abuse Prevention

Substance Abuse and
Mental Health Services
Administration
1 Choke Cherry Road
Rockville, MD 20857
Phone: 240-276-2420
Fax: 240-276-2430
Website:
http://www.samhsa.gov/
about/csap.aspx

Center for Substance Abuse Treatment

Substance Abuse and Mental
Health Services Administration
1 Choke Cherry Road
Rockville, MD 20857
Toll-Free: 800-662-HELP (800-662-4357)
Toll-Free TDD: 800-487-4889
Phone: 240-276-1660
Fax: 240-276-1670
Website: http://www.samhsa.gov/
about/csat.aspx
Substance Abuse Treatment Facility Locator:
http://www.findtreatment.samhsa.gov

Center on Alcohol Marketing and Youth

Johns Hopkins Bloomberg
School of Public Health
624 North Broadway, Suite 292
Baltimore, MD 21205
Phone: 410-502-6579
Website: http://www.camy.org
E-mail: info@camy.org

Centers for Disease Control and Prevention (CDC)

1600 Clifton Road
Atlanta, GA 30333
Toll-Free: 800-CDC-INFO
(800-232-4636)
Toll-Free TTY: 888-232-6348
Website: http://www.cdc.gov
Alcohol and Public Health:
http://www.cdc.gov/alcohol
E-mail: cdcinfo@cdc.gov

Do It Now Foundation

P.O. Box 27568
Tempe, AZ 85285-7568
Phone: 480-736-0599
Fax: 480-736-0771
Website:
http://www.doitnow.org
E-mail: email@doitnow.org

Drug Enforcement Administration

Office of Diversion Control
8701 Morrissette Drive
Mailstop: AES
Springfield, VA 22152
Toll-Free: 800-882-9539
Phone: 202-307-1000
Website:
http://www.justice.gov/dea
E-mail: ODE@usdoj.gov

FASD Center for Excellence

2101 Gaither Road, Suite 600
Rockville, MD 20850
Toll-Free: 866-STOPFAS
(866-786-7327)
Website:
http://www.fasdcenter.samhsa.gov
E-mail: fasdcenter1@ngc.com

Hazelden Foundation

P.O. Box 11
Center City, MN 55012-0011
Toll Free: 1-800-257-7810
Phone: 651-213-4200
Website: http://www.hazelden.org
E-mail: info@hazelden.org

Health and Human Development: Alcohol, Tobacco, and Other Drugs

Education Development Center, Inc.
43 Foundry Avenue
Waltham, MA 02453-8313
Toll-Free: 800-225-4276
Phone: 617-969-8313
Website:
http://hhd.edc.org/topics/
alcohol-tobacco-and-other-drugs
E-mail: HigherEdCtr@edc.org

International Center for Alcohol Policies

1519 New Hampshire Avenue NW
Washington, DC 20036
Phone: 202-986-1159
Fax: 202-986-2080
Website: http://www.icap.org
E-mail: info@icap.org

Join Together

The Partnership at
Drugfree.org
352 Park Avenue South
9th Floor
New York, NY 10010
Phone: 212-922-1560
Fax: 212-922-1570
Website:
http://www.drugfree.org/
join-together
E-mail: webmail@drugfree.org

Mothers Against Drunk Driving (MADD)

National Office
511 East John Carpenter Freeway
Suite 700
Irving, TX 75062
Toll-Free: 877-ASK-MADD
(877-275-6233)
Toll-Free Victim Services 24-Hour Help
Line: 877-MADD-HELP
(877-623-3435)
Phone: 214-744-6233
Fax: 972-869-2206 or 972-869-2207
Website: http://www.madd.org

National Association for Children of Alcoholics

10920 Connecticut Avenue, Suite 100
Kensington, MD 20895
Toll-Free: 888-55-4COAS
(888-554-2627)
Phone: 301-468-0985
Fax: 301-468-0987
Website: http://www.nacoa.net
E-mail: nacoa@nacoa.org

National Black Alcoholism and Addictions Council, Inc.

Administrative Office
1500 Golden Valley Road
Minneapolis, MN 55411
Toll Free: 877-NBAC-ORG
(877-622-2674)
Fax: 407-532-2815
Website: www.nbacinc.org
E-mail: information@nbacinc.org

National Center on Addiction and Substance Abuse (CASA) at Columbia University

633 Third Avenue
19th Floor
New York, NY 10017-6706
Phone: 212-841-5200
Fax: 212-956-8020
Website:
http://www.casacolumbia.org

National Council on Alcoholism and Drug Dependence

244 East 58th Street
4th Floor
New York, NY 10022
Toll-Free Hopeline:
800-NCA-CALL
(800-622-2255)
Phone: 212-269-7797
Fax: 212-269-7510
E-mail: national@ncadd.org
Website: http://www.ncadd.org

National Criminal Justice Reference Service

P.O. Box 6000
Rockville, MD 20849
Toll-Free: 800-851-3420
Toll-Free TTY: 877-712-9279
Phone: 301-519-5500
(international callers)
Fax: 301-519-5212
Website: http://www.ncjrs.gov

National Drug Control Policy

Website:
http://www.whitehousedrugpolicy.gov/
about/clearingh.html
Resources, Publications,
And Additional Information:
http://www.whitehouse.gov/ondcp/
publications-and-resources

National Highway Traffic Safety Administration

Headquarters
1200 New Jersey Avenue SE
West Building
Washington, DC 20590
Toll-Free: 888-327-4236
Toll-Free TTY: 800-424-9153
Phone: 202-366-4000
Website:
http://www.nhtsa.gov/Impaired

National Institute on Alcohol Abuse and Alcoholism

5635 Fishers Lane, MSC 9304
Bethesda, MD 20892
Toll-Free: 888-MY-NIAAA
(888-696-4222) (Publication Orders)
Website:
http://www.niaaa.nih.gov
Alcohol Policy Information System:
http://www.alcoholpolicy.niaaa
.nih.gov
NIAAA Publications:
http://pubs.niaaa.nih.gov/
publications/english-order.htm
E-mail: niaaaweb-r@exchange.nih.gov

National Institute on Drug Abuse

6001 Executive Boulevard
Room 5213, MSC 9561
Bethesda, MD 20892-9561
Phone: 301-443-1124
Phone: 240-221-4007 (Spanish)
Fax: 301-443-7397
Websites: http://www.nida.nih.gov
and http://www.drugabuse.gov
E-mail: information@nida.nih.gov

National Mental Health Information Center

Substance Abuse and Mental
Health Services Administration
P.O. Box 2345
Rockville, MD 20847
Toll-Free: 800-789-2647
Toll-Free TDD: 866-889-2647
Phone: 240-221-4021
TDD: 240-221-4022
Fax: 240-221-4295
Website: http://mentalhealth.samhsa.gov
E-mail: nmhic-info@samhsa.hhs.gov

National Organization on Fetal Alcohol Syndrome

1200 Eton Court NW
Third Floor
Washington, DC 20007
Toll-Free: 800-66-NOFAS
(800-666-6327)
Phone: 202-785-4585
Fax: 202-466-6456
Website: http://nofas.org
E-mail: information@nofas.org

Nemours Foundation

1600 Rockland Road
Wilmington, DE 19803
Phone: 302-651-4000
E-mail: info@kidshealth.org
Website: http://www.kidshealth.org

Office of Adolescent Health

1101 Wootton Parkway, Suite 700
Rockville, MD 20852
Phone: 240-453-2846
Website: http://www.hhs.gov/ash/oah
E-mail: oah.gov@hhs.gov

Office of National Drug Control Policy

Toll Free: 800-FED INFO
(800-333-4636) (Information Specialist)
Website: http://www.whitehouse.gov/ondcp
Above the Influence:
http://www.abovetheinfluence.com

Office of Safe and Healthy Students

(Formerly Safe and Drug-Free Schools)
U.S. Department of Education
Potomac Center Plaza
550 12th Street SW, 10th Floor
Washington, DC 20202-6450
Toll-Free: 800-872-5327
(Information Resource Center at
U.S. Department of Education)
Phone: 202-245-7896; Fax: 202-485-0013
Website: http://www2.ed.gov/about/offices/list/oese/oshs/index.html
E-mail: OESE@ed.gov

Office on Women's Health

200 Independence Avenue SW
Washington, DC 20201
Toll-Free: 800-994-9662
Website:
http://www.womenshealth.gov
Girl's health:
http://www.girlshealth.gov

Partnership at Drug-Free.org

352 Park Avenue South
9th Floor
New York, NY 10010
Phone: 212-922-1560
Fax: 212-922-1570
Website: http://www.drugfree.org
E-mail: webmail@drugfree.org

Phoenix House

164 West 74th Street
New York, NY 10023
Toll Free: 800-DRUG HELP
(800-378-4435)
Phone: 212-595-5810
Fax: 212-4966035
Website:
http://www.phoenixhouse.org

Stop Underage Drinking

Substance Abuse and Mental
Health Services Administration
1 Choke Cherry Road
Rockville, MD 20857
Toll-Free: 866-419-2514
Phone: 301-407-6798
Website:
http://www.stopalcoholabuse.gov

Students Against Destructive Decisions (SADD)

255 Main Street
Marlborough, MA 01752
Toll Free: 877-SADD-INC
(877-723-3462)
Fax: 508-481-5759
Website: http://www.sadd.org
E-mail: info@sadd.org

Substance Abuse and Mental Health Services Administration

(General Information and
Publications Ordering)
1 Choke Cherry Road
Rockville, MD 20857
Toll-Free: 877-SAMHSA-7
(877-726-4727)
Toll-Free: 800-729-6686
Toll-Free TDD: 800-487-4889
Phone: 240-276-2130
(Office of Communications)
Website: http://store.samhsa.gov/home

U.S. Bureau of Alcohol, Tobacco, Firearms, and Explosives

Office of Public and Governmental Affairs
99 New York Avenue NE
Room 5S 144
Washington, DC 20226
Toll Free: 800-800-3855
Phone: 202-648-7777
Website: http://www.atf.gov
E-mail: ATFTips@atf.gov

U.S. Food and Drug Administration (FDA)

10903 New Hampshire Avenue
Silver Spring, MD 20993
Toll-Free: 888-INFO-FDA
(888-463-6332)
Website: http://www.fda.gov

We Don't Serve Teens

Federal Trade Commission
Website:
http://www.dontserveteens.gov

World Health Organization (WHO)

Avenue Appia 20
1211 Geneva 27
Switzerland
Telephone: +41-22-791-21-11
Fax: +41-22-791-31-11
Website: http://www.who.int
E-mail: info@who.int

Index

Index

Page numbers that appear in *Italics* refer to tables or illustrations. Page numbers that have a small 'n' after the page number refer to information shown as Notes at the beginning of each chapter. Page numbers that appear in **Bold** refer to information contained in boxes on that page (except Notes information at the beginning of each chapter).

A

S

W, X